Chronic Pain

Chronic Pain

Edited by

Randal D. France, M.D.
and
K. Ranga Rama Krishnan, M.D.

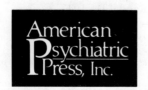

American
Psychiatric
Press, Inc.

1400 K Street, N.W.
Washington, DC 20005

Library of Congress Cataloging-in-Publication Data

Chronic Pain

 Includes bibliographies.
 1. Intractable pain. I. France, Randal D., 1947–
II. Krishnan, K. Ranga Rama, 1956– . [DNLM:
1. Chronic Disease. 2. Pain—diagnosis. 3. Pain—
therapy. WL 704 C557]
RB127.C475 1987 616′.0472 87-1480
ISBN 0-88048-206-0

Contents

CLINICAL CONCEPTS

ASSESSMENT

MANAGEMENT

CONTRIBUTORS

Csaba M. Banki, M.D.
Visiting Professor of Psychiatry,
Duke University Medical Center,
Durham, North Carolina

Scott T. Cain, Ph.D.
Postdoctoral Fellow,
Department of Psychiatry, Pharmacology, and
the Center for Aging and Human Development,
Duke University Medical Center,
Durham, North Carolina

Jonathan Davidson, M.D.
Associate Professor of Psychiatry,
Duke University Medical Center; and
Staff Psychiatrist,
Veterans Administration Medical Center,
Durham, North Carolina

Everett H. Ellinwood, M.D.
Professor of Psychiatry,
Duke University Medical Center,
Durham, North Carolina

Lars Erikkson, M.D.
Researcher in Neurobiology,
Duke University Medical Center,
Durham, North Carolina

Randal D. France, M.D.
Associate Professor of Psychiatry,
Duke University Medical Center,
Durham, North Carolina

Karen M. Gil, Ph.D.
Associate in the Department of Psychiatry,
Duke University Medical Center,
Durham, North Carolina

Jeffrey L. Houpt, M.D.
Professor and Chairman,
Department of Psychiatry,
Emory University School of Medicine,
Atlanta, Georgia

John S. Jordan, Ph.D.
Assistant Professor of Medical Psychology,
Department of Psychiatry,
Duke University Medical Center,
Durham, North Carolina

Francis J. Keefe, Ph.D.
Associate Professor of Medical Psychology;
Director, Pain Management Program,
Duke University Medical Center,
Durham, North Carolina

K. Ranga Rama Krishnan, M.D.
Assistant Professor of Psychiatry,
Duke University Medical Center,
Durham, North Carolina

Linda M. Lawrence, L.P.T.
Senior Physical Therapist,
Department of Physical Therapy,
Duke University Medical Center,
Durham, North Carolina

Allan A. Maltbie, M.D.
Associate Professor of Psychiatry,
Duke University Medical Center,
Durham, North Carolina

Ananth N. Manepalli, M.D.
Department of Psychiatry,
Duke University Medical Center,
Durham, North Carolina

Una D. McCann, M.D.
Department of Psychiatry,
Stanford University,
Stanford, California

Charles B. Nemeroff, M.D., Ph.D.
Associate Professor of Psychiatry,
Duke University Medical Center,
Durham, North Carolina

Merry Noel, M.D.
Department of Psychiatry,
Duke University Medical Center,
Durham, North Carolina

Suzanne L. Ross, M.A.
Psychology Intern,
Division of Medical Psychology,
Duke University Medical Center,
Durham, North Carolina

Mary Trainor, R.N.
Head Nurse, Clinical Specialty Unit,
Department of Nursing,
Duke University Medical Center,
Durham, North Carolina

Bruno J. Urban, M.D.
Professor of Anesthesiology
Assistant Professor of Neurosurgery;
and Director, Duke University Pain Clinic,
Duke University Medical Center,
Durham, North Carolina

LIST OF FIGURES

Foreword

Chronic pain affects 11 percent of the adult population, and acute pain affects a further 5 percent, at any given time. It is frequently, but not invariably, found in conjunction with psychiatric illness. Sometimes one's psychological state may cause the painful syndrome. More often, one's psychological state may promote pain or make it worse. Commonly, chronic pain from physical states generates psychiatric disorders.

There is a challenge to the psychiatrist—to try and understand, and help to resolve, these widespread and severe problems. Yet few have responded. The opportunities to do constructive work in this field exist, but the conditions of practice may be unattractive, or the psychiatrist may feel the lack of sufficient knowledge. Fortunately, the numbers of psychiatrists interested in this field are beginning to grow.

Drs. France and Krishnan are notable young psychiatrists who have already made valuable contributions to the international literature on pain and psychiatric illness, and especially on depression. With colleagues at Duke and elsewhere, they now present a first-rate survey of scientific knowledge and practical management which will be extremely useful to psychiatrists interested in this field.

The best work on pain is frequently multidisciplinary. Thus, in addition to the varied medical elements in this book, it is particularly pleasant to remark upon the masterly and instructive contributions from colleagues in psychology, physiotherapy, and nursing. Any psychiatrist wishing to extend his or her professional knowledge on pain will greatly benefit from this volume.

Harold Merskey, D.M.
London, Ontario, Canada

PREFACE

Pain is one of the most frequent presenting complaints of patients seen in a medical setting. Successful intervention or the healing process generally leads to resolution of the pain complaint. However, in some patients, pain continues despite treatment or apparent healing. In most cases, the use of the latest diagnostic procedures and tools fail to clarify the cause or quantify the severity of the chronic pain. The persistence of this pain is rarely understood by the patients, their families, or physicians.

By conceptualizing the chronic pain state as having a single etiological cause, one fails to fully appreciate the complex nature of chronic pain. The dilemma facing patients as well as clinicians in trying to conceptualize chronic pain is analogous to the parable of the blind men trying to describe the unseen elephant.

The interest in and investigation of pain dates back to antiquity. Historically, pain has been viewed as the opposite of pleasure. The polarity of these two states is described in religious as well as psychological writings. In the 19th and early 20th centuries, the knowledge base in neuroanatomy and pathophysiology of pain was greatly expanded. In recent years, the development in the fields of neurophysiology, pharmacology, and psychology has advanced our understanding of pain. The neuroanatomy and neurophysiology of pain now include an understanding and a study of pain pathways at cellular and subcellular levels, neurotransmitter systems in the peripheral and central nervous system, and neuroendocrine function. Drug therapy comprises a variety of medications that can modify the pain response by chemical manipulation of the functional activity in these pain pathways. The clinical characteristics of most pain states have been adequately described. Advances in cancer therapy have eased some of the suffering of these patients. In the last 20 years, analysis of the behavior of pain patients from the perspective of learning theory has led to the application of treatments for pain.

As our knowledge of chronic pain expands, it becomes increasingly clear that this illness is a complex syndrome. It is now advocated that comprehensive evaluation of chronic pain patients and application of multiple treatments be available to these patients. The multidisciplinary evaluation and multimodal treatments are now widely accepted by professionals working in the chronic pain field.

Among physicians, it is psychiatrists who are best equipped to deal with the psychosocial aspects of chronic pain. This book, we hope, will provide a knowledge base for the psychiatrist who desires to work comfortably and productively with chronic pain patients. Special emphasis will be placed on the psychiatric aspect of chronic pain, with a focus on its relationship to other processes involved. Because chronic pain is a complex problem, we have developed a systems model to help us understand this condition in order to develop rational assessment and management plans tailored to individual patients, and to provide guidelines and hypotheses for future investigation. The model is presented in Chapter 2. The conceptual multidimensional basis of chronic pain is neurobiological, behavioral, and psychological, which is elaborated in one section entitled Basic Concepts (Chapters 3–8). The section entitled Clinical Concepts (Chapters 9–15) provides a framework for identifying the clinical aspects relating both to the development and sequelae of chronic pain using the systems model. The third section, Assessment (Chapters 16 and 17), also uses the systems model and provides a rational, comprehensive, and multidimensional assessment scheme for evaluating the chronic pain patient. The components of the individualized management program for treating the chronic pain patient are examined in the last section, entitled Management (Chapters 18–25). An integrated approach is favored throughout the text.

Unfortunately, resolution of chronic pain eludes both patients and health professionals in many cases. However, the systematic integration and application of the various treatments can lead to effective management for the chronic pain patient.

Without the assistance and hard work of Ms. Elsie Priest, the manuscript of this text would still be an unorganized pile of handwritten pages. Her help on this text has been invaluable.

Randal D. France, M.D.
K. Ranga Rama Krishnan, M.D.

Introduction

Chapter 1

Overview

Randal D. France, M.D.
K. Ranga Rama Krishnan, M.D.
Jeffrey L. Houpt, M.D.

Pain is among the most common reasons for patients seeking medical treatment. Thus, the relief of pain is one of the physician's primary tasks, and the expectation of this relief often leads to patients' idealization of the physician. It is ironic that in this age of advanced medical technology, success often hinges on the relief of a symptom which cannot be measured, seen, percussed, or palpated. Physicians have their own experiences of pain, and patients must resort to analogies in order to communicate with their physician about their pain experience. Thus, the search for treatment begins with the patient's somewhat imprecise lexicon, shifts to the most advanced available technology for diagnosis and treatment, and then returns to the patient's lexicon to establish the effectiveness of that treatment.

While our understanding of the scientific basis of acute pain is minimal, our understanding of the scientific basis of chronic pain is even less. Chronic pain appears to serve no biological function, yet it remains recalcitrant to treatment. Rather than serving the patient in some protective function, chronic pain appears to inhibit the patient's capacity to function and to enjoy life. The patient gradually succumbs to changes in affect and behavior, which in themselves are undesirable. Then the affective and behavioral responses become prominent and require treatment. Finally, in addition to emotional turmoil, chronic pain adds significant economic and social stress to the patient, family, and society.

CONCEPTUALIZING PAIN

The concept of chronic pain and its puzzling phenomenology has been recognized since antiquity. Throughout history, explanations of chronic pain have been given within the framework of various mystical, spiritual, and religious structures. Religious explanations for chronic pain have greatly influenced Western thinking, where pain has often been viewed as a punishment inflicted by God for sins committed by the sufferer. The word pain is derived from the Latin word *poena,* meaning punishment. Aristotle believed the experience of pain to be a negative passion, a feeling state opposite to pleasure. He further postulated that the heart was the center of sensation and that pain was the result of an increase in the sensitivity to touch, which was carried by the blood to the heart. Aristotle's interpretation of pain predominated Western thinking until it was replaced by Descartes' postulation (1) that the brain was the center of sensation and that pain was transmitted by means of small threads running from the skin to the brain. This theory was, of course, verified and eventually extended when specific pain receptors in the periphery of the brain, along with pain pathways from the periphery to the brain, were identified.

Along with the expanded knowledge of pain mechanisms, there has been an increased focus on the psychological aspects of pain. Strong has

3

pointed out that pain has two components: the original sensation, and an accompanying psychological reaction to and processing of the sensation (1). Hardy and colleagues (2) state that pain perception is based on a neurophysiological process involving specialized neural receptors and conductive pathways for pain. While the receptor mechanism and pathway systems seem to be relatively similar and constant for all individuals, *reaction* to pain is influenced by past experience, social setting, and psychological factors, all of which account for the wide variability we see in responses to pain.

Szasz (3) describes pain as one component of a person's private data experience, which cannot be simultaneously shared and reported by anyone other than the person experiencing the pain. When collecting data concerning a patient's pain, the physician is totally dependent upon the report of the patient (4).

Engel (5) postulated that pain is evoked by appropriate stimulation of the peripheral sensory system. The capacity to experience pain develops initially from peripheral stimulation. However, later pain experiences may occur without the corresponding stimulation of the pain receptors. Melzack (6) states that pain is not a single quantitative experience that can be classified by a specified intensity or kind of stimulation. Pain, therefore, is a "category of experience."

In an attempt to define pain, Sternbach (7) describes three components: 1) personal and private sensation of hurt; 2) a harmful stimulation which signals current or impending tissue damage; and 3) a pattern of responses which operates to protect the organism from harm. The responses referred to in the third component are characterized by neurological, physiological, behavioral, and psychological factors. Merskey and Spear describe pain as "an unpleasant experience which we primarily associate with tissue damage or describe in terms of tissue damage or both" (8, p. 21). A subcommittee on taxonomy for the International Association for the Study of Pain set forth a similar definition of pain: "Pain is an unpleasant sensory and emotional experience associated with actual or potential tissue damage, or described in terms of such damage" (9, p. 5217). The committee further stated that experiences which resemble pain, such as "prickling," but which are not unpleasant, should not be classified as pain. Their definition attempts to account for early observations and concepts of pain, such as the subjective nature of pain, past learned experiences, and emotional and physical meanings. Established definitions for terms used to describe various aspects of pain are presented in Table 1. In addition, the committee developed a coding scheme and criteria for the diagnosis of various pain syndromes.

There is often the tendency to confuse the assessment and management of acute pain with that of chronic pain. It is important to understand some of the basic differences in the presentations, characteristics,

Table 1. Pain Terms*

Pain	An unpleasant sensory and emotional experience associated with actual or potential tissue damage, or described in terms of such damage
Allodynia	Pain due to a stimulus which does not normally provoke pain
Analgesia	Absence of pain in response to stimulation which would normally be painful
Anaesthesia dolorosa	Pain in an area or region which is anaesthetic
Causalgia	A syndrome of sustained burning pain, allodynia, and hyperpathia after a traumatic nerve lesion, often combined with vasomotor and pseudomotor dysfunction and later trophic changes
Central pain	Pain associated with a lesion of the central nervous system
Dysaesthesia	An unpleasant abnormal sensation, whether spontaneous or evoked
Hyperaesthesia	Increased sensitivity to stimulation, excluding the special senses
Hyperalgesia	An increased response to a stimulus which is normally painful
Hyperpathia	A painful syndrome, characterized by increased reaction to a stimulus, especially a repetitive stimulus, as well as an increased threshold
Hypoaesthesia	Decreased sensitivity to stimulation, excluding the special senses
Hypoalgesia	Diminished pain in response to normally painful stimulus
Neuralgia	Pain in the distribution of a nerve or nerves
Neuritis	Inflammation of a nerve or nerves
Neuropathy	A disturbance of function or pathological change in a nerve; in one nerve, mononeuropathy; in several nerves, mononeuropathy multiplex; if diffuse and bilateral, polyneuropathy
Nociceptor	A receptor preferentially sensitive to a noxious stimulus or to a stimulus which would become noxious if prolonged
Noxious stimulus	A noxious stimulus is one which is damaging to normal tissues
Pain threshold	The least experience of pain that a subject can recognize
Pain tolerance level	The greatest level of pain that a subject is prepared to tolerate
Paraesthesia	An abnormal sensation, whether spontaneous or evoked

* Recommended by the IASP Subcommittee on Taxonomy. Reprinted from Classification of Chronic Pain: Description of Chronic Pain Syndromes and Definitions of Pain Terms. Pain Supplement 3, 1986. Reprinted by permission of Elsevier Publishing Company.

and associated phenomenology of acute and chronic pain (other than duration).

ACUTE PAIN

Acute pain is of recent onset and of relatively short and variable duration. When associated with tissue damage or injury, the pain diminishes as the healing occurs. Acute pain may occur in several nonpathological states that are not the result of a disease process (such as "growing pain," labor pain during childbirth, fatigue, sleep-deprived states, and pain following periods of strenuous exercise). More commonly, pain is associated with a pathological state or tissue damage. On occasion, however, pain is not associated immediately with the tissue damage but develops during the healing process. Pain is the symptom of a disease or injury that most commonly motivates a person to seek medical care (8, 10). Acute pain can also be induced experimentally by blood-flow alterations, electrical stimulation, chemical irritation, mechanical changes, or temperature alterations. Pain induced by these changes is transient and therefore represents an acute pain model.

Acute pain warns a person that something is wrong. Acute pain signals one to initiate behavior that will eliminate the cause of the pain, the symptoms of the pain, or both. It also prepares an individual to cope with a disease or injury. In fact, Wall (11) states that pain may be associated with recovery, reinforcing rest in the injured person in order to promote healing. Pain-initiated behaviors are significantly influenced by past learned experiences, social-cultural settings in which pain and injury occur, the psychological state of the individual at the time of onset of pain, as well as the patient's personality. Data regarding the type, description, and location of the acute pain are useful to the physician when diagnosing pain, either as a symptom of a disease or as a response to a maneuver during a physical examination.

There is usually a strong correlation between the location, type, and severity of pain and the disease process and/or injury. The duration of acute pain in illness or injury can be predicted by the physician when the cause of the pain is known. Both the patient and the physician expect that the pain will diminish, for example, as the underlying illness resolves. Acute pain also serves as a coping mechanism (defense mechanism) in patients with various forms of psychopathology (such as personality disorders or major depression).

Anxiety uniformly occurs in acute pain states. The autonomic responses of sympathetic hyperactivity in acute pain and anxiety are identical. The autonomic changes include tachycardia, tachypnea, increased peripheral blood flow, increased systolic and diastolic blood pressure, increased striated muscle tension, pupillary dilatation, palmar sweating, decreased gut motility, decreased salivary flow, and release of catecholamines. The intensity of the autonomic activity is usually proportional to the extent of nociception. Methods to reduce anxiety (that is, hypnosis, relaxation, antianxiety drugs, explanation, reassurance, and self-control of painful stimulus) reduce the intensity of pain as well as the magnitude of the pain response. This effect occurs in both experimental and clinical pain.

CHRONIC PAIN

Chronic pain is most often defined as the daily occurrence of pain over an extended period of time (more than six months). Chronic pain occurs most commonly in headache, back pain, arthritis, cancer, and certain psychiatric disorders—major depression, anxiety disorders, somatoform disorders, hypochondriasis, and psychogenic pain disorder. All of these conditions will be described in greater detail in the third section of this book, Clinical Concepts.

Chronic pain persists despite the intervention of medical treatment and the passage of time. Patient and physician alike are unable to give a satisfactory explanation for the presence and continuation of the pain. The time course of chronic pain is unknown. The physiological, anatomical, and biochemical pathology identified by physical examination and diagnostic tests usually do not adequately uncover the cause of the pain.

Patients with chronic pain display little autonomic hyperactivity. They exhibit neurovegetative symptoms such as disrupted sleep, altered appetite and weight, decreased libido and energy, diminished concentration, and irritability. Such patients usually have a history of multiple medical and surgical interventions aimed at relieving the cause of the pain. The associated emotional distress, family disturbance, economic hardship, and altered lifestyle secondary to the persistent pain become significant problems in themselves. Generally, the longer a patient suffers from chronic pain, the more psychological and social factors influence the course of the syndrome. In addition to exhibiting increased irritability, as just mentioned, chronic pain patients show signs of social withdrawal. They become increasingly inactive as their pain persists. In addition to the emotional distress, inactivity, and social isolation experienced by these patients, they often believe, despite reassurance, that their persistent pain arises from a serious disease (12, 13). Pilowsky describes this behavior as "abnormal illness behavior" (14; see also Chapters 7 and 11 of this volume).

THE DICHOTOMY BETWEEN ORGANIC AND PSYCHOGENIC PAIN

Another quandary surrounds the attempt to dichotomize the etiology of pain as either organic or psychogenic. This attempt tends to ignore that the development and continuation of pain are most often secondary to a

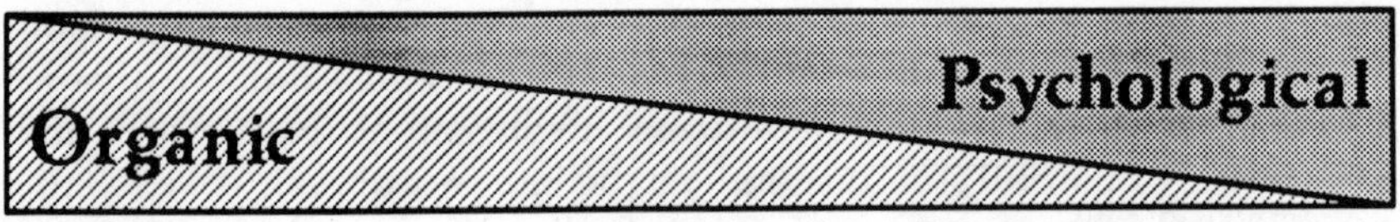

Organic		Psychological
Neuropathies	Low back	Depression
Trigeminal neuralgia	Atypical facial	Conversion disorder
Cancer	TMJ	Psychogenic pain
Thalamic syndrome	Chronic pelvic	disorder
Central pain	Myofascial pain	Somatization disorder
Deafferent pain	Headache	Hypochondriasis
Arthritis	Causalgia	Dementia
Phantom limb		Generalized anxiety
Peripheral nerve injury		disorder

Figure 1. Classification based on predominant etiological factors in chronic pain.

complex interplay of organic and psychological factors (Figure 1). The notion that pain is secondary to or influenced by multiple factors is supported by several studies.

BIOLOGICAL AND PSYCHOLOGICAL FACTORS INFLUENCING THE LEVEL OF NOCICEPTION, PAIN THRESHOLD, AND PAIN TOLERANCE

Nociception is defined as the perception that tissue damage is taking place or has already occurred (9). Pain threshold refers to the degree of pain just noticeably different from the neutral or pain-free sensation. Pain tolerance means the most intense pain—in both magnitude and duration—that one can endure. Pain complaints and pain behavior are physical expressions of the experiences of nociception, pain threshold, and pain tolerance. Nociception, pain threshold, and pain tolerance have biological determinants, but can also be influenced by psychological processes. A brief summary of the various factors influencing pain threshold is given in Table 2.

A person's pain threshold can be altered by certain psychological states such as anxiety (15) and depression (15, 16, 17), and by certain disorders such as bipolar disorder (18), and psychosis (19, 20, 21) [see Table 2]. In addition, fatigue (21), insomnia (21), and suggestion (22, 23) can alter pain threshold. Certain medications—including benzodiazepines (24), barbiturates (24), meprobamate (24), narcotics (25), and, possibly, antidepressants (26)—can also affect the pain threshold. It has been re-

Table 2. Factors Affecting Pain Threshold

Factors	Pain Threshold
Psychological state	
depression	↑
anxiety	↓
bipolar depressed phase	↑
bipolar manic phase	↑
psychosis	↑
stress	↑
fatigue	↓
suggestion	↑
Medical disorders	
osteoarthritis	↓
myofascial syndrome	↓
Medications	
barbiturates	↓
meprobamate	↓
antidepressants	↑
benzodiazepines	?
(diazepam IV)	↑
opioid analgesics	
low dose	↑↓
moderate dose	↑
high dose	↑

↑ = increases pain threshold   ↑↓ = variable
↓ = decreases pain threshold   ? = questionable

ported that myofascial pain syndrome and osteoarthritis can lower pain threshold (27, 28).

It should be noted that a factor that alters pain threshold may not necessarily alter pain behavior or complaints in the same direction. A notable example of this occurs in depression. Several studies (15, 16, 17) have shown that major depression increases a patient's pain threshold. However, pain complaints are frequent symptoms of the depressive syndrome (29, 30) [Table 3]. Pain complaints are also common in patients with anxiety disorder (31, 32) and substance use disorder (33). The manic phase of bipolar disorder is associated with a decrease in pain complaints (34), while the depressed phase is associated with an increase in pain complaints (35). The presence of secondary gain factors (36), fatigue (21, 37), and insomnia (38) will increase pain complaints. Reassurance (39, 40), distraction (41, 42), and elation (34) will minimize pain complaints. Control of pain stimuli (43, 44), placebo response, sug-

Table 3. Factors Affecting Pain Complaints

Factors	Pain Complaints
Psychiatric disorders	
depression	↑
generalized anxiety disorder	↑
bipolar disorder	
manic	↓
depressed	↑
substance/use disorder	↑
Psychological/physical state	
anxiety	↑
fatigue	↑
insomnia	↑
distraction	↓
reassurance	↓
control of painful stimuli	↑↓
placebo response	↑↓
secondary gain	↑↓
elation	↓
depression	↓
uncertainty	↑
cognitive strategies	↑↓
advanced age	↑
Medications	
antidepressants	↓
opioid analgesics	↓
antianxiety agents	↓
sedative/hypnotics	
acute	↓
chronic	↑

↑ = increases pain complaints   ↑↓ = variable
↓ = decreases pain complaints

gestion (22, 23), and cognitive strategies (45, 46) may have conflicting effects on pain complaints. Uncertainty (39, 40) and anxiety will increase pain complaints. Increasing age is associated with increased pain complaints (15). The use of antidepressants/antianxiety agents (31) and opioid analgesics (25) will decrease pain complaints. Acute administration of sedative/hypnotics will decrease pain complaints, but prolonged use will increase pain complaints. The significance of the relationship among pain threshold, pain complaints, and behavior may be limited in clinical practice. If pain does not elicit the associated response of anxiety, fear, or suffering, then the patient's ability to tolerate pain may be increased, even when the capacity to perceive this sensation is relatively unaltered (47, 48).

THE ECONOMIC IMPACT OF CHRONIC PAIN

So far, we have addressed the conceptual and nosological aspects of chronic pain as they relate to individual patients. We would now like to address the economic impact of chronic pain.

The chronic pain syndromes that involve the clinician fall into three categories. The first category includes those disorders in which the pain persists beyond the usual course for an acute disease, beyond a reasonable time for an injury to heal, or recurs at intervals for months or years. Chronic low back pain would be a prime example of this type of disorder. A second category includes pain that persists in the face of obvious underlying pathology, but for which the underlying pathology itself cannot be altered. This would include cancer pain. The third category includes those disorders that occur in greater frequency or with greater severity than normal. These would include migraine headaches or arthritis.

Data are not available from a single national comprehensive survey on the prevalence of chronic pain; rather, available evidence is extrapolated for national and regional surveys of specific disorders drawn from both private and federal sources. These data suggest that acute and chronic pain cost the national economy between $85 and $90 billion annually, and that approximately $60 billion of that total is attributed to the cost from chronic pain (49). It is estimated that one-third of all Americans suffer from one form or another of chronic pain. Furthermore, it is likely that 50 million individuals are partially or totally disabled and that 700 million work days are lost each year because of chronic pain.

Among the most frequent and debilitating forms of chronic pain that are so costly to the nation's economy are headache, low back pain, cancer pain, pain related to arthritis, posttraumatic pain, and burn pain.

Headache

It is estimated that 42 million American men and 48 million American women experience headache (50). Of this group, about 40 million individuals are severely affected, as defined by requiring medications or by absence from work because of their need for bed rest (51). Approximately 13 percent of men and 15 to 25 percent of women are absent from work at least four days a year for bed rest secondary to headache (50). For migraine headache alone, 65 million work days are lost and $4 billion are spent on medication (51).

Low Back Pain

Approximately 15 percent of the adult population in the United States has had low back pain at some time (50). Fifteen million individuals are affected at any one time, with 5 million Americans qualifying for at least partial disability as a result of chronic low back pain (50, 51). Two million Americans are so severely disabled that they cannot work (50). Ninety-three million work days a year are lost as a result of people falling into these two groups, and costs for direct medical care alone are estimated to be $5 billion (51).

Cancer Pain

The exact number of patients suffering from cancer pain has not been clearly established. It is thought that cancer affects at least one million Americans annually (51). Some hospital-based studies have found that up to 50 percent of hospitalized cancer patients have unrelieved pain (50), leading us to suspect that a significant number of Americans suffer pain from this disease.

Arthritis

Twenty million individuals suffer from arthritis, and of this group, some three to four million require intensive medical care or hospitalization (51). Three million arthritis sufferers are disabled, and $4 billion in productivity and health care costs are lost each year as a result of arthritis pain (51).

Posttraumatic Pain

One-third of the 50 million accidental injuries that occur annually are associated with moderate to severe pain (50).

Burn Pain

One hundred and sixty thousand people each year sustain burns that produce continuous pain (50).

The above categories highlight the dramatic impact that pain has on our nation's economy. Harder to delineate, however, but just as dramatic, are the other costs that these people endure. Many chronic pain patients develop depression, somatic preoccupation, and anxiety. Some attempt suicide. Depression is estimated to occur in more than 50 percent of these chronic pain patients, and some form of abnormal behavioral functioning is estimated to occur in about 70 percent (50). Data from one clinic suggest that 95 percent of these patients use narcotics regularly; 90 percent use psychotropics regularly; 90 percent are estimated to misuse drugs; and 80 percent suffer withdrawal symptoms from one or more of the drugs they are taking (50).

In this chapter we have introduced some of the basic concepts and nosology of pain; we have discussed the differences between acute and chronic pain; and we have addressed the major economic impact of chronic pain.

In the next chapter we present a systems model which will provide a framework for refining the conceptual basis of chronic pain, as well as a tool for assessment and management.

REFERENCES

1. Bonica JJ: Neurophysiologic and pathologic aspects of acute and chronic pain. Arch Surg 112:750–761, 1977
2. Hardy JD, Wolff HD, Goodell H: Pain Sensations and Reactions. Baltimore, Williams & Wilkins, 1952
3. Szasz TS: Pain and Pleasure. A Study of Bodily Feelings. New York, Basic Books, 1957
4. Engel GL: Psychogenic pain. Med Clin North Am 42:1481–1496, 1958
5. Engel GL: 'Psychogenic' pain and the pain-prone patient. Am J Med 26:899–918, 1959
6. Melzack R: The Puzzle of Pain. New York, Basic Books, 1973
7. Sternbach RA: Pain: A Psychophysiological Analysis. New York, Academic Press, 1968
8. Merskey H, Spear FG: Pain, Psychological and Psychiatric Aspects. London, Bailliere, Tindall and Cassel, 1967
9. IASP Subcommittee on Taxonomy: Classification of Chronic Pain: Description of Chronic Pain Syndromes and Definitions of Pain Terms. Pain Supplement 3, 1986
10. Douglas-Wilson I: Somatic manifestations of psychoneurosis. Br Med J 1:413–415, 1944
11. Wall PD: On the relation of injury to pain. Pain 6:253–264, 1969
12. Pilowsky I, Chapman CR, Bonica JJ: Pain, depression, and illness behavior in a pain clinic population. Pain 4:183–192, 1977
13. Pilowsky I, Spence ND: Illness behavior syndromes associated with intractable pain. Pain 2:61–71, 1976
14. Pilowsky I: Abnormal illness behavior. Br J Med Psychol 42:347–351, 1969
15. Hall KRL, Stride E: The varying response to pain in psychiatric disorders: a study in abnormal psychology. Br J Med Psychol 27:48–60, 1954
16. Hemphill RE, Hall KRL, Crookes TG: A preliminary report on fatigue and pain tolerance in depressive and psychoneurotic patients. Journal of Mental Science 98:433–440, 1952
17. Davis GC, Buchsbaum MS, Bunney WE: Analgesia to painful stimuli in affective illness. Am J Psychiatry 136:1148–1151, 1979
18. Marchand WE, Shrota B, Marble HC: Occurrence of painless acute surgical disorder in psychotic patients. N Engl J Med 260:580–585, 1959

19. Geschwind N: Insensitivity to pain in psychiatric patients. N Engl J Med 296:1480, 1977
20. Torrey EF: Headaches after lumbar puncture and insensitivity to pain in psychiatric patients. N Engl J Med 301:110, 1979
21. Sternbach RA: Acute versus chronic pain, in Textbook of Pain. Edited by Wall PD, Melzack R. London, Churchill, Livingstone, 1984
22. Wolff BB, Harland AA: Effect of suggestion upon experimental pain: a validation study. J Abnorm Psychol 72:402–407, 1967
23. Blitz B, Dinnerstein AJ: Effects of different types of instruction on pain parameters. J Abnorm Psychol 73:276–280, 1968
24. Harvey SC: Hypnotics and sedatives, in The Pharmacological Basis of Therapeutics. Edited by Goodman AF, Goodman LS, Gilman A. New York, MacMillan, 1980
25. Jaffe JH, Martin WR: Opioid analgesics and antagonists, in The Pharmacological Basis of Therapeutics. Edited by Goodman AF, Goodman LS, Gilman A. New York, MacMillan, 1980
26. Sternbach RA, Janowsky DS, Huey LY, et al: Effects of altering brain serotonin activity on human chronic pain, in Advances in Pain Research and Therapy, vol. 1. Edited by Bonica JJ, Albe-Fessard D. New York, Raven Press, 1976
27. Smythe HA: Fibrositis as a disorder of pain modulation. Clin Rheum Dis 5:823–832, 1979
28. Lamo T: The role of activity in the central of membrane and contractile properties of skeletal muscle, in Motor Innervation of Muscle. Edited by Thesleff S. New York, Academic Press, 1976
29. Sternbach RA: Pain Patients: Traits and Treatment. New York, Academic Press, 1974
30. Weisenberg M: Pain and pain control. Psychol Bull 84:1008–1044, 1977
31. Craig KD: Emotional aspects of pain, in Textbook of Pain. Edited by Wall PD, Melzack R. London, Churchill Livingstone, 1983
32. Merskey H: The effects of chronic pain upon the response to noxious stimuli by psychiatric patients. J Psychiatr Res 8:405–419, 1965
33. Maruta T, Swanson DW, Finlayson RE: Drug abuse and dependency in patients with chronic pain. Mayo Clin Proc 54:241–244, 1979
34. Compton-Smith RN: Psychological factors in pain. Br Med J 2:535, 1965
35. Cassidy WL, Flanagan ND, Spellman M, et al: Clinical observations in manic-depressive disease. JAMA 164:1535–1546, 1957
36. Fordyce WE: Behavioral Methods for Chronic Pain and Illness. St. Louis, C. V. Mosby, 1976
37. Moldofsky H, Scaresbrick P, England R, et al: Musculoskeletal symptoms and non-REM sleep disturbance in patients with fibrositis syndrome and healthy subjects. Psychosom Med 37:341–351, 1975
38. Moldofsky H, Scaresbrick P: Induction of neurasthenic musculoskeletal pain syndrome by selective sleep stage deprivation. Psychosom Med 38:35–44, 1976
39. Kendall PC, Watson D: Psychological preparation for stressful medical procedures, in Medical Psychology: Contributions to Behavioral Medicine. Edited by Prokop CK, Bradley LA. New York, Academic Press, 1981

40. Reading AE: The short term effects of psychological preparation for surgery. Soc Sci Med 13A:641–654, 1979
41. Horan JA, Dellinger DK: 'In vivo' emotive imagery: a preliminary test. Percept Mot Skills 39:359–362, 1974
42. Chaves JF, Barber TY: Cognitive strategies, experiment modeling, and expectation in the attenuation of pain. J Abnorm Psychol 83:356–363, 1974
43. Straub E, Turskey B, Schwartz GE: Self-control and predictability: their effects or reactions to aversive stimulation. J Pers Soc Psychol 18:157–162, 1971
44. Glass DC, Singe JE, Leonard HS, et al: Perceived control of aversive stimulation. J Pers 41:577–595, 1973
45. Turk DC: Cognitive behavioral techniques in the management of pain, in Cognitive Behavior Therapy: Research and Application. Edited by Foreyt JP, Rathjen DP. New York, Plenum Press, 1978
46. Tan SY: Cognitive and cognitive behavioural methods of pain control: a selective review. Pain 12:201–228, 1982
47. Wolff BB: Behavioural measurement of human pain, in The Psychology of Pain. Edited by Sternbach RA. New York, Raven Press, 1978
48. Beecher HK: The Measurement of Subjective Responses: Quantitative Effects of Drugs. New York, Oxford University Press, 1959
49. Bonica JJ: Preface—New Approaches to Treatment of Chronic Pain, in A Review of Multidisciplinary Pain Clinics and Pain Centers. Research Monograph. Edited by Ng LKY. Washington, DC, NIDA, 1981
50. Bonica JJ: Pain research and therapy: past and current status and future needs, in Pain, Discomfort and Humanitarian Care. Edited by Ng LKY, Bonica JJ. New York, Elsevier North Holland, 1980
51. Report of the Panel on Pain to the National Advisory Neurological and Communicative Disorders and Stroke Council, NIH Publication No. 79-1912. Washington, DC, DHEW, 1979

Chapter 2

Systems Approach to Chronic Pain Syndromes

K. Ranga Rama Krishnan, M.D.

Randal D. France, M.D.

Bruno J. Urban, M.D.

Multiple factors are involved in the development of chronic pain syndromes. As we have noted in Chapter 1, these include organic, psychological, and socioenvironmental factors. Chronic pain syndrome is not only the sum of the interaction of all of these factors, but is also influenced by the sequelae of chronic pain, which again are organic, psychological, and socioenvironmental in nature.

A systems approach is probably the best way to assess the role of all of these factors. A basic systems model for chronic pain syndromes is presented in Figure 1. In this figure we show 1) the role of multiple factors in the development of a chronic pain state; 2) the sequelae to chronic pain; 3) the factors that interact in the development of these sequelae; 4) the progression of the sequelae; and, 5) the effect of the sequelae on the chronic pain syndrome. Although the basic model as described appears static, the dynamic nature of the processes described must be kept in mind.

The system that we describe in this chapter focuses on the individual, but it can be developed to interrelate with systems at other levels. Furthermore, this approach can provide a framework for understanding chronic pain syndrome, for assessing chronic pain syndrome, for the rational management of chronic pain syndrome, and for the development and testing of hypotheses.

CLASSIFICATION OF ORGANIC FACTORS

Some chronic pain syndromes have primarily an organic etiology (Figure 2). These include trigeminal neuralgia, chronic gastric ulcer pain,

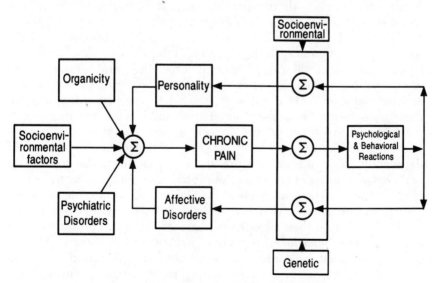

Figure 1. Systems model for chronic pain

17

chronic arthritis pain, angina, some types of cancer pain, and central pain syndromes. It must be noted that even in these primarily organic conditions, the patient's personality, sociocultural, and psychological factors may also play a role in the development of chronic pain.

Bonica (1) has provided a framework that classifies organic factors responsible for chronic pain into three groups based on the origin of the nociceptive input: a) peripheral, b) central, and c) peripheral-central.

Peripheral Origin

Biochemical, mechanical, or thermal stimuli acting upon pain receptors can generate a chronic pain state. This mechanism may be responsible for the chronic pain of arthritis, peptic ulcer, angina, and some types of cancer pain.

Central Origin

Lesions of the central nervous system often produce a condition that has been referred to as "central pain." The lesions can occur in the spinal cord (pain in paraplegics), thalamus (thalamic syndrome), and cortical areas (trauma). The mechanism of this disorder is unknown, but evidence suggests a loss of descending inhibitory influences or a loss of sensory inputs (2). Central pain is discussed in detail in Chapter 10.

Peripheral-Central Origin

Abnormalities of both the peripheral and central portions of the somatosensory system can generate chronic pain (1). Examples of chronic pain that have both a peripheral and central abnormality of the somatosensory system include phantom limb pain, causalgia, migraine, paresthesias associated with peripheral nerve injury, and surgical lesions of rhizotomies and cordotomies, diabetic neuropathy, toxic neuropathy, and herniated disc (1). As Bonica has noted, the pathophysiology of these abnormalities is not well understood and it is possible that several mechanisms are involved (1). In this group, psychological and sociocultural mechanisms probably play a major role in the development of the chronic pain syndrome (Figure 2). The development of chronic pain in these conditions depends on multiple factors, with the role and importance of each factor in a given individual usually impossible to assess.

Patients with pain in whom no clearly identifiable psychological factors can be found often show a history of repeated childhood hospitalizations as well as illness behavior patterns that are abnormal (3). Green (4) points out that children have difficulty communicating and understanding pain. The experience of illness requiring hospitalization during a period when the child's linguistic and interpersonal skills are not well developed

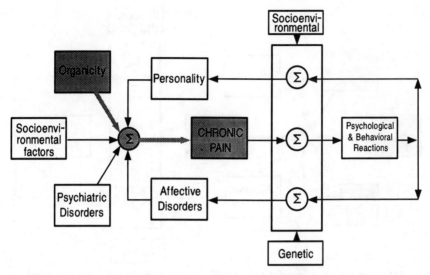

Figure 2. Systems model for chronic pain: chronic pain of organic etiology

may lead to the subsequent development of abnormal illness behaviors, including chronic pain and the behavior associated with it.

PSYCHOLOGICAL MECHANISMS CAUSING OR MODIFYING CHRONIC PAIN

Psychological, behavioral, and psychiatric factors can influence pain and pain behavior even when the mechanism is primarily of an organic origin. In some cases the pain can be explained to a considerable extent by psychological mechanisms (Figure 3). For instance, pain is a common complaint in patients with generalized anxiety (5). On the other hand, pain is a relatively rare complaint of manic and schizophrenic patients (6). Chronic pain may occur as part of the symptom complex of: a) major depression, especially when associated with anxiety; b) generalized anxiety disorder; c) dementia; and d) occasionally, psychosis (7).

Pain as a symptom of depression is found in 30 to 60 percent of patients with affective disorder (8, 9, 10). Studies by von Knorring found that 57 percent of patients with depression reported pain as a symptom (9, 10). Depressed patients with pain complaints also showed significant degrees of anxiety, agitation, sleep disturbance, suicidal thoughts, and muscle tension (10). Pain as a symptom of depression is discussed further in Chapter 9.

Pain may also be part of the symptom complex of somatoform disorder, conversion disorder, malingering, and Munchausen syndrome. It is also more commonly seen in patients with certain types of personality

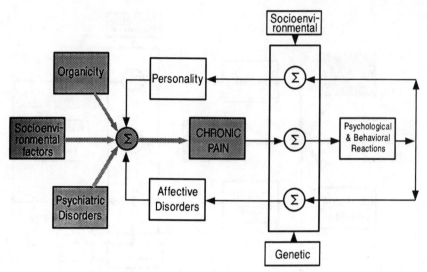

Figure 3. Systems model for chronic pain: chronic pain of idiopathic etiology

traits and/or disorders, such as histrionic personality disorder (11). Personality (as shown in Figure 4) refers not only to the core personality of the individual but also to the effects of superimposed illness behavior and psychological functioning.

SOCIOENVIRONMENTAL FACTORS

Socioenvironmental factors play a role in almost all types of chronic pain syndromes. Patients whose income is primarily derived from manual labor, who have limited education, and whose personality styles involve denial of emotional distress are prone to developing chronic pain following an injury (6). In certain patients, complaints and pain behavior are strongly influenced by socioenvironmental factors, and their behavior is usually inconsistent. These patients may appear to be in severe pain during the physical examination, while they appear quite calm and relaxed in the waiting room beforehand. Although this behavior can be viewed from several perspectives, including psychodynamic, one useful approach is based on operant mechanisms; that is, patients adopt a chronic pain life-style because they find it highly reinforcing. Operant theorists maintain that pain behavior patterns of chronic low back pain develop slowly over time (12). For example, in the acute stage of back pain, patients learn to assume stiff postures to reduce the pain, endure forced inactivity, and increase their medication intake. They may also discover that their pain enables them to avoid unwanted work and home responsibilities as well as family conflicts. In some patients who go on to

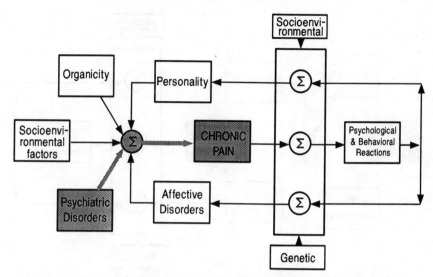

Figure 4. Systems model for chronic pain: chronic pain in psychiatric disorders

develop chronic back pain, the pain complaints may become controlled primarily by their positive social and environmental consequences (operant mechanisms). Figure 5 summarizes these mechanisms.

Patients with clear organic disease origins for pain—such as those with "learned pain disease" as described by Fordyce (13, 14), Sternbach (15), and Brena (16)—suffer prolonged disability, emotional disorder, and illness behavior patterns (17) that make these patients similar in appearance to patients whose pain behavior is adequately accounted for by the behavioral model. However, once the organic cause of the chronic pain is treated, the pain behavior reduces and eventually disappears.

Another socioenvironmental factor that assumes a role in the development of chronic pain is that of compensation. One condition in which this is a major factor is compensation neurosis (18). The pain in this condition often becomes a symbol, not only of pain, but also of feelings (19).

Effects of Chronic Pain

Chronic pain may affect the intrapsychic functioning of the individual and may engender feelings of helpless anxiety that are frequently followed by despair and depression. Chronic pain may also disrupt the patient's interpersonal functioning, both at the familial and societal levels. In some cases the helplessness is reinforced and the pain behavior is encouraged: in other cases the patient is rejected and consequently suffers despair. These styles of functioning are based upon the complex

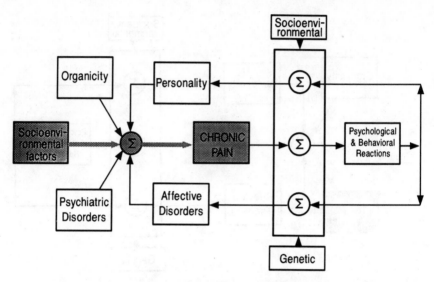

Figure 5. Systems model for chronic pain: chronic pain of socioenvironmental etiology

interaction between premorbid personality and the illness. As shown in figures, personality encompasses both the core personality—which is probably developed as a result of the interaction between the innate characteristics of the individual and the environment—and the effects of the superimposed illness behavior and psychological functioning. The occurrence of maladaptive styles of functioning and behavior patterns are often secondary to social and environmental factors. Behaviors that reinforce pain, both in the family and in society, play a role in the persistence of chronic pain (see Figure 1).

Major depression, intermittent depressive disorder, and minor depression are common sequelae of chronic pain. These affective disorders in turn (see Figure 1) exacerbate chronic pain (20). The occurrence of major depression and other psychiatric sequelae again result from a complex interplay of family, genetic, social, and environmental factors. An increased familial incidence of depression in chronic pain patients who become depressed indicates the possibility of a genetic component (21). Psychological and behavioral sequelae are further discussed in Chapters 7 and 13.

Assessment

The systems approach outlined in Figure 1 provides a rational and systematic method for assessing chronic pain patients. The presence of organic factors, personality and psychiatric disorders, as well as socioenvironmental factors has to be evaluated. Thus, a careful clinical, laboratory, and radiological evaluation (Figure 6), coupled with a detailed assessment for the presence of psychiatric disorders, must be performed (Figure 7). The presence of psychiatric disorders secondary to chronic pain should also be recognized. The dexamethasone suppression test (DST) may be helpful in identifying major depression in these patients, although it will be useful only as an adjunct (22, 23). Details of the assessment procedures are provided in Chapters 16 and 17.

The patient's history and an evaluation of family interaction patterns should be done where possible, preferably by interviewing the family. The Minnesota Multiphasic Personality Inventory (MMPI) can be useful in assessing the role of various psychological factors. However, as noted by Sternbach (15), there are no differences on MMPI between patients with and without organic findings. Most patients experiencing chronic pain, and especially those with chronic low back pain, show elevations on three scales—hypochondriasis, hysteria, and depression. Another scale that is sometimes useful in assessing the role of psychological factors is the Hendler Pain Inventory (24). These scales are not diagnostic instruments by themselves but serve to complement clinical and diagnostic assessments.

It is also necessary to assess the *effects* of chronic pain. Thus, maladaptive styles of functioning and operant mechanisms should be sought and identified through the use of a videotape assessment of body movements and pain behavior. A review of the patient's activity records will also

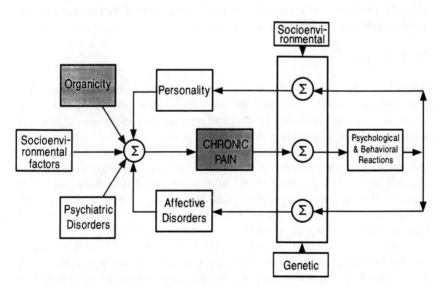

Figure 6. Systems model for chronic pain: physical assessment

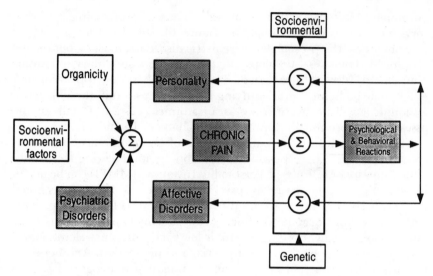

Figure 7. Systems model for chronic pain: psychiatric assessment

provide valuable assessment data. A behavioral interview with the patient, spouse, and other family members regarding their activities, the nature of any changes in the activities of family members, and the nature of any changes in family relationships will give the clinician an understanding of the operant mechanisms (Figure 8). Similarly, standardized behavioral assessments of pain behavior and daily activity diaries also provide information regarding both environmental factors and behavioral activities related to pain.

Management

After a careful assessment of the chronic pain patient, management of the pain should be individually tailored to that patient. At the very beginning, it needs to be clearly understood in the minds of both the patient and the physician that the pain is real. If any specific treatable organic factor is found, then treatment should be directed first toward that (for example, treatment of ulcer, trigeminal neuralgia, or depression). The rest of the treatment should then be based upon an assessment of the various components of the system described in Figure 1. We will discuss the various management methods in relation to selected components of the system in Chapters 18 to 25 (Figure 9).

Given the complexity of chronic pain syndromes, the best treatment can be given only in multidisciplinary settings. Toward this end, several programs, both inpatient and outpatient, have been started that include psychiatrists, psychologists, nurses, physical therapists, neurosurgeons, and orthopedic surgeons as part of the multidisciplinary treatment teams.

Pain patients are very accepting of the concept of pain clinics and, within the context of the clinic, they are more willing to accept psychological intervention than they are when such recommendations are made

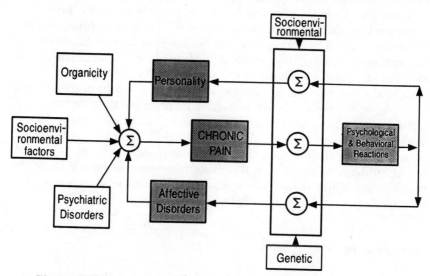

Figure 8. Systems model for chronic pain: behavioral assessment

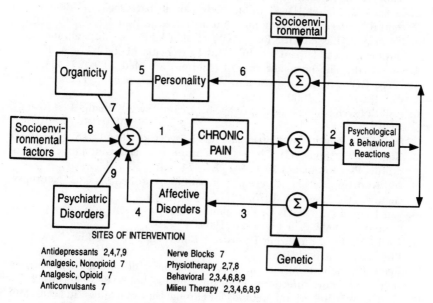

Figure 9. Systems model for chronic pain: management

by their personal physicians. Since the time Bonica and colleagues started the pain clinic concept, the number of such clinics has rapidly grown (25, 26). Psychiatrists who intend to be part of such a team will find it useful to gain an understanding of chronic pain from the multidisciplinary point of view. Furthermore, we have found that it is a multidisciplinary approach that best serves the patient.

It must be clearly understood that the systems approach provides a framework in which theories can be tested. The systems approach is not a theory by itself. The framework that we have outlined is based on our current understanding of chronic pain. It must also be understood that the systems approach allows us to understand and evaluate the role of each of the components involved in chronic pain *in a given* patient. For example, in a patient with psychogenic pain disorder, the role of organic factors might be minimal or nonexistent. In patients with chronic organic back pain, the role of psychological factors may vary—in one patient being a major factor, in another being almost inconsequential.

The subsequent chapters will provide more details about each of the components of the system: the mechanisms, clinical aspects, assessment methodologies, and management techniques.

REFERENCES

1. Bonica JJ: Neurophysiologic and pathologic aspects of acute and chronic pain. Arch Surg 112:750–761, 1977
2. Melzack R, Loeser JD: Phantom body pain in paraplegics: evidence for a central "pattern generating mechanism" for pain. Pain 4:195–210, 1978
3. Pilowsky I, Bassett DL, Begg MW, et al: Childhood hospitalization and chronic intractable pain in adults. Int J Psychiatry Med 12:75–84, 1982
4. Green DE: The hospitalization of children. NZ Med J 89:323–354, 1979
5. Large RG: The psychiatrist and the chronic pain patient: 172 anecdotes. Pain 9:253–263, 1980
6. Paul L: Psychosomatic aspects of low back pain. Psychosomatics 12:116–124, 1959
7. Spear FG: Pain in psychiatric patients. J Psychosom Res 11:187–193, 1967
8. Gentry WD, Shous WD, Thanas M: Chronic low back pain: a psychological profile. Psychosomatics 15:174–177, 1974
9. von Knorring L: The experience of pain in depressed patients. Neuropsychobiology 1:155–165, 1975
10. von Knorring L, Perris C, Eisemann M: Pain as a symptom in depressive symptomatology. Pain 15:19–26, 1983
11. Ford CV: The Somatizing Disorders: Illness As a Way of Life. New York, Elsevier Biomedical, 1983
12. Keefe FJ: Behavioral assessment and treatment of chronic pain: current status and future directions. J Consult Clin Psychol 50:896–899, 1982
13. Fordyce WE: Behavioral methods for chronic pain and illness. St. Louis, MO, C.V. Mosby, 1976

14. Fordyce WE, Fowler RS, Lehmann JF: Some implications of learning in problems of chronic pain. J Chronic Dis 21:179–190, 1968
15. Sternbach RA: Pain Patients: Traits and Treatment. New York, Academic Press, 1974
16. Brena SF: Chronic Pain: America's Hidden Epidemic. New York, Atheneum, 1978
17. Pilowsky I, Chapman CG, Bonica JJ: Pain, depression and illness behavior in a pain clinic population. Pain 4:183–192, 1977
18. Ross WD: How to get a neurotic worker back on the job successfully. Occup Health Saf 46:20–23, 1977
19. Pokorny AD, Moore FJ: Neuroses and compensation: psychiatric disorders following injury in compensable situations. Archives of Industrial Hygiene and Occupational Medicine 8:547–563, 1953
20. Krishnan KRR, France RD, Pelton S, et al: Chronic pain and depression, I: clarification of depression in chronic low back pain patients. Pain 22:279–287, 1985
21. Krishnan KRR, France RD, Houpt JL: Chronic low back pain and depression. Psychosomatics 26:299–302, 1985
22. France RD, Krishnan RKK, Houpt JL, et al: Differentiation of depression from chronic pain using the DST and DSM–III. Am J Psychiatry 141:1577–1579, 1987
23. France RD, Krishnan KRR: Biological markers of depression in chronic pain using the DST. Pain 21:49–55, 1985
24. Hendler NA, Viernstein M, Gruncer P, et al: A preoperative screening test for chronic back pain patients. Psychosomatics 20:801–805, 1979
25. Bonica JJ: Organization and function of a pain clinic. Adv Neurol 4:433–443, 1974
26. Hudson JS, Pratt TH: Pain clinics: their value to the general practitioner. South Med J 72:845–847, 1979

Basic Concepts

Chapter 3

Neuroanatomy and Neurophysiology of Chronic Pain

K. Ranga Rama Krishnan, M.D.

Randal D. France, M.D.

Lars Erikkson, M.D.

Everett H. Ellinwood, M.D.

Mechanisms of Pain and Pain Control

As we have already noted, pain can result from a number of factors. In this chapter, we describe the mechanisms—the nociceptors and the ascending pathways—involved in the perception of nociception (which we have defined in Chapter 1 as the perception that tissue damage is taking place or has already occurred), the mechanisms that modulate pain, and various theories of pain.

Nociceptors

Nociceptors are primary neurons consisting of: a receptor terminal in the periphery; an afferent fiber connecting the terminal to the neuronal cell body; an efferent connecting the cell to other neurons, with the cell body probably receiving efferents from other neurons.

Several types of nociceptors have been described. In the skin an unencapsulated, unmyelinated mechanoreceptor with a myelinated fiber capable of responding to mechanical, thermal, and chemical noxius stimuli has been described.

The central terminations of myelinated afferent fibers (enpassant enlargements) serve as synapses with neurons of the spinal cord. Mechanical nociceptive fibers branch on entry into the spinal cord and have terminals in lamina I, lamina II, lamina V, close to central canal (lamina X), and occasionally on lamina V on the opposite side of the dorsal column of the spinal cord. The central terminations of unmyelinated afferent fibers from nociceptors are usually seen in the substantia gelatinosa. The areas where nociceptors terminate are complex structures. Neurons from lamina I, lamina V, and substantia gelatinosa give rise to the ascending pathways of pain transmission (1–5). Figure 1, which shows a cross-section of the spinal cord with the various laminae, will help orient the reader to the description given above.

Spinal Dorsal Horn and the Ascending Pathways

The primary nociceptive afferents terminate in the dorsal horn, which also has long projection neurons, local circuit neurons, and axon terminals of neurons originating mainly from brainstem pathways. The long projection neurons conveying painful stimuli run mainly in the spinothalamic tract. These neurons are, for the most part, found in laminae I and V. Contemporary evidence suggests a single (rather than two) spinothalamic pathway that is multimodal, and that is without distinct separation between noxious and non-noxious components (6, 7).

The terminations in the thalamus can be grouped into two systems—a lateral and a medial. The lateral system terminates in the ventroposterolateral nucleus. The medial system terminates in the medial divi-

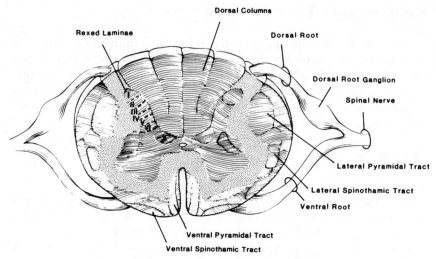

Figure 1. Spinal cord cross-section

sion of the posterior group and the medial thalamus (see Figure 2 for two views of thalamic nuclei). The lateral system is considered to be involved primarily in the transmission of acute pain, while the medial system is involved only in patients with deafferentation pain. The ventroposterolateral nucleus of the thalamus projects to the primary somatosensory cortex, including areas 3a and 12. Neurons responding to noxius stimuli are found in these areas. The entire pathway is illustrated in Figure 3 and Figure 4.

Other pathways that might play a role include the spinoreticular, spinomesencephalic, spinocervical, and the second order dorsal column tract.

Modulation of Pain Pathways

The pathways for pain that we have described so far can be modulated at several different levels and by multiple mechanisms (Figure 5). A three-tiered pain modulation system was described by Basbaum and Fields (8, 9). The major components were the midbrain periaqueductal gray (PAG), several nuclei of the rostral ventral medulla (nucleus raphe magnus [NRM] and raphe magnocellularies), and the spinal dorsal horn.

In brief, the PAG has excitatory connections to the NRM, which, in turn, projects via a pathway in the dorsal part of the lateral funiculus of the spinal cord to the spinal dorsal horn, selectively inhibiting the nociceptive neurons and interneurons. The intrinsic circuitry of the PAG is largely unknown. Furthermore, the PAG is chemically heterogeneous

and contains substance-P, vasoactive intestinal polypeptide (VIP), enkephalin, and serotonin. The PAG receives significant inputs from the
frontal and insular cortex, the amygdala, and the hypothalamus. Cognitive factors probably can activate this analgesic system through these
routes. The brain stem inputs to the PAG originate from the locus
coeruleus, pontine reticular formation, and the nucleus cuneiformis.
The locus coeruleus projection may be responsible for the norepinephrine antagonism of opiate induced analgesia. The neurons of the PAG
are known to project to the rostral medulla and also directly to the spinal
dorsal horn (10).

The NRM is also a complex structure. Serotonergic neurons are found
in large numbers. In addition, enkephalin, substance-P, somatostatin,

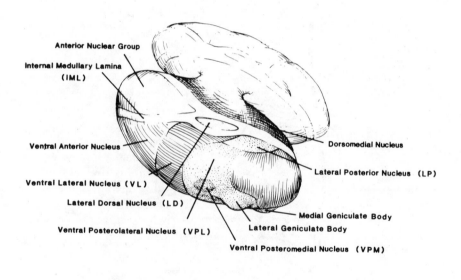

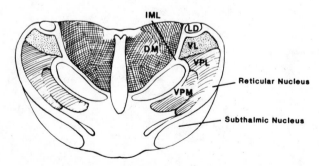

Figure 2. Thalamic nuclei: dorsolateral view of the thalamus (top); cross-section of the thalamus (bottom)

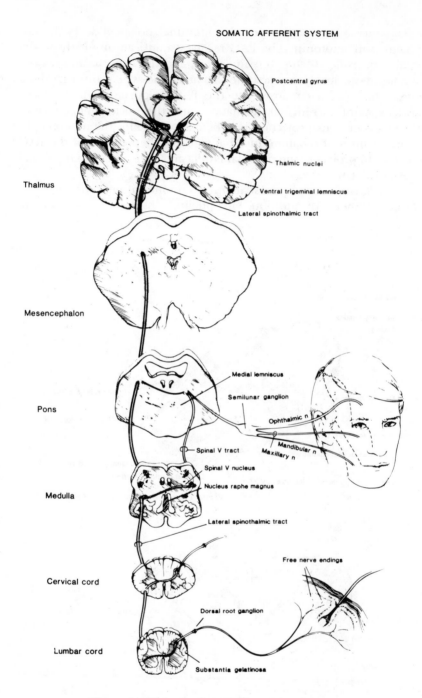

Figure 3. Diagram of ascending pain pathways

THEORIES OF PAIN PERCEPTION

Specificity and Intensity Theories

Aristotle was the first to describe the physiology of pain perception. He postulated that pain resulted when there was an excess of "vital heat" causing an increase in the sensation of touch. He believed that this "vital heat" was conveyed by the blood to the heart, where the signal was experienced as pain. Aristotle's view prevailed for a long time despite attempts on the part of anatomists and physiologists to demonstrate that the brain is the organ where pain is perceived. For a more detailed discussion of the evolution of the concept of pain, refer to Melzack (16), Bonica (17), Dallenbach (18), and others (19).

Descartes believed that there was a connection between the skin and the brain, analogous to the connection between the pulling of a rope in a church tower and the ringing of a bell in a belfry (16). And the pain, like the bell ringing, serves to transmit a message. The person feels the pain and a reaction results.

Magendie and Bell, in the early 19th century, identified ventral roots of the spinal nerves involved in motor function and the dorsal roots involved in sensory function (20). Mueller, in 1840, stated that the brain received information about external stimuli and body structure by way of the sensory nerves, and that each sensory nerve from the five classical senses had specific qualities of energy for each sensation (16). Von Frey (1890) thought that pain arose from specific receptors in the periphery, and that various sensations (touch, temperature) had specific types of receptors.

These views comprise the "specificity theory," which states that pain is a sensation with a specific receptor in the periphery and that the pain signal is transmitted by specific nerve pathways to the brain, where the message is interpreted. This theory was challenged by Darwin, Henle, Weber, and Goldscheider in the late 19th century (20). Goldscheider stated that there were no specific receptors for pain and that pain was a result of summation. Any stimulus, if it reached a certain threshold, could produce the sensation of pain. This is the "intensity theory."

The specificity theory is supported by the specialization of the peripheral nervous system and specific pain pathways, with localized interpretation of the pain message in the brain. This theory does not account for the lack of success in the diminution of pain by surgical lesions in certain pain states such as phantom limb pain, neuralgia, and causalgia. In addition, non-noxious stimuli (touching, vibration) can produce excruciating pain and can occur for long periods of time after removal of the apparent stimuli.

The intensity theory is supported by studies demonstrating a relationship between the intensity of input and the degree of the painful sensation. However, this theory ignores the specificity of the peripheral nerves and pain pathways.

Neither theory explains the phenomena of "referred pain." In this condition, pain is mislocated, light touch applied to the painful area increases the pain, and local anesthetics decrease the pain.

Gate Control Theory

The theory of pain mechanisms that is now in favor, the gate control theory of Melzack and Wall, explains the phenomenon of referred pain (16). This theory proposes that a mechanism in the spinal cord acts like a gate which can modulate the flow of nerve impulses from the periphery to the brain. The modulation of the sensory input occurs both by local mechanisms as well as by descending influences from the brain.

Injury produces signals which are transmitted by two types of fibers: the large diameter and the small diameter fibers. The large diameter fibers are beta fibers; the small diameter fibers are delta fibers and C-fibers. Nerve impulses from the delta fibers and the C-fibers terminate on what are called transmission cells or 'T' cells in lamina 5 of the dorsal horn of the spinal cord. Fibers also impinge on cells in the substantia gelatinosa. The large diameter fibers impinge upon the 'T' cells. Large fiber activity activates cells in the substantia gelatinosa, which act as modulators. Activity of the large fibers inhibits transmission of activity from the small fibers to the 'T' cells. It is believed that this inhibition is mediated by substantia gelatinosa cells. Further inhibitory effects and transmission from afferent fibers to 'T' cells are exerted by the descending control systems described in Figure 2.

According to the gate control theory, the large diameter fibers are also believed to activate selective cognitive processes, which then, by way of descending fibers, modulate the spinal gating mechanisms. In the output of the spinal cord, transmission cells exceed the critical level and activate the complex patterns of behavior and experience that are characteristic of pain. Figure 6 is a schematic diagram of the gate control theory of pain.

Certain parts of the gate control theory are accepted; others are not. Gate control theory is able to explain some of the puzzling aspects of pain. It explains the finding that pain does not always occur following peripheral stimulation; it explains the influence of psychological factors on pain; and it explains the clinical phenomenon of the persistence of pain after healing.

In summary, the signal from noxious stimulation as it passes from the peripheral nerves into the spinal cord is modified by a "gating" mechanism located in the dorsal horn of the spinal cord. If the gate is open, information from the periphery is transmitted to the brain; if the gate is partially open or closed, less information or no information reaches the

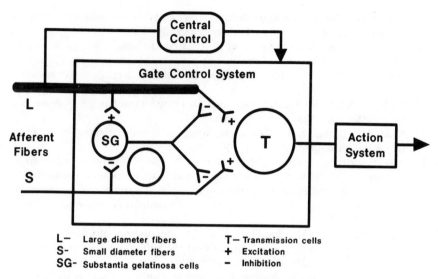

Figure 6. Gate control theory

interpreting centers in the brain. The gate is controlled by afferents coming in from the periphery and descending pathways from the brain stem.

Interested readers should refer to references 21–29 for a discussion of the gate control theory of pain and to the controversy surrounding it. Another theory, the "unified theory of pain," incorporates recent findings on enkephalins, endogenous opioid peptides, serotonin, and other neurotransmitters into the traditional theories (30). The roles of these neurotransmitters in nociception are described in the ensuing chapters.

REFERENCES

1. Perl ER: Myelinated afferent fibers innervating the primate skin and their response to noxious stimuli. J Physiol 197:593–615, 1968
2. Perl ER: Sensitization of nociceptors and its relation to sensation, in Advances in Pain Research and Therapy, vol. 1. Edited by Bonica JJ, Fessard AB. New York, Raven Press, 1976
3. Ranson SW: Unmyelinated nerve fibers as conductors of protopathic sensation. Brain 38:381–389, 1965
4. Light AR, Perl ER: Differential termination of large diameter and small diameter primary afferent fibres in the spinal dorsal gray matter as indicated by labelling with horseradish peroxidase. Neurosci Lett 6:59–63, 1979
5. Snyder R: The organization of the dorsal root entry zone in cats and monkeys. J Comp Neurol 174:47–69, 1977

6. Kerr FWL: The ventral spinothalamic tract and other ascending systems of the ventral funiculus of the spinal cord. J Comp Neurol 159:335–356, 1976
7. Ralson HJ: Synaptic organization of the spinothalamic tract: projection to the thalamus with special reference to pain, in Advances in Pain Research and Therapy, vol. 6. Edited by Kruger L, Liebeskind JC. New York, Raven Press, 1984
8. Basbaum AI, Fields HL: Endogenous pain control mechanisms: review and hypothesis. Ann Neurol 4:451–462, 1984
9. Fields HL, Basbaum AI: Brainstem control of spinal transmission neurons. Annu Rev Physiol 40:193–221, 1978
10. Albe-Fessard D, Condres LM, Sanderson P, et al: Tentative explanation of the special role played by the areas of paleo spinothalamic projection in patients with deafferentation pain syndrome, in Advances in Pain Research and Therapy, vol. 6. Edited by Kruger L, Liebeskind JC. New York, Raven Press, 1984
11. Gibson SJ, Polate JM, Bloom SR, et al: The distribution of nine peptides in rat spinal cord with special emphasis on the substantia gelatinosa and on Lamina X. J Comp Neurol 201:65–69, 1981
12. Wall PD: Mechanisms of acute and chronic pain, in Advances in Pain Research and Therapy, vol. 6. Edited by Kruger L, Liebeskind JC. New York, Raven Press, 1984
13. Basbaum AI, Fields HL: Endogenous pain control systems: brainstem spinal pathways and endorphin circuitry. Annu Rev Neurosci 7:309–338, 1984
14. Tasker RR, Organ LW, Hawrylyshyn PA: The Thalamus and Midbrain of Man: A Physiological Atlas Using Electrical Stimulation. Springfield Ill, Charles C Thomas, 1981
15. Melzack R, Loeser JD: Phantom body pain in paraplegics: evidence for a central pattern generating mechanism for pain. Pain 4:195–210, 1978
16. Melzack R: The Puzzle of Pain. New York, Basic Books, 1973
17. Bonica JJ: The Management of Pain. Philadelphia, Lea & Febiger, 1953
18. Dallenbach KM: History and present status. AmJ Psychol 52:331–347, 1939
19. Procacci P, Maresca M: Pain concept in western civilization: a historical review, in Advances in Pain Research and Therapy, vol. 7. Edited by Benedetti C, Chapman CR, Moricca G. New York, Raven Press, 1984
20. Bonica JJ: Neurophysiologic and pathologic aspects of acute and chronic pain. Arch Surg 112:750–761, 1977
21. Melzack R, Wall PD: Pain mechanisms: a new theory. Science 150:971–979, 1965
22. Melzack R, Wall PD: The Challenge of Pain. New York, Basic Books, 1983
23. Iggo A: Peripheral and spinal pain mechanisms and their modulation, in Advances in Pain Research and Therapy, vol. 1. Edited by Bonica JJ, Albe-Fessard D. New York, Raven Press, 1975
24. Melzack R, Loesser JD: Phantom body pain in paraplegics—evidence for a central pattern generating mechanism for pain. Pain 4:195–210, 1978
25. Wall PD: The substantia gelatinosa: a gate control mechanism set across a sensory pathway. Trends in Neurosciences 3:221–224, 1980
26. Wall PD: The role of substantia gelatinosa as a gate control, in Pain. Edited by Bonica JJ. New York, Raven Press, 1980

27. Wall PD: Modulation of pain by non-painful events, in Advances in Pain Research and Therapy, vol. 1. Edited by Bonica JJ, Albe-Fessard D. New York, Raven Press, 1976
28. Lourie H, King RB: Sensory and neurohistological correlates of cutaneous hyperpathia. Arch Neurol 14:313–320, 1966
29. Nathan PW: Critical review of gate control theory. Brain 99:123–158, 1976
30. Luce CM, Thompson TL, Getto GF, et al: New concepts of chronic pain and their implications. Hosp Pract 14:113–123, 1979

Chapter 4

Catecholamines and Indolamines: Role in Nociception and Chronic Pain

Scott T. Cain, Ph.D.

Charles B. Nemeroff, M.D., Ph.D.

Csaba M. Banki, M.D.

Randal D. France, M.D.

K. Ranga Rama Krishnan, M.D.

It is now well established that noxious stimuli activate afferents—either small (A delta) or lightly myelinated (C-fibers)—to the dorsal horn of the spinal cord. Input to the dorsal horn is, in turn, modified by both interneurons within the spinal cord and descending projections from supraspinal neurons. The latter circuits originate in a variety of reticular and medullary nuclei. In addition, spinal cord neurons project both ipsilaterally and contralaterally to a number of brainstem and thalamic nuclei. The major ascending pathways are the spinoreticular, paleo- and neospinothalamic, propriospinal, spinal cervical, and the dorsal columns (see Chapter 3, Figures 1, 2, and 3). For a comprehensive discussion of the anatomical substrates of nociception, the reader is referred to recent reviews by Melzack and Wall (1) and Yaksh (2). A brief overview is presented in Chapter 3.

In this chapter we present an overview of the role of catecholamines and indolamines in nociception. We also briefly present the putative role of histamine in nociception. The first part of this chapter focuses on animal studies, while the second half focuses on the sparse human studies of the role of these neurotransmitters in nociception. The possible role of these neurotransmitters as candidates for analgesic effects of antidepressants is explored.

ANIMAL STUDIES

This section emphasizes the descending serotonergic and catecholaminergic modulation of nociception. Some of the experimental evidence linking serotonin (5-HT), norepinephrine (NE), dopamine (DA), and histamine to nociception is described.

First, an important caveat: much of the experimental laboratory evidence relating biogenic amine-containing neural circuits to the modulation of nociception has been gathered using *acute* noxious stimulation, such as the hot-plate or tail-flick paradigms. As previously suggested by Loeser (3), the anatomical and biochemical substrates subserving chronic pain may differ from those involved in the processing of acute noxious stimulation. Thus, one must clearly proceed cautiously when trying to extrapolate mechanisms of chronic pain in humans from acute nociceptive mechanisms in laboratory animals. Progress in this field is also limited by the humanitarian and ethical considerations involved in experimental animal models of chronic pain. The deafferentation syndrome of Albe-Fessard and colleagues (4, 5) and the stereotyped behavioral response of rats to subcutaneous formalin injections (1) may prove to be valid animal models of chronic pain.

Serotonin (5-HT)

A wide variety of biochemical, behavioral, and electrophysiologic evidence implicates descending serotonergic supraspinal systems in the modulation of pain perception. In this chapter an overview is provided and some of the controversy in this research area, particularly as it pertains to chronic pain mechanisms, is discussed. Recent, comprehensive reviews are available (6, 7).

In general, experimental treatments that stimulate 5-HT turnover (activate serotonergic circuits) inhibit nociception and increase pain threshold (Table 1). In particular, interest has focused on the nucleus raphe magnus (NRM) located in the rostral ventral medulla as a central relay between the periaqueductal gray (PAG) and the spinal cord. NRM contains a significant number of 5-HT containing cells, receives input from the PAG, and projects via the dorsolateral funiculus (DLF) to the dorsal horn of the spinal cord (see Chapter 3, Figure 2) (8). Electrical stimulation of NRM or PAG results in an increase in nociceptive threshold, which has been termed stimulation-produced analgesia (SPA) (8, 9).

During analgesia resulting from either intra-PAG morphine or electrical stimulation, 5-HT is released into cerebrospinal fluid (CSF), suggesting a role for 5-HT in modulating nociception in the spinal cord (10). The 5-HT is presumably released from terminals of 5-HT perikarya located in NRM (11). Consistent with this model are the effectiveness of 5-HT perfusion of the spinal cord in producing analgesia (12), and the inhibitory effect of ionophoretically applied 5-HT on spinal cord neurons (13, 14). In addition, intra-NRM morphine induces both analgesia and increased 5-HT turnover in the spinal cord (15). The analgesia is

Table 1. Serotonergic and Catecholaminergic Modulation of Pain Based on Animal Studies

Neurotransmitter	Pathways	Neurophysiological Effect	Nociceptive Effect
Serotonin	NRM to spinal cord	Tonic inhibition	Analgesia
	PAG to NRM	Tonic inhibition	Analgesia
	PAG to spinal cord	Tonic inhibition	Analgesia
Norepinephrine	Bulbospinal to spinal cord	Tonic inhibition	Analgesia
	Pathways originating from A5 catecholamine neurons to NRM	Tonic inhibition	Hyperalgesia

NRM = nucleus raphe magnus
PAG = periaqueductal gray

blocked by depletion of spinal cord 5-HT. Further evidence for a modulatory descending 5-HT pathway was obtained by showing that analgesia induced by spinal cord superfusion with morphine did not alter 5-HT turnover and was not suppressed by 5-HT depletion (15).

Intrathecal administration of 5-HT (16, 17) or stimulation of 5-HT release in the spinal cord (18) produces analgesia in the tail-flick test; that is, response to noxious heat stimulation. This antinociceptive effect associated with increased spinal cord 5-HT release is blocked by inhibition of 5-HT synthesis (18). In contrast, the hind-paw lick response in the hot-plate test (17) and the analgesia induced by hind-paw foot shock (19) do not appear to be altered by manipulation of spinal cord 5-HT metabolism in the rat. However, depletion of spinal cord 5-HT with 5,6-dihydroxytryptamine (5,6-DHT) suppresses morphine-induced analgesia in the hot-plate test, but not in the tail-flick or tail-pinch tests (20). Morphine-induced analgesia in the hot-plate test, but not in the tail-flick test, is also attenuated by infusion of the 5-HT neurotoxin, 5,7-dihydroxytryptamine (5,7-DHT) into the NRM (21). There is, however, no effect of this treatment on baseline nociceptive threshold, indicating that the 5-HT system in the NRM does not exert a tonic inhibitory influence, but, instead, apparently modulates opiate analgesia. Further support for this hypothesis is provided by the finding that blockade of 5-HT receptors in the NRM reduces the analgesic effect of intra-NRM morphine (22) and PAG stimulation (6), but has no effect by itself on nociceptive threshold. Additionally, inhibition of 5-HT uptake in the NRM potentiates the effect of a subanalgesic dose of morphine (22).

Certain evidence also supports the notion of a 5-HT nociceptive modulatory pathway between the PAG and NRM and/or between the PAG and the spinal cord. In cats, electrical stimulation of the PAG inhibits the response of dorsal horn neurons to noxious heating of the skin. This inhibition, but not that obtained with stimulation of the midbrain reticular formation, is prevented by systemic administration of a 5-HT antagonist (23).

Dorsal horn neurons are inhibited after noxious stimulation such as tail immersion in hot water or nose pinch. This phenomenon (Diffuse Noxious Inhibition) is under supraspinal control and is potentiated by administration of a 5-HT precursor and blocked by 5-HT antagonism (24, 25).

In summary, stimulation of 5-HT turnover is often effective in producing antinociception (Table 1). This effect may be mediated through 5-HT pathways between NRM and the spinal cord, between PAG and NRM, and/or between PAG and spinal cord. Some of the data support the notion that 5-HT exerts a tonic inhibitory influence. Other evidence supports the notion of a serotonergic modulation of opiate analgesia. The type of noxious stimulation also appears to be important, though the evidence is not consistent in this regard. Further investigation is particularly important because 5-HT seems to be more effective in modulating 'reflex' response to pain (tail-flick, hot-plate) than in mediating nociceptive responses to stimuli (formalin test) (26), which appear to be more closely related to chronic pain. One must also be aware of experimental results that are not consistent with a role for 5-HT in pain inhibition. For example, one report indicates that the 5-HT concentration is *inversely* related to footshock-induced analgesia (27).

Norepinephrine (NE)

The prevailing evidence to date indicates that NE exerts a biphasic modulation of nociception, producing analgesia at spinal cord sites and hyperalgesia in the brain (Table 1). In the spinal cord, ionophoretically administered NE depresses spontaneous firing of dorsal horn cells and also inhibits the excitation resulting from peripheral stimulation (13, 28). Whether the inhibitory effect of NE is limited to excitation elicited by noxious stimulation is uncertain (29). Norepinephrine also reduces the excitability of C-fiber afferents to the dorsal horn (30). Again, it is unknown if this is a direct action on the C-fibers or is mediated through dorsal horn interneurons.

Bulbospinal NE metabolism is activated by noxious stimulation and by morphine (31). In most experimental situations, the intrathecal administration of NE or NE agonists produces analgesia or potentiates the analgesic action of morphine. Both tonically (17) and in conjunction with morphine (20), NE is a more effective inhibitor of mechanical nociception (for example, tail-pinch) than it is of thermal nociception (for example, hot-plate or tail-flick). As with 5-HT, spinal cord NE plays a role in front paw footshock-induced analgesia, but not in hind paw analgesia (19). The effectiveness of intrathecal NE antagonists in producing a decrease in nociceptive threshold is correlated with the potency of the antagonists for the alpha-2 receptor (32).

The origin of at least part of the bulbospinal NE pathway appears to be the locus coeruleus. Stimulation of this NE-rich nucleus inhibits the evoked discharge of dorsal root cells. This inhibition is attenuated by alpha-adrenergic receptor antagonists (33).

In contrast to the inhibitory role of NE in the spinal cord, intraventricular infusion of NE antagonizes morphine-induced analgesia (34). An interaction of NE with the descending 5-HT modulatory system has been proposed by Proudfit and colleagues (35, 36, 37). Infusion of the alpha-adrenergic antagonist phentolamine into the NRM produces an increase in pain threshold which is prevented by intrathecal serotonergic antagonism (35). These results have demonstrated that an NE system tonically inhibits the 5-HT inhibitory system. Adding support to this theory is the finding that iontophoretically applied NE inhibits NRM neurons (38).

A layer of complexity has been added by the subsequent demonstration that intrathecal administration of phentolamine and depletion of spinal cord NE and/or 5-HT also block the hypoalgesic effect of intra-NRM phentolamine (36, 37). NE, therefore, appears to promote nociception by inhibiting both the 5-HT descending pathway and an NE bulbospinal pathway. The origin of the responsible NE neurons may be the A5 catecholamine group (39).

Of potential relevance to chronic pain is the potential interaction of NE and peptides in the periphery. For example, combined depletion of peripheral peptides with capsaicin and NE sympathetic blockade with guanethidine reduces sensitivity to both heat pain and inflammatory pain induced by formalin (40).

Dopamine (DA)

Limited data are available implicating dopaminergic neurons in pain perception. In one series of reports (41, 42, 43), the intrathecal administration of DA or the DA agonist, apomorphine, to spinal rats increased the latency of the tail-flick response. This effect was blocked by dopamine receptor antagonists. In intact animals, apomorphine increased tail-flick latency only in conjunction with either 5-HT and/or NE blockade. The implication of these results is that descending 5-HT/NE pathways inhibit DA mediation of spinal reflexes. That the relevant supraspinal pathways descend in the DLF was shown by the apomorphine-induced analgesia following a DLF lesion. The origin of the spinal DA is unknown, as is the relevance of spinal dopamine-mediated analgesia in normal physiologic function.

Contradictory reports have appeared concerning the nociceptive responses after manipulation of CNS DA systems. In one study, reduced concentrations of brain DA decreased the efficiency of SPA evoked by PAG stimulation (44). Consistent with that finding is the reduced morphine-induced antinociception following lesions of the dopaminergic nigrostriatal pathway (45). In addition, a number of neurons in the striatum (46) and substantia nigra (47) are responsive to nociceptive stimulation. It is curious, however, that only five percent of the nigrostriatal neurons are responsive to nociceptive stimuli (47).

In contrast to the above results, potentiation of DA transmission by inhibition of DA reuptake results in hyperalgesia, which seems to be mediated through a D_1 receptor mechanism (48, 49). Stress-induced analgesia is potentiated by the dopaminergic receptor antagonist haloperidol and antagonized by apomorphine (50).

Clearly, the study of dopaminergic modulation of nociception is in an early stage. The conflicting results may ultimately be resolved by evaluation of the contribution of each of the known DA-containing pathways, which may have different influences on pain perception.

Histamine

Peripheral injections of a number of histamine H_1 receptor antagonists produce antinociception in rats and also potentiate the antinociceptive action of morphine (51). In monkeys, H_1 receptors are co-localized with opiate receptors in a subpopulation of sensory fibers (52).

Histaminergic H_2 receptor blockade prevents hind-paw foot shock-induced analgesia through a non-naloxone sensitive mechanism (53). Evidence that a histaminergic modulation of nociception may occur centrally is provided by the fact that histamine injections into the PAG or the dorsal raphe produce analgesia, which is antagonized by an H_2 receptor antagonist (54).

Future elucidation of the contrasting functions of H_1 and H_2 receptors in terms of a possible spinal/higher CNS dichotomy may be important to the understanding of pain perception.

HUMAN STUDIES

Only a few studies are available which relate changes in monoamine metabolism to chronic pain in patients. These studies can be divided, basically, into cerebrospinal fluid (CSF) studies of chronic pain patients versus pain-free controls, and studies which involve the pharmacological pertubation of the monoamine system in chronic pain patients. France and colleagues recently studied 40 patients with chronic low back pain of organic origin and 21 pain-free controls (55). All subjects were drug-free. Cerebrospinal fluid was collected at the same time of day and at the same spinal level. The mean CSF 5-hydroxyindoleacetic acid (5-HIAA) level was 22.69 ± 8.2 ng/ml. This was significantly higher than the level found in controls (15.68 ± 5.63 mg/ml) [$p < 0.001$]. Cerebrospinal fluid homovanillic acid (HVA), a metabolite of dopamine, was also increased in patients as compared to controls. There was no significant difference in the CSF 5-HIAA or HVA between patients with major depression versus patients without major depression. Ghia and colleagues (56) also showed elevated levels of CSF 5-HIAA in chronic pain patients. A positive relationship between the levels of fraction I endorphins and 5-HIAA has also been found in chronic pain patients (57). This suggests that there is an interaction between serotonin and endorphin systems in the modulation of pain in humans.

Additional evidence is obtained from studies using drugs that potentiate the serotonergic systems in pain patients. Stimulation of the serotonergic system can be accomplished both by using specific reuptake inhibitors of serotonin, such as zimelidine (58), and also by using serotonergic precursors, such as L-tryptophan (59, 60, 61) or 5-hydroxytryptophan (62). Further, zimelidine-induced reduction in pain levels in chronic pain patients has been shown to correlate highly with significant reductions in the concentrations of 5-HIAA in fraction I in the CSF of chronic pain patients. Neither the decrease in pain nor the changes in the CSF correlate to a decrease in depressive symptomatology. In contrast, DeBenedittis and colleagues have shown that pain relief with 5-hydroxytryptophan was correlated with increases in the CSF concentrations of 5-HIAA. The role of serotonin in human chronic pain remains unresolved.

Animal studies suggest that serotonin plays primarily an inhibitory role in nociception (analgesia), norepinephrine having a biphasic role inhibiting at the spinal level (analgesia) and excitatory at higher levels (hyperalgesia).

Interaction with opiate peptides, histamine, and other neuropeptides such as substance-P, modulate nociception in ascending and descending neural pathways. The role of these neurotransmitters has been sparsely studied in humans. As pointed out earlier, caution needs to be exercised in applying animal data (especially from acute pain studies) to chronic pain in humans.

Antidepressants, which are known to affect both norepinephrine and serotonin transmission, are widely used to treat chronic pain (63). However, the mechanism of action may not involve just these neurotransmitters. For a further discussion, see Chapter 18.

REFERENCES

1. Melzack R, Wall PD: The Challenge of Pain. New York, Basic Books, 1983
2. Yaksh TL: Pain transmission in Handbook of Neurochemistry, vol. 8. Edited by Lajtha A. New York, Plenum Press, 1985
3. Loeser JD: Definition, etiology, and neurological assessment of pain originating in the nervous system following deafferentation. Advances in Pain Research and Therapy 5:701–711, 1983
4. Lombard MC, Nashold BS, Albe-Fessard D: Deafferentation hypersensitivity in the rat after dorsal rhizotomy: a possible animal model of chronic pain. Pain 6:163–174, 1979
5. Albe-Fessard D, Lombard MC: Use of an animal model to evaluate the origin of and protection against deafferentation pain. Advances in Pain Research and Therapy 5:691–700, 1983
6. Roberts MHT: 5-hydroxytryptamine and antinociception. Neuropharmacology 23:1529–1536, 1984
7. Basbaum AI, Moss MS, Glazer EJ: Opiate and stimulation-produced analgesia: the contribution of the monoamines. Advances in Pain Research and Therapy 5:323–339, 1983
8. Basbaum AI, Fields HL: Endogenous pain control systems: brainstem spinal pathways and endorphin circuitry. Annu Rev Neurosci 7:309–338, 1984

9. Fields HL: Brainstem mechanisms of pain modulation. Advances in Pain Research and Therapy 6:241–252, 1984

10. Yaksh TL, Tyce GM: Microinjection of morphine into the periaqueductal gray evokes the release of serotonin from spinal cord. Brain Res 171:176–181, 1979

11. Rivot J-P, Weil-Fugazza J, Godefroy F, et al: Involvement of serotonin in both morphine and stimulation-produced analgesia: electrochemical and biochemical approaches. Advances in Pain Research and Therapy 6:135–150, 1984

12. Yaksh TL, Wilson PR: Spinal serotonin terminal system mediates antinociception. J Pharmacol Exp Ther 208:446–453, 1979

13. Headley PM, Duggan AW, Griersmith BT: Selective reduction by noradrenaline and 5-hydroxytryptamine of nociceptive responses of cat dorsal horn neurons. Brain Res 145:185–189, 1978

14. Randic M, Yu HH: Effects of 5-hydroxytryptamine and bradykinin in cat dorsal horn neurons activated by noxious stimuli. Brain Res 3:197–203, 1976

15. Vasko MR, Pang I-H, Vogt M: Involvement of 5-hydroxytryptamine minecontaining neurons in antinociception produced by injection of morphine into nucleus raphe magnus or onto spinal cord. Brain Res 306:341–348, 1984

16. Hylden JLK, Wilcox GL: Intrathecal serotonin in mice; analgesia and inhibition of a spinal action of substance-P. Life Sci 33:789–795, 1983

17. Kuraishi Y, Hirota N, Satoh M, et al: Antinociceptive effect of intrathecal opioids, noradrenaline and serotonin in rats: mechanical and thermal analgesic tests. Brain Res 326:168–171, 1985

18. Berge OG, Fasmer OB, Jorgensen HA, et al: Test-dependent antinociceptive effect of spinal serotonin release induced by intrathecal p-chloroamphetamine in mice. Acta Physiol Scand 123:35–41, 1985

19. Watkins LR, Johannessen JN, Kinscheck IB, et al: The neurochemical basis of footshock analgesia: the role of spinal cord serotonin and norepinephrine. Brain Res 290:107–117, 1984

20. Kuraishi Y, Harada Y, Aratani S, et al: Separate involvement of the spinal noradrenergic and serotonergic systems in morphine analgesia: the differences in mechanical and thermal algesic tests. Brain Res 273:245–252, 1983

21. Mohrland JS, Gebhart GF: Effect of selective destruction of serotonergic neurons in nucleus raphe magnus on morphine-induced antinociception. Life Sci 27:2627–2632, 1980

22. Llewelyn MB, Azami J, Roberts MHT: The effect of modification of 5-hydroxytryptamine function in nucleus raphe magnus on nociceptive threshold. Brain Res 306:165–170, 1984

23. Carstens E, Fraunhoffer M, Zimmerman M: Serotonergic mediation of descending inhibition from midbrain periaqueductal gray, but not reticular formation, of spinal nociceptive transmission in the cat. Pain 10:149–167, 1981

24. Chitour D, Dickenson AH, Bars DL: Pharmacological evidence for the involvement of serotonergic mechanisms in diffuse noxious inhibitory controls. Brain Res 236:329–337, 1982

25. Dickenson AH, Chitour D, Bars DL: Influence of serotonergic receptor blockade on diffuse noxious inhibitory controls in the rat. Advances in Pain Research and Therapy 5:155–160, 1983

26. Dennis SG, Melzack R: Pain modulation by 5-hydroxytryptaminergic agents and morphine as measured by three pain tests. Exp Neurol 69:260–270, 1980

27. Tricklebank MD, Hutson PH, Curzon G: Analgesia induced by brief footshock is inhibited by 5-hydroxytryptamine but unaffected by antagonists of 5-hydroxytryptamine or by naloxone. Neuropharmacology 21:51–56, 1982

28. Belcher G, Ryall RW, Schaffner R: The differential effects of 5-hydroxytryptamine, noradrenaline and raphe stimulation on nociceptive and non-nociceptive dorsal horn interneurons in the cat. Brain Res 151:307–321, 1978

29. Satoh M, Kawajiri S-T, Ukai Y, et al: Selective and nonselective inhibition by enkephalin and noradrenaline of nociceptive responses of lamina V type neurons in the spinal dorsal horn of the rabbit. Brain Res 177:384–387, 1979

30. Jeftinija S, Semba K, Randic M: Norepinephrine reduces excitability of single cutaneous primary afferent C and A fibers in the cat spinal cord. Advances in Pain Research and Therapy 5:271–276, 1983

31. Takagi H, Shiomi H, Kuraishi Y, et al: Pain and the bulbospinal noradrenergic system: pain-induced increase in normetanephrine content in the spinal cord and its modification by morphine. Eur J Pharmacol 54:99–107, 1979

32. Sagen J, Proudfit HK: Effect on intrathecally administered noradrenergic antagonists on nociception in the rat. Brain Res 310:295–301, 1984

33. Mokha SS, McMillan JA, Iggo A: Descending influences on spinal nociceptive neurons from locus coeruleus: actions, pathway, neurotransmitters and mechanisms. Advances in Pain Research and Therapy 5:387–392, 1983

34. Sparkes C, Spencer P: Antinociceptive activity of morphine after injection of biogenic amines in the cerebral ventricles of the conscious rat. Br J Pharmacol 42:230–241, 1971

35. Hammond DL, Levy RA, Proudfit HK: Hypoalgesia induced by microinjection of a norepinephrine antagonist in the raphe magnus: reversal by intrathecal administration of a serotonin antagonist. Brain Res 201:475–479, 1980

36. Sagen J, Proudfit HK: Hypoalgesia induced by blockade of noradrenergic projections to the raphe magnus: reversal by blockade of noradrenergic projections to the spinal cord. Brain Res 223:391–396, 1981

37. Sagen J, Winker MA, Proudfit HK: Hypoalgesia induced by the local injection of phentolamine in the nucleus raphe magnus: blockade by depletion of spinal cord monoamines. Pain 16:253–263, 1983

38. Behbehani MM, Pomeroy SL, Mack CE: Interaction between central gray and nucleus raphe magnus: role of norepinephrine. Brain Res 226:361–364, 1981

39. Takagi H, Yamamoto K, Shiosaka S, et al: Morphological study of noradrenaline innervation in the caudal raphe nuclei with special reference to fine structure. J Comp Neurol 203:15–22, 1981

40. Coderre TJ, Abbott FV, Melzack R: Behavioral evidence in rats for a peptidergic–noradrenergic interaction in cutaneous sensory and vascular function. Neurosci Lett 47:113–118, 1984

41. Jensen TS, Smith DF: Role of 5-HT and NE in spinal domaminergic analgesia. Eur J Pharmacol 86:65–70, 1983

42. Jensen TS, Smith DF: Stimulation of spinal dopaminergic receptors: differential effects on tail reflexes in rats. Neuropharmacology 22:477–483, 1983

43. Jensen TS, Schroder HD, Smith DF: The role of spinal pathways in dopamine mediated alteration in the tail-flick reflex in the rats. Neuropharmacology 23:149–153, 1984

44. Akil H, Liebeskind JC: Monoaminergic mechanisms of stimulation-produced analgesia. Brain Res 95:279–296, 1975

45. Price MTC, Fibiger HC: Ascending catecholamine systems and morphine analgesia. Brain Res 99:189–193, 1975

46. Lin MT, Vang WN, Chan HK: Both thermal and nociceptive afferents influence the unit activity of the neurons in the corpus striatum. Experientia 41:120–122, 1985

47. Barasi S, Pay S: Influence of striatal and limbic afferents on nociceptive nigral neurons. Advances in Pain Research and Therapy 5:169–177, 1983

48. Gonzalez JP, Sewell RDE, Spencer PSJ: Evidence for central selective dopamine receptor stimulation in the mediation of nomifensine-induced hyperalgesia and the effects of opiate antagonists. Neuropharmacology 20:1039–1045, 1981

49. Gonzalez JP, Littler ME, Sewell RDE: Stereoselective opiate antagonist-induced hyperalgesia: evidence for a dopaminergic involvement. J Pharm Pharmacol 34:334–336, 1982

50. Snow AE, Tucker SM, Dewey WL: The role of neurotransmitters in stress-induced antinociception (SIA). Pharmacol Biochem Behav 16:47–50, 1982

51. Sun CLJ, Hui FW, Hanig JP: Effect of H_1 blockers alone and in combination with morphine to produce antinociception in mice. Neuropharmacology 24:1–4, 1985

52. Ninkovic M, Hunt SP, Gleave JRW, et al: Autoradiographic localization of neurotransmitter receptors on sensory neurons. Advances in Pain Research and Therapy 5:257–263, 1983

53. Hough LB, Glick SD, Su K: A role for histamine and histamine H_2-receptors in non-opiate footshock-induced analgesia. Life Sci 36:859–866, 1985

54. Glick SD, Crane LA: Opiate-like and abstinence-like intracerebral histamine administration in rats. Nature 273:547–549, 1978

55. France RD, Urban BJ, Krishnan KRR, et al: Monoamine metabolites in chronic pain and depression. Paper presented at the Fourth World Congress of Biological Psychiatry, Philadelphia, 1985

56. Ghia JN, Mueller RA, Duncan GH, et al: Serotonergic activity in man as a function of pain, pain mechanisms, and depression. Anesth Analg 60:854–861, 1981

57. Almay BGL, Johansson F, vonKnorring L, et al: Relationships between CSF levels of endorphins and monoamine metabolites in chronic pain patients. Psychopharmacologia 67:139–142, 1980

58. Johansson F, vonKnorring L: A double-blind controlled study of a serotonin

uptake inhibitor (zimelidine) versus placebo in chronic pain patients. Pain 7:69–78, 1979

59. King RB: Pain and tryptophan. J Neurosurg 53:44–52, 1980
60. Seltzer S, Marcus R, Stoch R: Perspectives in the control of chronic pain by nutritional manipulation. Pain 11:141–148, 1981
61. Warfield CA, Stein JM: The nutritional treatment of pain. Hosp Pract 18:100N–100P, 1983
62. DeBenedittis G, DiGiulio AM, Massei R, et al: Effects of 5-hydroxytryptophan on central and deafferentation chronic pain: a preliminary clinical trial. Advances in Pain Research and Therapy 5:295–304, 1983
63. Rosenblatt RM, Reich J, Dehring D: Tricyclic antidepressants in treatment of depression and chronic pain: analysis of the supporting evidence. Anesth Analg 63:1025–1032, 1984

Chapter 5

Endogenous Opiates in Chronic Pain

Merry Noel, M.D.
Charles B. Nemeroff, M.D., Ph.D

Biological mechanisms of pain have received increasing attention in recent years, and a group of endogenous morphine-like compounds are now the focus of much of this research. Discovery of opiate receptors in the brain by three independent groups (1, 2, 3) stimulated the search for endogenous morphine-like substances that might act as natural ligands for these receptors. These efforts led to the identification of endogenous morphine-like substances, which were named endorphins (4, 5). Much research has now been conducted on the distribution and function of endogenous opioids and their receptors (Figure 1). The endogenous opioids that have been structurally identified to date have been peptides, but a number of other uncharacterized opioids have been identified as well. Because endogenous opioids are expected to have pharmacological properties similar to morphine, a considerable portion of this research has emphasized evaluation of the role of these compounds in nociception.

Since the initial discovery of the opiate receptors and the endogenous ligands (opioids) for these receptors, research in this area has expanded exponentially. This research has taken several distinct routes: study of the biochemistry and pharmacology of both the peptides and the partially characterized endogenous opioids, correlation of these substances with abnormal physiological states such as pain, and characterization of the receptor. It is now known that the opioid peptides belong to three genetically distinct peptide families, and much has been learned about their distribution and biosynthesis (Figure 1). Several partially characterized opioids have been shown to be correlated with pain states. In addition, multiple opioid receptors have now been identified. Indeed, endogenous opioid systems now appear to be a very complex system of neurochemicals with many potential interactions with other neuroregulators.

Opioid peptides are now known to derive from three precursors: the β-endorphin/ACTH precursor (proopiomelanocortin or POMC), the enkephalin precursor (proenkephalin A), and the dynorphin/neo-endorphin precursor (prodynorphin or proenkephalin B). Cleavage by proteolytic enzymes of each of these precursors yields biologically active peptide fragments (Figure 2).

The long chain (31-amino acid) peptide β-endorphin derives from the immediate precursor β-lipotropin, which in turn derives from the much larger precursor POMC. POMC also contains the sequences of ACTH (corticotropin) and three melanotropins (α-, β-, γ-MSH). The β-endorphin molecule contains the peptide sequence of met-enkephalin, but the synthesis of both enkephalins has clearly been shown to originate from a different precursor than β-endorphin. The pentapeptides methionine-enkephalin (Tyr-Gly-Gly-Phe-Met) and leucine-enkephalin (Tyr-Gly-Gly-Phe-Leu) were first identified in pig brain extracts (6), and now are known to be widely distributed in the central nervous system (CNS).

Receptor Subtype	μ	δ	κ	ε	σ
Endogenous Agonist	β-endorphin [Met] enkephalin	[Leu] enkephalin	Dynorphin$_{1-17}$	β-endorphin	
Endogenous Agonist Precursor	Proopiomelanocortin (POMC) Proenkephalin A	Proenkephalin A	Prodynorphin (Proenkephalin B)	Proopiomelanocortin (POMC)	
Prototype Agonist	Morphine	[Leu] enkephalin	Ketocyclazocin	β-endorphin	N-allylnormetazocine (SKF 10,047)
Selective Agonists	Morphiceptin Tyr-D-Ala-Gly-NMe-Phe Gly-ol (DAGO)	D-Ala^2-D-Leu^{5}enkephalin (DADL) D-Pen^2-D-Pen^{5}enkephalin	U50,488 Dynorphin$_{1-17}$	β-endorphin	Phencyclidine
Selective Antagonists	Naloxonazine β-funaltrexamine Naloxone	Naloxone ICI 154,129 ICI 174,864	Naloxone WIN-44,441-3 MR-2266	Naloxone	
In-vitro Assay System	Guinea-pig Ileum	Mouse Vas deferens Guinea-pig Ileum	Rabbit Vas deferens Guinea-pig Ileum	Rat Vas deferens	Guinea-pig Ileum

Figure 1. Opiate receptor subtypes: receptor pharmacology

Also, these pentapeptides form the active core of several slightly larger peptides. Neo-endorphin and dynorphin A and B are leu-enkephalin-containing peptides which are derived from prodynorphins. These biosynthetic processes have been elucidated by several investigators and these findings have recently been reviewed in detail (7, 8, 9). Multiple opiate receptors were first postulated by Martin and colleagues (10). Based on his studies with spinal dogs, Martin defined a mu or morphine receptor, and a kappa receptor specific for other narcotic analgesics, with ketocyclazocine as the prototype. Opioid peptides have been found to interact with both the mu-receptor and an additional delta or enkephalin receptor.

All of the pro-enkephalin related peptides have been found to show delta receptor activity, with varying proportions of mu-receptor activity. All of the dynorphins and neo-endorphins show a kappa receptor preference (11), but dynorphin A(1–8) also binds the delta-receptor (12) while dynorphin A(1–13) is very potent at both mu and kappa receptors. Finally, the POMC family gives rise to only one opioid peptide, β-endorphin, which is potent at both mu and delta receptors with a slight preference for the latter group. These receptor affinities are based on *in vitro* assays but may differ *in vivo* (7).

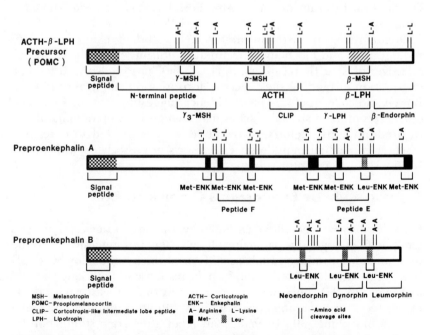

Figure 2. Structural relationship of POMC, preproenkephalin A, and preproenkephalin B cleavage points and their peptide fragments.

DISTRIBUTION OF ENDORPHINS

Enkephalin-containing neurons have been demonstrated with immunohistochemical methods in various CNS sites: the ventrolateral periaqueductal gray matter of the midbrain, the nucleus raphe magnus and adjacent ventromedial reticular giganto-cellular region in the medulla oblongata, the substantia gelatinosa of the spinal dorsal horn, and the descending trigeminal nucleus (13, 14). These areas have been implicated in sensory integration and nociception. Relatively high concentrations of enkephalins have also been found in the globus pallidus, hypothalamus, thalamus, amygdala, and nucleus accumbens.

Distribution of β-endorphin does not parallel that of the enkephalins. The areas of highest β-endorphin immunoreactivity are the hypothalamus, thalamus, and substantia nigra (15–18). β-endorphin is found in the periaqueductal gray and other areas implicated in nociception. β-endorphin and its immediate precursor, β-lipotropin, are also found in high concentrations in the pituitary. The origin of most of the β-endorphin-containing nerve terminals in the CNS is the arcuate nucleus of the hypothalamus.

A number of laboratories have reported the existence of other compounds with opiate action which are definitely not identical with known endogenous opioids (19–22) in brain extracts of animals and humans. Distribution in brain of these substances has not yet been studied in detail.

Opiate receptor distribution has been studied using both autoradiographic and biochemical techniques utilizing radiolabeled ligands selective for specific receptors. Such studies have shown a differential distribution of binding sites selective for mu and delta ligands (23, 24). Bowen and colleagues (25) have evidence suggesting that the subtype of opiate receptors in striatal patches may change from predominantly mu to predominantly delta sites. Further work is needed to determine whether individual peptide systems always are associated with unique relationships to receptor subtypes.

RELATIONSHIP OF ENDOGENOUS OPIOIDS TO PAIN

Considerable evidence links endogenous opioids to nociception. Existence of an endogenous pain-controlling system was suggested by studies on stimulation-produced analgesia (SPA), in which stimulation of specific brain regions led to a reduction in pain response in both lower animals and man (26, 27). This analgesia can be reversed, at least partly, by the opiate receptor antagonist naloxone (28, 29) and produces cross-tolerance to morphine (30). In man, pain relief after brain stimulation has been shown to be accompanied by an increase in enkephalin-like material and β-endorphin immunoreactivity in the cerebrospinal fluid (CSF) (31–34). Moreover, intraventricular and intrathecal administration of opioids such as β-endorphin have been reported to produce analgesia in laboratory animals and humans (35), though in the latter group troublesome side effects have been reported.

The narcotic antagonist naloxone has been used to determine whether blockade of opioid receptors produces physiological alterations. For example, Jacob and colleagues (36) provided such evidence in regard to nociception when they demonstrated that mice and rats exhibit hyperalgesia after naloxone treatment. These findings have been confirmed by some (37, 38) but not by others (39), suggesting that the tonic activity of the endogenous opioid system may be low, or alternatively that endogenous opioid systems may vary in their sensitivities to naloxone. Different types of painful stimuli may differentially activate endogenous opioid systems.

Naloxone has also been administered to persons in pain. In 1965, Lasagna (40) observed naloxone-induced hyperalgesia in patients with postoperative pain. Levine and colleagues (41) later confirmed this enhancement of postoperative clinical pain by naloxone in a double blind crossover experiment of postsurgery dental patients. However, Lindblom and Tegner (42) observed no change in spontaneous pain or heat-pain thresholds of chronic pain patients given naloxone in a subsequent double blind study. Similar null effects of naloxone were reported by Grevert and Goldstein (43) in chronic pain patients.

An unusual and rare syndrome characterized by congenital insensitivity to pain has been described (44). Administration of naloxone to these subjects greatly lowers their pain threshold while exerting little effect on normal subjects (45, 46). Such findings have been interpreted as revealing hyperactivity of endorphin stems in this unusual group of subjects.

Acute stress has been shown to be accompanied by increases in brain concentrations of endogenous opioids, as well as analgesia. Akil and colleagues (28) reported that intermittent footshock led to insensitivity to pain that was partially but significantly naloxone-reversible. After repeated footshock, this stress no longer produced analgesia. Stress-induced analgesia was shown to be accompanied by an increase in the concentration of brain endogenous opioids (47). When activated by stress, both the anterior pituitary and the adrenal medulla have been shown to release endogenous opioids (48–52) as well. Further research has shown that there are at least two types of stress-induced analgesia. Short durations of stress result in a nonopioid-mediated analgesia, while longer durations of stress produce opioid-mediated analgesia (53).

The ability of acupuncture to relieve pain has been hypothesized to result from the endorphin release. Mayer (54), in a double blind study, reported that naloxone reversed acupuncture analgesia to experimental pain in humans given electrical shock to a tooth. Pert (55) demonstrated that acupuncture in rats' ears was associated with endorphin release in periaqueductal gray, medial thalamus, and basomedial thalamus, areas that contain a high density of opiate receptors.

Plasma levels of β-endorphin have been found to be elevated during pregnancy and further elevated during labor (56, 57). However, no statistically significant correlation has been found between β-endorphin elevation and pain perception (58).

In addition to these models of acute pain and pain relief, chronic pain conditions have been studied by several groups to discover the role of endogenous opioids. Chronic pain patients have been reported to have lowered levels of met-enkephalin-like immunoreactivity in ventricular CSF (32).

As noted earlier, other partially characterized opioids have been identified in the CSF. Terenius and Wahlstrom (19, 20) have identified two fractions of opioid activity in CSF (Fractions I and II) after chromatography. Fraction II may be similar to enkephalin (59, 60). Fraction I appears to have clinical significance in pain: this substance is present in significantly lower concentration in CSF of chronic pain patients with organic, but not psychogenic, pain; also, pain threshold and tolerance have been found to be greater in patients with high levels of Fraction I (59). Moreover, pain relief by acupuncture in chronic pain patients is correlated with an increase in CSF Fraction I in approximately one-half of the patients studied (60). Similarly, another partially characterized endogenous opioid in CSF, labeled Peak B, has been found to be present in lower concentration in chronic pain patients (22).

The placebo response in pain patients may be partially mediated through endogenous opioids. Levine and colleagues (41, 61) found that the opiate antagonist naloxone had a greater pain-intensifying effect in placebo-responding postoperative dental patients. However, these findings are in conflict with those of Mihic and Binkert (62), who found that naloxone neither reversed nor prevented placebo analgesia. Direct evidence for endogenous opioid mediation of the placebo response in chronic pain has been obtained through measurement of opioids in CSF. Placebo-responding pain patients demonstrate a rise in the partially characterized opioid Peak B that has been correlated with pain relief (63).

Clinical trials with endogenous opioids have been undertaken. β-endorphin has been administered intravenously to three cancer patients, as well as directly into the CSF (64). Pain relief was observed only after intraventricular administration. However, in a recent study, Pickar and colleagues (35) observed a significant decrease in pain in a patient with adenocarcinoma of the pancreas after intrathecal β-endorphin (3 mg) administration; unfortunately, he exhibited confusion, disorientation, and agitation as well as auditory and visual hallucinations.

A biologically stable analogue of met-enkephalin, FK 33-824, has been administered to humans and increases pain tolerance, but also produced oppressive feelings, drowsiness, and dysphoria (65).

The research literature concerning endogenous opioids continues to grow at a rapid pace. Although some results are contradictory, the physiological significance of this system in nociception is likely. Multiple endogenous opioids appear to interact with a variety of opiate receptors (Figure 1). The ability of stress or placebo to elicit both endorphin release and pain relief suggests some interesting parallels between the psychology and biochemistry of pain. As knowledge of the biochemistry, anatomy, and pharmacology of the endogenous opioids expands, a better understanding of nociception and the links between nociception, brain mechanisms, and behavior will result. This understanding will almost certainly play a significant role in the clinical management of pain.

REFERENCES

1. Pert CB, Snyder SM: Opiate receptor: demonstration in nervous tissue. Science 179:1011–1014, 1973
2. Simon EJ, Hiller JM, Edelman I: Stereospecific binding of the potent narcotic analgesic 3H-etorphine to rat brain homogenate. Proc Natl Acad Sci USA 70:1949–1957, 1973
3. Terenius L: Stereospecific interaction between narcotic analgesics and a synaptic plasma membrane fraction of rat cerebral cortex. Acta Pharmacol Toxicol 32:317–319, 1973
4. Hughes JT: Isolation of an endogenous compound from the brain with the pharmacological properties similar to morphine. Brain Res 88:295–308, 1975
5. Terenius L, Wahlstrom A: Search for an endogenous ligand for the opiate receptor. Acta Physiol Scand 94:74–81, 1975
6. Hughes J, Smith TW, Kosterlitz NW, et al: Identification of two related pentapetides from the brain with potent opiate agonist activity. Nature 258:577–579, 1975
7. Akil H, Watson SJ, Young E, et al: Endogenous opioids: biology and function. Annu Rev Neurosci 7:223–255, 1984
8. Kosterlitz NW, McKnight AT: Endorphins and enkephalins, in Advances in Internal Medicine, vol. 26. Edited by Siperstein MD, Stokerman GH. Chicago, Yearbook Medical Publishers, 1980
9. Kosterlitz NW, McKnight AT: Opioid peptides and sensory function, in Progress in Sensory Physiology, vol. 1. Edited by Ottoson D. Berlin, Springer, 1981

10. Martin WR, Eades CG, Thompson JA, et al: The effects of morphine and nalorphine-like drugs in nondependent and morphine-dependent chronic spinal dog. J Pharmacol Exp Ther 197:517–532, 1976
11. Chavkin C, James IF, Goldstein A: Dynorphin is a specific endogenous ligand of the kappa opioid receptor. Science 215:413–415, 1982
12. Corbett AD, Patterson SJ, McKnight AT, et al: Dynorphin (1–8) and dynorphin (1–19) are ligands for the kappa subtype of opiate receptor. Nature 299:79–81, 1982
13. Hokfelt T, Ljungdahl A, Terenius L, et al: Immunohistochemical analysis of peptide pathways possibly related to pain and analgesia: enkephalin and substance-P. Proc Natl Acad Sci USA 74:3081–3085, 1977
14. Luttinger D, Hernandez DE, Nemeroff CB, et al: Peptides and nociception. Int Rev Neurobiol 25:185–241, 1984
15. Bloom FE, Rossier J, Battenberg E, et al: Beta-endorphin: cellular localization, electrophysiological and behavioral effects. Adv Biochem Psychopharmacol 18:88–109, 1978
16. Akil H, Watson S, Berger P, et al: Endorphins, beta-LPH and ACTH: biochemical, pharmacological and anatomical studies. Adv Biochem Psychopharmacol 18:125–137, 1978
17. Matsukura S, Yoshimi H, Sueoka S, et al: The regional distribution of immunoreactive beta-endorphin in the monkey brain. Brain Res 159:228–233
18. Rossier J, Vargo T, Minick S, et al: Regional dissociation of beta-endorphin and enkephalin contents in rat brain and pituitary. Proc Natl Acad Sci USA 74:5162–5165, 1977
19. Terenius L, Wahlstrom A: Morphine-like ligands for opiate receptors in human CSF. Life Sci 16:1759–1764, 1975
20. Terenius L, Wahlstrom A, Johansson L: Endorphins in human cerebrospinal fluid and their measurement, in Endorphins in Mental Health Research. Edited by Usdin E, Bunney WE, Kline N. New York, Oxford University Press, 1979
21. Sarne Y, Azov R, Weissman BA: A stable enkephalin-like immunoreactive substance in human CSF. Brain Res 151:399–403, 1978
22. Miller BE, Codd EE, Ungar AL, et al: Partial purification of endorphins from human cerebrospinal fluid from chronic back pain and elective surgery patients, in Endogenous and Exogenous Opiate Agonists and Antagonists. Edited by Way EL. New York, Pergamon, 1980
23. Goodman RR, Snyder SH, Kuhar MJ, et al: Differentiation of delta and mu opiate receptor localizations by light microscopic autoradiography. Proc Natl Acad Sci USA 77:6239–6243, 1980
24. Lewis ME, Pert A, Pert CB, et al: Opiate receptor localization in rat cerebral cortex. J Comp Neurol 216:339–358, 1983
25. Bowen WD, Gentleman S, Nerkenham M, et al: Interconverting mu and delta forms of the opiate receptor in rat striatal patches. Proc Natl Acad Sci USA 78:4818–4822, 1981
26. Mayer DJ, Wolfle TL, Akil H, et al: Analgesia from electrical stimulation in the brainstem of the rat. Science 174:1351–1354, 1971
27. Richardson DE, Akil H: Pain reduction by electrical brain stimulation in

man (part 2): chronic self-administration in the periventricular gray matter. J Neurosurg 47:184–194, 197

28. Akil H, Madden J, Patrick RL, et al: Stress-induced increase in endogenous opiate peptides: concurrent analgesia and its partial reversal by naloxone, in Opiates and Endogenous Opioid Peptides. Edited by Kosterlitz H. Amsterdam, Elsevier, 1976

29. Akil H, Mayer DG, Liebeskind JC: Antagonism of stimulation produced analgesia by naloxone, a narcotic antagonist. Science 191:961–962, 1976

30. Mayer DJ, Hayes RL: Stimulation-produced analgesia: development of tolerance and cross-tolerance to morphine. Science 188:841–943, 1975

31. Akil H, Hughes J, Richardson DE: Enkephalin-like material elevated in ventricular cerebrospinal fluid of pain patients after analgetic focal stimulation. Science 201:463–465, 1978

32. Akil H, Watson SJ, Sullivan S, et al: Enkephalin-like material in normal human CSF: measurement and levels. Life Sci 23:121–126, 1978

33. Amano K, Tanikawa T, Kawamura H, et al: Endorphins and pain relief: further observations on electrical stimulation of the lateral part of the periaqueductal gray matter during rostral mesencephalic retculotomy for pain relief. Appl Neurophysiol 45:123–135, 1982

34. Hosobuchi Y, Rossier J, Bloom F, et al: Electrical stimulation of periaqueductal gray in pain relief in humans is accompanied by elevation of immunoreactive beta-endorphin in ventricular fluid. Science 203:279–281, 1979

35. Pickar D, Dubois M, Cohen MK: Behavioral change in a cancer patient following intrathecal beta-endorphin administration. Am J Psychiatry 141:103–104, 1984

36. Jacob JJ, Tremblay EC, Colombel MC: Facilitation de reactions nociceptives pain la nalosone chez la souris et chez le rat. Psychopharmacologia 37:217–223, 1974

37. Goldfarb J, Hu JW: Enhancement of reflexes by naloxone in spinal cats. Neuropharmacology 15:785–792, 1976

38. Walker JM, Bernstrom G, Sandman C, et al: An analog of enkephalin having prolonged opiate like effects in vivo. Science 196:85–87, 1977

39. Goldstein A, Pryor GT, Otis LD, et al: On the role of endogenous opioid peptides: failure of naloxone to influence shock escape threshold in the rat. Life Sci 18:599–604, 1976

40. Lasagna L: Drug interaction in the field of analgesic drugs. Proceedings of the Royal Society of Medicine 58:978–983, 1965

41. Levine JD, Gordon NC, Fields HL: The mechanism of placebo analgesia. Lancet 2:654–657, 1978

42. Lindblom U, Tegner R: Are the endorphins active in clinical pain stress? Narcotic antagonism in chronic pain patients. Pain 7:65–68, 1979

43. Grevert P, Goldstein A: Effects of naloxone on experimentally induced ischemic pain and/or mood in human subjects. Proc Natl Acad Sci USA 74:1291–1294, 1977

44. Thrush DC: Congenital insensitivity to pain: a clinical, genetic and neurophysiological study of four children from the same family. Brain 96:369–386, 1973

45. Dehen H, Willer J, Boureau F, et al: Congenital insensitivity to pain, and

endogenous morphine-like substances. Lancet 2:293–294, 1977

46. Dehen H, Willer J, Prier S, et al: Congenital insensitivity to pain and "morphine-like" analgesic system. Pain 5:351–358, 1978

47. Madden J, Akil H, Patrick RL, et al: Stress-induced parallel changes in central opioid levels and pain responsiveness in the rat. Nature 265:358–360, 1977

48. Guillemin R, Vargo T, Rossier J, et al: Beta-endorphin and adrenocorticotropin are secreted concomitantly by the pituitary gland. Science 197:1367–1369, 1977

49. Viveros OH, Diliberto EG Jr, Hazum E, et al: Opiate-like materials in the adrenal medulla: evidence for storage and secretion with catecholamines. Mol Pharmacol 16:1101–1108, 1979

50. Costa E, Guidotti A, Hanbauer I, et al: Regulation of acetylcholine receptors by endogenous cotransmitters: studies of adrenal medulla. Federation Proceedings of the American Society of Experimental Biology 40:160–165, 1981

51. Saria A, Wilson SP, Molnar A, et al: Substance P and opiate-like peptides in human adrenal medulla. Neurosci Lett 20:195–200, 1980

52. Livett BG, Dean DM, Whelan LG, et al: Co-release of enkephalin and catecholamines from cultured adrenal chromaffin cells. Nature 289:317–319, 1981

53. Lewis JW, Cannon JT, Liebeskind JC: Opioid and non-opioid mechanism of stress analgesia. Science 208:623–625, 1980

54. Mayer DJ, Price DD, Rafii A: Antagonism of acupuncture analgesia in man by the narcotic antagonist naloxone. Brain Res 121:368–372, 1977

55. Pert A, Dionne R, Ng L, et al: Alterations in rat central nervous system endorphins following transamricular electro-acupuncture. Brain Res 224:83–93, 1981

56. Thomas TA, Fletcher JE, Hill RG: Influence of medication pain and progress in labour on plasma beta-endorphin-like immunoreactivity. Br J Anaesthesiol 54:401–408, 1982

57. Pilkington JW, Nemeroff CB, Mason GA, et al: Increase in plasma beta-endorphin-like immunoreactivity at parturition in normal women. Am J Obstet Gynecol 145:111–113, 1983

58. Cahil CA, Akil H: Plasma beta-endorphin-like immunoreactivity, self-reported pain perception and anxiety levels in women during pregnancy and labor. Life Sci 32:1879–1882, 1982

59. von Knorring L, Almay BGL, Johansson F, et al: Pain perception and endorphin levels in cerebrospinal fluid. Pain 5:359–365, 1978

60. Sjolund B, Terenius L, Eriksson M: Increased cerebrospinal fluid levels in endorphins after electro-acupuncture. Acta Physiol Scan 100:382–384, 1977

61. Levine JD, Gordon NC, Bornstein JC, et al: Role of pain in placebo analgesia. Proc Natl Acad Sci 76:3528–3531, 1979

62. Mihic D, Binkert: Is placebo analgesia mediated by endorphines?, in Abstracts, Second World Congress on Pain, Montreal, 1978

63. Lipman JJ, Miller BE, Mays KS, et al: CSF endorphin levels in chronic pain patients and in patients before and after a placebo pain relief, in Advances in Endogenous and Exogenous Opioids. Edited by Takagi H, Simon EJ. Tokyo, Kodansha Ltd, 1981

64. Foley KM, Kourides IA, Inturrissi CE, et al: Beta-endorphin: analgesia and hormonal effects in man. Proc Natl Acad Sci USA 76:5377–5381, 1979
65. Stacher G, Bauer P, Steinringer H, et al: Effects of the synthetic enkephalin analogue FK 33-824 on pain threshold and pain tolerance in man. Pain 7:159–172, 1979

Chapter 6

Nonopioid Neuropeptides in Chronic Pain

Charles B. Nemeroff, M.D., Ph.D.

The author is supported by NIMH MH-39415, MH-40524 and a Nanaline Duke Fellowship from Duke University Medical Center.

In spite of the intensive research conducted on the endogenous opiate-like peptides for more than a decade, relatively little is known about their role in the *physiology* of nociception or the pathophysiology of acute and chronic pain (1, 2) (see Chapter 5). Although the results are still not unequivocal, naloxone, the opiate receptor antagonist, produces little if any effect on the perception of pain in humans. This may not simply be a reflection of a lack of any meaningful role for opioid peptides in pain perception, but instead may represent the activation of compensatory mechanisms involving nonopioid peptides or more classical neurotransmitters. These findings, as well as the growing literature on the role of nonopioid peptides in pain physiology and neurobiology, have stimulated study of nonopioids in chronic pain. The purpose of this chapter is to provide a brief review of what is known about the neurobiology of nonopioid peptides and, moreover, to describe what little is known about these neuropeptides as putative candidates for involvement in the physiology of chronic pain. Of clinical interest is the possibility that certain of the nonopioid peptides or structural analogs of one or more of them might be used to develop a novel analgesic agent without abuse or dependence liability.

More than 40 neuropeptides have been isolated from the mammalian central nervous system (CNS) (Table 1) and advances in molecular genetics using recombinant DNA techniques have provided data that more than 200 neuropeptides are present, but not yet chemically identified, in brain. It is likely that one or another of these peptides acts to alter pain processes by one of the following mechanisms of action: 1) modulation of pain perception transmitted by primary afferent fibers to the spinal cord; 2) alteration in sympathetic nervous system activity which is known to be involved in certain pain syndromes, for example, causalgia; and 3) inhibition of pain processes at higher CNS centers (3, 4). Elsewhere (5), we have comprehensively reviewed the preclinical and clinical literature on peptides and pain. The interested reader may refer to that work for more experimental detail. In this chapter, the data are briefly summarized with an emphasis on recent findings for each nonopioid peptide.

SUBSTANCE P

Of all the nonopioid peptides, substance P, an undecapeptide, is considered the best candidate as a mediator of the transmission of noxious stimuli in primary afferent neurons. The evidence for this has been reviewed by our group (5) and by Sweet (6). Elegant immunocytochemical studies of Hokfelt and his colleagues (7) have unequivocally demonstrated the presence of substance P in primary afferent fibers that innervate the substantia gelatinosa of the spinal cord and trigeminal nerve nucleus. The cell bodies of these neurons are localized in the spinal dorsal root and trigeminal ganglia, and the peripheral distribu-

Table 1. Nonopioid Neuropeptides Identified in Mammalian Brain

Thyrotropin-releasing hormone (TRH)
Gonadotropin-releasing hormone (GnRH, LHRH)
Somatostatin (SRIF, GHIH)
Corticotropin-releasing factor (CRF)
Growth hormone-releasing factor (GRF, GHRH)
Thyroid-stimulating hormone (thyrotropin, TSH)
Adrenocorticotropin (ACTH)
Luteinizing hormone (LH)
Prolactin (PRL)
Growth hormone (GH)
α-melanocyte-stimulating hormone (α-MSH)
β-melanocyte-stimulating hormone (β-MSH)
Neurotensin
Substance P
Bombesin
Gastrin
Cholecystokinin
Secretin
Gastrin-releasing peptide
Calcitonin
Carnosine
Insulin
Glucagon
Neuromedin N
Neuropeptide Y
Vasoactive intestinal peptide (VIP)
Vasopressin
Oxytocin
Vasotocin
Delta-sleep inducing peptide (DSIP)
Melanocyte stimulating hormone-release inhibiting factor (MIFI)
Angiotensin
Kallikrein
Bradykinin

tion of these fibers has been found in dental pulp and in skin, presumably associated with nociceptors. Results from lesion studies are consistent with the hypothesis that substance P is the neurotransmitter of unmyelinated primary afferent neurons that transmit pain information. For example, capsaicin, which acutely causes release of substance P, produces pain; however, once it results in substance P depletion, pain sensitivity is reduced (8). In addition, direct application of substance P to the spinal cord elicits nociceptive behavior in rats (9) and the peptide selectively excites nociceptive units in the spinal cord (10). Finally, Kuraishi and colleages (11) recently demonstrated release of substance P from the rat dorsal horn after noxious mechanical or thermal stimuli. Opiates may partially act to inhibit nociception by an action on substance P neurons. Opiates such as morphine and opioids such as beta-endorphin inhibit potassium-induced substance P release from rat trigeminal nucleus (12). Substance P is also present in neurons in higher CNS centers such as the periaqueductal gray and nucleus raphe magnus. Whether it mediates pain processes in these supra-spinal centers is still unclear.

Depending on the dose employed and the route of administration, substance P has been reported to produce both analgesia and hyperalgesia. Low doses, administered intraventricularly, produce analgesia that is naloxone-reversible, whereas hyperalgesia can be seen at very high doses (5).

BRADYKININ

Bradykinin, a nonapeptide, has been reported to possess algesic (pain-producing) properties when applied to a blister base preparation or administered intra-arterially. Several workers have identified a bradykinin-like substance in the superfusate from exposed tooth pulp following noxious stimulation. Electrophysiological data support the hypothesis that bradykinin is physiologically involved in the response to noxious stimuli. Taken together, the data suggest that in the periphery bradykinin, or a closely related peptide, is released from damaged tissue and produces pain. Its role in the CNS, where it is distributed heterogeneously and fulfills some but not all of the requisite neurotransmitter criteria, is obscure (5).

NEUROTENSIN

Neurotensin (NT), a tridecapeptide, was first identified in extracts of bovine hypothalamus by Carraway and Leeman (13). Immunohistochemical and radioimmunoassay (RIA) studies have revealed a differential distribution of the peptide in the CNS, with high concentrations in several brain regions known to be involved in nociception, including the substantia gelatinosa of the spinal cord, the periaqueductal gray, and the amygdala (14, 15). The peptide is not contained in primary afferent spinal cord fibers, but in interneurons (16). The peptide is released from brain slices and synaptosomes by depolarizing agents, degraded by peptidases found in brain, and alters the firing rate of CNS neurons after iontophoretic application. Biochemical and autoradiographic techniques have revealed the presence of high affinity neurotensin receptors in the CNS. In short, neurotensin fulfills many other criteria to be considered a neurotransmitter candidate, as these data have recently been reviewed (17, 18).

Intraventricular or intracisternal administration of neurotensin produces antinociception in rats and mice (19, 20). This peptide produces analgesia in a variety of standard laboratory tests, including the hot plate, tail immersion, and acetic acid writhing test. However, in mice, the minimally effective dose of neurotensin in these tests differs markedly; as little as 250 picograms is effective in the acetic acid writhing test, whereas considerably higher doses (> 25 nanograms) are necessary in the hot plate test. In a comprehensive study, our group (21) implanted rats with bilateral injection cannulae to determine the loci where neurotensin produces its analgesic effects. Of all the brain regions studied, the peptide produces analgesia only in the central nucleus of the amygdala, the caudal diagonal band of Broca, the rostral medial perioptic area, the rostral mesencephalic periaqueductal gray, the medial pontine reticular formation, and the ventral thalamus. All of these areas contain substantial quantities of neurotensin.

The analgesia produced by neurotensin after microinjection into the central nucleus of the amygdala has been studied in some detail. The effect is dose-dependent and is abolished by lesions of the stria terminalis, a major efferent and afferent fiber tract of the amygdala (22). Although some controversy still surrounds this issue, most investigators have found no effect of the opioid receptor antagonist, naloxone, on the antinociception produced by centrally administered neurotensin. Clineschmidt and colleagues (23) reported that drugs that block muscarinic cholinergic, histaminergic, beta-adrenergic, alpha-adrenergic, or serotonergic receptors did not alter neurotensin-induced analgesia. However, recently Behbebani and Pert (24) reported that destruction of the nucleus raphe magnus, a major source of serotonin-containing neuronal perikarya, by an electrolytic lesioning method, abolished the analgesic effects observed after neurotensin was injected into the periaqueductal gray. From these data, as well as electrophysiological findings, they concluded that neurotensin produces analgesia by excitation of periaqueductal gray neurons, which activates a pain inhibitory system that originates in the nucleus raphe magnus.

Recently, Nicolaides and colleagues (25) studied the structure–activity relations (SAR) of neurotensin-induced analgesia in the acetic acid writhing test. Neurotensin, administered intraventricularly, was quite a potent analgesic in the mouse; the C-terminal hexapeptide was three to four times less active than neurotensin, and neurotensin 6–8 was inactive. These findings are consistent with previous SAR studies, as well as with receptor bindings studies.

ADRENOCORTICOTROPIC HORMONE (ACTH)

This peptide, composed of 39 amino acids, is known to be produced in the adenohypophysis from the precursor peptide, POMC. After release from the anterior pituitary, it is transported in the systemic circulation to the adrenal cortex, which causes increased synthesis and release of glucocorticoids such as cortisol. Recently, ACTH has been found in extrapituitary sites including the CNS, adrenal medulla, and lymphocytes. Several researchers (5) have reported that ACTH has activity at opiate binding studies, resembling a partial opiate agonist–antagonist. After intraventricular administration in rats, ACTH has been reported to produce hyperalgesia in two different laboratory paradigms. The peptide also has been reported to inhibit morphine-induced analgesia.

SOMATOSTATIN (SRIF)

Somatostatin is a tetradecapeptide that was discovered a little more than a decade ago in extracts of ovine hypothalamus. Like thyrotropin-releasing factor (TRF), luteinizing hormone releasing hormone (LHRH), and corticotropin releasing factor (CRF), it appears to act not only as a hypothalamic hypophysiotropic hormone but also in extrahypothalamic sites. In its former role, it is known to inhibit growth hormone secretion, as well as that of other pituitary hormones including thyroid-stimulating hormone (TSH) and ACTH. Its latter role remains obscure, but the evidence for involvement of SRIF in both depression and Alzheimer's disease is compelling. The peptide appears to interact with opiate receptors; it inhibits radio-labelled naloxone binding. The peptide has analgesic properties after intraventricular administration in rats that are blocked by naloxone. Others have suggested that SRIF inhibits enkephalin degradation. These findings have been reviewed recently (5).

CHOLECYSTOKININ (CCK)

This peptide, first discovered in the small intestine and later in the brain, is believed to be physiologically involved in the regulation of satiety, as well as acting as a bona fide gastrointestinal hormone. There is at least one report that CCK inhibits the binding of radiolabelled naloxone to opiate receptors in rat brain. When administered subcutaneously, CCK produces naloxone-reversible analgesia in rats in two laboratory tests. Direct injection of low dose of the peptide into the periaqueductal gray, caudate, ventromedial thalamus, and cuneiform nucleus produces significant analgesia; this analgesia is reversed by naloxone. It would appear that CCK acts to alter responses to noxious stimuli by either directly interacting with opiate receptors or releasing endogenous opioids.

VASOPRESSIN

This neurohypophyseal peptide released from nerve terminals in response to changes in plasma osmolarity, is also found in extrahypothalamic brain areas. When administered intraventricularly to rats, lysine vasopressin produces analgesia that is not reversed by naloxone. Similar findings have been reported in mice. Clinical trials with vasopressin have been conducted. In patients with acute herpes zoster, intramuscular injections of lysine vasopressin reduced both superficial and deep pain (26). There was no tolerance to the effects of repeated injections and the duration of action was 12–24 hours. The peptide was more effective in acute than in chronic pain.

OTHER PEPTIDES

A variety of other peptides have been implicated in pain processes or have been identified as potential novel analgesic agents. Tuftsin, a tetrapeptide, synthesized in the spleen, produces an analgesia after intraventricular administration that is not reversed by naloxone. Calcitonin is a 32-amino acid containing peptide that is believed to function physiologically in the regulation of calcium metabolism. It is present in the C-cells of the thyroid and in the CNS. High affinity binding sites exist for calcitonin in brain, and these as well as the other peptides are found in substantial concentrations in brain areas known to be involved in pain processes. The peptide produces analgesia after central injection in rabbits and mice. This analgesia is not reversed by naloxone. Bombesin, an amphibian tetra-decapeptide homologous to mammalian gastrin releasing peptide, produces analgesia in rats after direct injection into the periaqueductal gray.

DISCUSSION

It is evident from the foregoing text that several nonopioid neuropeptides are candidates as neuromodulators of pain transmission. One hypothesis that must be considered is that all of the substances modulate nociception by an interaction with endogenous opioid systems. This hypothesis has been discussed (27) but is unlikely because of the number of reports which claim that certain neuropeptides can produce a naloxone-insensitive analgesia; for example, neurotensin or vasopressin. The greatest part of the problem is our ignorance of neuropeptide neurobiology and, hence, our inability to selectively alter peptide transmission. As our understanding of neuropeptide synthesis and degradation increases, specific synthesis and breakdown inhibitors will be developed. Selective neuropeptide receptor antagonists will also be helpful. The paucity of clinical studies on neuropeptides other than opiates is striking. This leaves the preclinical literature, which is somewhat confusing. This is partly because of the myriad of animal models of acute and chronic pain, none of which are entirely satisfactory (28).

Table 2. Criteria for Involvement of Endogenous Neuropeptides in Nociception

Peptide present in the organism
Peptide released when the system is physiologically activated by noxious stimulation
Access of the peptide to anatomical sites of action
Administered peptide produces physiological activation at the postulated site of action
System for peptide inactivation
Antagonists of administered peptides should also antagonize the physiological activation of the system

When we last reviewed the literature on peptides and nociception (5), we recommended six criteria that must be fulfilled for a substance to be considered to be physiologically involved in pain transmission (Table 2). At this time no peptides fulfill these criteria, though certain opioids and substance P come close. There seems little doubt that neuropeptides are important regulators of neutrotransmission in the CNS, and they appear to play a role in nociception. Further study is essential to determine the role of each of these peptides in the pathophysiology of acute and chronic pain states.

REFERENCES

1. Kosterlitz HW, McKnight AT: Pain and opiate-like peptides, in Disorders of Neurohumoral transmission. Edited by Crow TJ. London, Academic Press, 1982
2. Herz A: Role of multiple opioid receptors and corresponding legands in pain modulations. Arzneimittelforsch 34:1080–1083, 1984
3. Fields H: Neurophysiology of pain and pain modulation. Am J Med 77:2–8, 1984
4. Zimmerman M: Basic concepts of pain and pain therapy. Arzneimittelforsch 34:1053–1059, 1984
5. Luttinger D, Hernandez DE, Nemeroff CB, et al: Peptides and nociception. Int Rev Neurobiol 25:185–241, 1984
6. Sweet WH: Neuropeptides and pain: neurosurgical implications. Clin Neurosurg 26:657–672, 1979
7. Hokfelt TQ, Ljugdahl A, Terenivs L, et al: Immunohistochemical analysis of peptide pathways possibly related to pain and analgesia: enkephalin and substance P. Proc Natl Acad Sci USA 74:3081–3085, 1977
8. Hayes AG, Tyfers MB: Effects of capsaicin on nociceptive heat, pressure and chemical thresholds and on substance P levels in the rat. Brain Res 189:561–564, 1980

9. Seybold VS, Hylden JLK, Wilcox GL: Intrathecal substance P and somatostatin in rats: behaviors indicative of nociception. Peptides 3:49–54, 1982

10. Henry JL: Effects of substance P on functionally identified units in cat spinal cord. Brain Res 114:439–451, 1976

11. Kuraishi Y, Hirota N, Sado Y, et al: Evidence that substance P and somatostatin transmit separate information related to pain in the spinal dorsal horn. Brain Res 325:294–298, 1985

12. Jessell TM, Iversen LL: Opiate analgesics inhibit substance P release from rat trigeminal nucleus. Nature 208:549–551, 1977

13. Carraway RE, Leeman SE: The isolation of a new hypothalamic peptide, neurotensin, from bovine hypothalamus. J Biol Chem 284:6854–6861, 1973

14. Uhl GR, Goodman RH, Snyder SH: Neurotensin containing cell bodies, fibers and nerve terminals in the brainstem of the rat: immunohistochemical mapping. Brain Res 167:77–91, 1979

15. Manberg PJ, Youngblood WW, Nemeroff CB, et al: Regional distribution of neurotensin in human brain. J Neurochem 38:1777–1780, 1982

16. Leranth C, Csilik B, Knyihar-Csilik E: Depletion of substance P and somatostatin in the upper dorsal horn after blockade of axoplasmic transport. Histochemistry 81:391–400, 1984

17. Nemeroff CB: The interaction of neurotensin with dopaminergic pathways in the central nervous system: basic neurobiology and implications for the pathogensis and treatment of schizophrenia. Psychoneuroendocrinolgy 11:15–37, 1986

18. Nemeroff CB, Cain ST: Neurotensin–dopamine interactions in the central nervous system. Trends in Pharmacological Sciences 6:201–205, 1985

19. Clineschmidt BV, McGuffin JC: Neurotensin administered intracisternally inhibits the responsiveness of mice to noxious stimuli. Eur J Pharmacol 46:395–396, 1977

20. Nemeroff CB, Osbahr AJ III, Manberg PJ, et al: Alterations in nociception and body temperature after intracisternally administered neurotensin, beta-endorphin, other endogeneous peptides and morphine. Proc Natl Acad Sci USA 76:5368–5371, 1979

21. Kalivas PW, Jennes L, Nemeroff CB, et al: Neurotensin: topographic distribution of brain sites involved in hypothermia and antinociception. J Comp Neurol 210:225–238, 1982

22. Kalivas PW, Gau BA, Nemeroff CB, et al: Antinociception after microinjection of neurotensin into the central amygdaloid nucleus of the rat. Brain Res 243:279–286, 1982

23. Clineschmidt BV, McGuffin JC, Bunting PB: Neurotensin: antinocisponsive action in rodents. Eur J Pharmacol 54:129–139, 1979

24. Behebani NN, Pert A: A mechanism for the analgesic effect of neurotensin as revealed by behavioral and electrophysiological techniques. Brain Res 324:35–42, 1984

25. Nicolaides ED, Lunney EA, Katterbronn JS, et al: Anti-writing activity of some peptides related to neurotensin and tuftsin. Int J Pept Protein Res 25:435–441, 1985

26. Forssman O, Leczinsky CG, Mulder J: Synthetic lysine vasopressin in herpetic neuralgia. Acta Derm Venereol (Stockh) 53:359–362, 1973

27. Thamandas KH: Opioid–neurotransmitter interactions: significance in analgesic tolerance and dependence. Prog Neuropsychopharmacol Biol Psychiatry 8:565–570, 1984

28. Wood PL: Animal models in analgesic testings, in Analgesics: Neurochemical, Behavioral and Clinical Perspectives. Edited by Kuhar M, Pasternak G. New York, Raven Press, 1984

Chapter 7

Personality and Chronic Pain

Randal D. France, M.D.

K. Ranga Rama Krishnan, M.D.

Jeffrey L. Houpt, M.D.

Allan A. Maltbie, M.D.

Physicians have long recognized the importance of personality and psychodynamic factors in a patient's response to pain. Interest has expanded from a general interest in emotional factors to more specific formulations of personality types, psychodynamic conflicts, affective syndromes, and somatoform disorders in relation to pain syndromes. The variance in response to pain from one patient to another fuels this interest, as does the lack of response of certain individuals to treatment.

This chapter focuses on the role of personality and psychodynamic conflicts in chronic pain.

PERSONALITY VARIABLES IN CHRONIC PAIN

As early as 1911, Cabot stated that "psychoneurotic backache is recognizable by its obvious connection with psychic and especially emotional states. A depressing emotion will produce it, a joyful event will correct it; but one must be aware of doing the patient injustice by dubbing the pain imaginary or unreal, either in this or any other type of psychoneurotic trouble. What the facts show is that a certain direction and morbid concentration of attention is followed by pain, and that a new habit of life, physical and mental, leading to a more profitable direction, is followed by relief" (1, p. 80).

In 1954 Brown, Nemiah, and others extended this formulation by suggesting that six characteristics indicate the presence of complicating psychological factors. These are: 1) a vague history of present illness with confused chronology and irrelevant information; 2) expression of either open or veiled resentment toward the medical personnel for supposed neglect; 3) dramatic description of and reactions to symptoms; 4) difficulty in localization and description of pain; 5) failure of the usual forms of treatment to give significant relief from pain; and 6) accompanying neurotic symptoms (anxiety, depression, and the like) (2).

At about the same time that Brown and colleagues were studying complicating psychological factors, investigators began exploring the relationship of psychological factors to chronic low back pain by using the Minnesota Multiphasic Personality Inventory (MMPI). Hanvik, in 1951, compared low back pain patients with clear physical findings to those without clear findings. His sample included 30 male Veterans Administration hospital patients in each group. Those without physical findings showed increased scores in hypochondriasis and hysteria, but a lower depression scale. This has come to be called a conversion V (3).

Gentry and colleagues' 1974 MMPI data suggested that patients with chronic low back pain had a strong need to interpret their situations in a logically and socially acceptable manner, and displaced emotional conflicts onto somatic concerns. They had a contrasting personality style—they were externally extroverted and sociable, yet internally demanding, self-centered, and dependent (4). Thus, we observe the correlation of pain with Axis I (DSM-III-R) symptomatology (for example, depression, hypochondriasis), personality style, and psychodynamic formulations.

Interest grew to compare acute and chronic pain on the assumption that the length of pain symptomatology might also be related to personality. Philips, in 1964, showed that female patients with low back pain had significantly elevated scores on hysteria, depression, and hypochondriasis, whereas females with fractures had only slightly elevated scores (5). Sternbach, in 1973, obtained similar results when he reported that patients with increased hypochondriasis and hysteria scores generally had a chronic form of pain syndrome, were often involved in litigation, and that patients with acute pain seldom had these elevations (6).

Minnesota Multiphasic Personality Inventory profiles have also been correlated with outcome. In 1973, Wilfing showed that patients who scored significantly lower on the hysteria, hypochondriasis, and depression scales had greater success from spinal fusions than the group that scored higher on these scales (7). Similarly, Beals and Hickman reported in 1972 that patients with polysurgeries scored higher on hysteria and hypochondriasis scales than did patients having had one surgery, acute pain, extremity injury, or normals (8).

Sternbach has suggested that the specific profile on the MMPI is important. Sternbach pointed out that low back pain patients who have an elevated depression scale can be expected to have a favorable response to treatment, whereas those with a dominant hysteria component respond poorly to surgery and psychological treatment. He went on to argue that those with a classic conversion may or may not respond favorably (6).

These studies bring to light a major problem. Does the personality as assessed at the time of evaluation of chronic pain reflect the premorbid personality, or does the personality as assessed reflect change secondary to the chronic pain? Or, does the personality as assessed at that time reflect both premorbid personality as well as change secondary to the chronic pain, as we contend in Chapter 2? At this time, we are unaware of any studies that have attempted to answer these questions. Before we examine the various psychodynamic theories of chronic pain, it would be worthwhile to discuss the possible psychological reactions to chronic pain in a temporal fashion and view them as adaptive mechanisms. The concept of illness behavior as introduced by Pilowsky will be considered (9).

PSYCHOLOGICAL REACTIONS TO CHRONIC PAIN

The psychological reactions to chronic pain syndromes vary, depending upon the duration of pain, the type of illness, and the severity of disability. Chronic pain patients employ their adaptive defensive mechanisms and use social supports to cope with persistent pain (Table 1). The adaptative mechanisms vary from patient to patient and depend upon the premorbid personality.

As pain persists, its impact on a patient's psychological and social well-being increases. The persistence of pain, as tissue heals, leaves the patient confused. The cycle of continual pain and treatment failure often leads to psychological distress: depression, anxiety, irritability, social isolation, lowered self-esteem, and fearfulness. Repetition of this cycle intensifies the psychological sequelae of chronic pain. The changes affect not only the patient but family, friends, and healthcare providers. Patients' adaptive responses may vary from a rather nonchalant attitude to an excessive response to the persistent pain. Some patients with crippling intractable pain display little, if any, concern for the severity and extent of their disability. This reaction can be seen in chronic pain patients whose pain may be secondary to malignancy, or whose pain may be of nonmalignant origin. Conversely, in other patients, mild intractable pain can result in significant psychological reactions, leading to an exaggeration of the clinical condition and disability imposed by the chronic pain state.

The control of the disproportionate pain complaint by the patient may vary from no conscious awareness to conscious manipulation of symptoms and complaints. The secondary gain of the former involves issues of unmet dependency needs, enhancement of self-esteem and social identity, stabilization of weak ego functions and immature personality, and conflict resolution of sexual and aggressive drives. Generally, the more chronic the pain complaints, the more extensive the secondary gain issues become. As secondary gain issues become prominent in reinforc-

Table 1. Problems Facing the Chronic Pain Patient

Interpersonal issues	Spouse relationship
decreased autonomy	role reversal
extended social isolation	increased dependency
impaired interpersonal skills	change in sexual interactions
increased dependency	issue of separation/divorce
Family relations	Personal issues
change in role of spouse	loss of control
increased dependency on family	impaired cognitive functions
withdrawal from family members	altered coping/adaptive skills
limited role in functions of family	psychological distress
change in family structure	physical changes
change in financial resources	change in body image
absences from family	loss of mobility

ing the chronic pain complaints, the patient becomes increasingly resistant to treatment. The general consensus among clinicians seems to be that if the level of disability from a chronic pain syndrome is continually reinforced beyond a two-year period, the reversal of this pattern is rare. To the outside observer, it may make little sense that the patient's secondary gain from chronic pain and disability is commensurate with the extent of the suffering. This apparent discrepancy can be understood in the context of the patient's personality structure, ego functioning, and interpersonal skills. In most instances, the degree of the discrepancy can provide insight into the adaptive mechanisms that can be utilized by the chronic pain patient.

Effects of Premorbid Personality

The patient's premorbid personality often predicts his or her response to chronic pain. Emotionality may either decrease or increase in patients with chronic pain, depending upon the preexisting personality of the patient as well as on the severity of the pain. As pain is relieved, the emotionality will return to normal (10). A patient will have the potential for successful adjustment to chronic pain with a history of a stable supportive marriage, good sexual adjustment, steady employment and good work record, negative history of acting out behavior (suicide, arrest, drug and alcohol abuse, and the like), supportive and stable family, good interpersonal skills, and supportive friends.

An unsuitable marital relationship may produce either overprotective behavior or rejection of the chronic pain patient by the spouse. The overprotective spouse will unknowingly view the ill mate as being more disabled than the physical condition warrants. The response of the spouse becomes fixed to the patient's pain behavior rather than to the pain itself. As this relationship develops, pain behavior and the spouse's response to it dominate the marital relationship. The uninvolved spouse resists support and participation in the management of the pain. Such a spouse does not support changes in lifestyle due to the concomitant disability. Typically, the uninvolved spouse supports treatment of a curative nature despite a past history of unsuccessful treatment. Lack of a supportive family and social network promotes social withdrawal and isolation in the chronic pain patient as the level of psychological distress increases.

A patient with a prior history of drug or alcohol abuse will have the tendency to abuse prescribed medications, especially opioid analgesics and minor tranquilizers. In addition, the reemergence of drug or alcohol abuse may occur in a chronic pain patient whose substance use had been under control prior to the development of the chronic pain. This type of patient with addictive personality traits typically refuses self-reliant techniques for pain control (such as physical therapy, diversion, and biofeedback) in favor of pain relief by medication. These patients often try to manipulate physicians into prescribing pain medications in excess of normal dose ranges. When physicians refuse to comply with these requests, these patients frequently doctor shop in order to procure the pain medications they desire.

Types of Psychological Reactions

The type of psychological reaction and distress experienced by a chronic pain patient depends in part upon the stage and duration of the pain. Hendler has drawn a parallel between the psychological reactions of the chronic pain patient and the emotional reactions of the dying patient (11). In the acute stage of the pain, the patient, family, and health caregivers all expect that the pain will abate as the pathophysiological process resolves. Opioid medications are extremely effective in reducing acute pain. Patients and physicians share this knowledge. The psychological reaction associated with acute pain is an anxiety reaction that is prominent only during the acute phase of the pain. This anxiety is reduced as adequate treatment of the pain proceeds. When the pathological process is identified and appropriate treatment instituted, the physician and other health caregivers convey a sense of hope and confidence, either implicitly or explicitly, in the diagnosis and treatment. This message is reassuring to both the patient and the family. In most cases, pain resolves as the illness remits.

However, in some patients, pain continues after the acute pathological process is resolved. Physicians and patients then begin to have difficulty explaining the persistence of the pain. Many patients deny the persistence of the pain and the potential meaning of the chronic illness. This denial causes patients to pursue the same level of activity, lifestyle, and adaptive function that they pursued prior to the onset of the pain. This denial process allows patients to overextend themselves, leading to activities which may, in turn, reinjure or perpetuate the pathophysiological process causing the pain.

It is in this phase that the abuse of pain medication usually begins. The patient uses the pain medication to overextend the safe limit of activity, and the cycle of pain intensification and medication use is initiated. The use of pain medication may become associated with the pain behaviors rather than with the pain itself. The patient's interest is directed toward curative therapies despite repeated treatment failures. In some patients, the passage of time and repeated treatment failures are not sufficient to lessen the denial process, as we have already noted. Chronic pain patients often deny the presence of any sort of psychological distress despite observations by family members of the presence of emotional distress. Patients become restless, irritable, and withdrawn from family and friends.

Many chronic pain patients seek medical care from additional physicians, tending to idealize new physicians and discredit the physicians who were unable to find the cure for their chronic pain. This pattern of idealization and disqualification may be repeated as the patient searches for a cure for chronic pain. This emotional reaction and behavior is also seen in patients with severe premorbid personality disturbances such as borderline or narcissistic personality disorders. In patients whose psychological defenses are splitting, idealization, regression, projection, denial, or omnipotence, the emotional reaction to pain treatment failures is greatly intensified. As these patients rely on such primitive psychological defenses, they are unable to achieve an acceptance of the chronic pain and disability.

As the patient begins to accept the chronic pain condition, the motivation for seeking a cure and the ambivalence toward physicians decreases. As the denial in these patients abates, psychological distress begins to appear. At this stage, social and job pressures begin to develop. Patients and their employers usually need to make temporary arrangements for the patients' jobs. (However, chronic pain patients with poor job records or employment problems will find it more difficult to return to their former jobs or to be retrained for other jobs.) Issues of temporary disability payments, workmen's compensation payments, and disability retirement begin to surface. Patients on long-term disability or extended medical leave of absence believe that they will return to their previous occupations.

During the period of adjustment to the condition of chronic pain, patients may begin to experience changes in their marriage. Sexual activity may be reduced, financial responsibility often shifts, and lifestyle of the family unit may be altered, causing the patient to become more isolated and withdrawn. Self-esteem can be affected, and the patient may begin to question at times whether the pain is present. The patient may become bitter, self-pitying, and jealous toward family, friends, and health caregivers, frequently asking, "Why me?" These reactions may become pronounced and fixed in some patients, especially in cases where the chronic pain interferes with the person's adaptive functions responsible for maintaining self-esteem (an example is the gifted athlete, whose self-esteem is derived mainly from physical prowess, who can no longer be as physically active because of chronic pain).

The reactions of bitterness, diminished self-esteem, and self-pity also defend against the reaction to loss (grief) brought about by the chronic pain and disability. In some patients the pain may be exaggerated and serve as a defense against the loss. During this period the neurovegetative symptoms appear (insomnia, weight change, altered concentration, altered level of energy, and decreased sexual interest). Patients report feelings of hopelessness, helplessness, and periods of depression. The extent of the depressive reaction varies; approximately

10 to 20 percent of chronic pain patients will experience major depression (12, 13, 14), while 60 percent of the patients will develop a chronic intermittent depression (dysthymia) with mild to moderate depressive symptomatology (14). Endogenous depression occurs in a small number of patients (14).

The suicide rate in chronic pain patients appears to be higher than the rate found in other medically ill patients (15). Since the frequency of major depression is relatively low, the suicide potential in chronic pain patients must be due to other factors. The chronic pain patient has to contend not only with disability, but often with social isolation and significant lifestyle change. If a chronic pain patient is unable to adjust psychologically and socially to the illness, and if the patient experiences social isolation, limited social support systems, and marital separation, the potential for suicide is present.

The depressed state resolves as the chronic pain patient successfully adapts to the illness. The degree of adaptation is again dependent upon the severity of the disorder, premorbid personality, and the patient's social support system. Part of the adaptive process is the resolving of the grief reaction caused by personal losses. At the stage of successful adaptation, the patient may have little need for pain medications. At the same time, the patient shows renewed interest in social activities. The chronic pain patient engages in work or recreation that is appropriate for his or her level of physical ability and self-esteem and a sense of well-being can be enhanced by these new activities.

Appropriate adjustment in the family system occurs along with the patient's adjustment. The roles of family members change to accommodate the disabled member. This does not mean that healthy family members view the chronic pain patient as ill and dysfunctional, but ill and functional appropriate to the level of his or her capabilities. In addition, the marital relationship undergoes similar adjustment. Financial responsibilities often shift to the healthy spouse since disability payments rarely can support an average size family. The chronic pain patient and spouse adjust their sexual relationship given the physical and pain limitations. The chronic pain patient realizes that each increase of this pain pattern does not indicate a reoccurrence of the original problem, but that the pain level will fluctuate. The chronic pain patient maintains constant contact with one physician to monitor any change in condition or medical treatment, as opposed to consulting a number of physicians and receiving multiple treatments.

In summary, a successful adaptation to chronic pain requires the patient to deal with the losses caused by the illness. He or she must develop or modify preexisting coping skills. Adjustment in marriage, family, and social support systems must also occur. Failure to successfully work through the emotional reaction to chronic pain leaves the patient with persistent psychological and behavioral symptoms which, at times, can be more incapacitating than the pain itself. Because a patient's ability to cope with chronic pain depends upon premorbid personality, social support systems, and severity of the pain, the level of adaptation varies from one patient to another.

Illness Behavior

Pain experiences and pain behavior may be seen as one aspect of illness behavior (9). Pilowsky has classified the illness behavior that accompanies pain into those behaviors that are adaptive and those that are pathological. He terms the pathological behavior abnormal illness behavior (AIB), or dysnosognosia (16), and categorizes them as follows: cognitive, affective, and behavioral.

Cognitive: A person's thoughts about the pain will influence his or her feelings and behavior. These thoughts can be viewed as the sum of multiple determinants, some of which are listed in Table 2. It is important to remember these determinants when assessing the illness behavior in a given patient.

Affective: An individual's feelings are based not only on conscious thought processes but also on unconscious thought processes. Thus, pain and pain behavior may be of symbolic significance.

Behavioral: The illness behavior is related not only to cognition and affect, but also to other factors such as the role of the doctor, family, work place, and society.

Table 2. Multiple Determinants of Cognitive Aspects of Pain

Developmental history
    past experiences of pain, especially childhood experiences
    past experiences of illnesses, especially childhood illnesses
    past experiences of pain in a close relative or family member

Personality traits
    obsessive personality
    histrionic personality
    narcissistic/borderline personality

Sociocultural
    ethnic
    economic strata
    family structure amd relationship

Information about disease and pain

Pathological, or abnormal, illness behavior is usually related to an abnormal psychopathological state. The abnormalities that determine this state include those listed in Table 2. In abnormal illness behavior, there is a disagreement between the physician and the patient regarding the degree and nature of the patient's sick-role (16). Abnormal illness behavior, when it is conscious, is the same as malingering. When it is unconscious, it may be a manifestation of any of the disorders described in Chapter 9, which include both psychoses and neuroses. Pilowsky has described a self-rating instrument as well as an observer-rating method for calculating illness behavior (17, 18).

Thus far we have examined the role of premorbid personality and noted the classification of illness behavior in chronic pain patients. In this section we have addressed primarily psychological reactions to chronic pain in patients with an organic basis for their pain complaints. Sometimes pain may be a result of psychological conflicts. We will now address some of the psychodynamic concepts relating to chronic pain.

PSYCHODYNAMIC CONCEPTS OF CHRONIC PAIN

In his paper, "Inhibitions, Symptoms, and Anxiety," Freud (19) defined pain as an affective response to an actual loss or injury. He conceived of chronic pain as producing an emotional investment or preoccupation with the pain that can be so all-consuming as to drain the individual of the capacity to function. He noted a psychodynamic similarity between the experience of mourning and that of pain: in the case of mourning, an actual *loss* has occurred; in the case of pain, an actual *injury* has occurred. In both situations an adaptation of the ego to an actual event is required. This adaptation is clearly more complex and potentially more intractable with pain than it is with mourning. The actual loss of an external object is both obvious and irreversible, and requires active adaptation directed toward acceptance (grief), or a clearly pathologic response denying that reality. In chronic pain the experience is perceived as a physical injury to the body that might be repaired or healed and hence relieved. This persistent hope for and pursuit of cure serves to reinforce the denial of the chronic nature of the illness. In this manner, acceptance of the injury and its associated change in self-perception is avoided. This denial and avoidance of reality obstructs or even prevents effective adaptation and coping.

Rangell (20) explained the normal emotional responses of an individual to pain as having two phases. The first phase includes the ability to tolerate and utilize small amounts of pain as warning signals, accompanied by appropriate responses designed to avoid pain. The second phase applies to pain that is persistent and unavoidable, a condition to which an individual must react appropriately and adaptatively. He discusses deviations from the normal reaction, noting that some individuals with psychogenic pain seem to seek and produce pain rather than avoid it. Masochism is an example of pain-seeking behavior, in which a neurotic component of the pain exists, or in which the pain may satisfy a feeling of guilt or need for punishment. In addition, the pain may be sought for and suffered with so that accompanying gratification will continue. Such gratification might include enhanced affection or attention from others, or an elevation in self-esteem if one's shortcomings are attributed to painful illness.

Rangell (20) made the additional observation that pain adaptation reflects the historical development of the individual, taking into account his or her total personality structure. Experience of pain or illness may activate a latent unconscious longing to provide a neurosis, or it may become incorporated into a preexisting neurotic or psychotic defensive structure. In this way the experience of pain is utilized in a psychologically defensive manner. Freud (19) and Rangell (20) both emphasized that the psychologic, defensive use of pain serves to maintain an individual's psychological equilibrium. Concomitantly, the relinquishing of the pain poses a potential threat to that equilibrium. Psychotic reactions or suicide attempts following relief of pain, or even in anticipation of that relief, are well known (21).

Engel, in a study of headache, postulated that pain is associated with the experience of guilt resulting from overt hostility (22).

According to Engel, patients who experience chronic headache are characterized by repeated chronic suffering from one or multiple painful disabilities. They may or may not have physical findings. Engel has stated that these patients do not constitute a homogeneous group, but the expression of pain is based on a psychodynamic process common to all such patients. He has stated that these patients have excessive guilt feelings for which the experience of pain serves as punishment. According to Engel, the pain may be unconsciously initiated in these patients by several situations: 1) lack of external circumstances to satisfy the unconscious need to suffer; 2) response to a threatened, fantasized, or real loss; and 3) guilt from intense, aggressive, or forbidden sexual feelings. Characteristically, such patients are unable to express anger directly and usually turn anger on themselves. This leads to a chronically guilt-ridden person who appears depressed, pessimistic, and has self-deprecating attitudes. Sexual adjustment is poor, with sexual fanatasies being sadomasochistic in nature. An episode of pain may develop in association with the loss of a loved one; the pain can occur on the anniversary of a loss.

Engel has pointed out that when such patients are free of pain or when their life situation improves, their painful symptoms may develop or intensify. These patients are described as being unusually tolerant of pain inflicted upon them by either a true illness or by physicians in the course of treatment. A review of the life history of these patients reveals poor tolerance for success and repeated episodes of suffering and defeat. They frequently have a history of physical abuse as children with punishment being used to discipline. Commonly, parents of these patients were attentive only when their children were sick or hurt.

If there is no physical basis, Engel has stated that the patient will usually assign a location to the pain. He believes that the location will be determined by one of the following: pain that has been experienced by the patient at some other time, identification with pain actually experienced by another person; or pain that the patient imagines or wishes another person had. Engel has said that the pain-prone patient may have received one of the following psychiatric diagnoses: conversion hysteria, depression, hypochondriasis, or schizophrenia. He further has stated that this specific psychodynamic pattern can also be seen in patients during brief periods in their lives, and not necessarily be part of a chronic masochistic somatizing patient.

Clinicians need not work long in this area to appreciate the masochistic style of some pain patients. Engel never suggested that all pain patients suffer in the manner just outlined, and it is important to recognize that the psychodynamics can logically operate in a variety of personality disorders or styles. Finally, it is necessary to acknowledge that there has never been an empirical validation of Engel's theory. A clearer understanding of the role of personality and psychological conflicts in the development of chronic pain as well as the psychological reactions to it can be understood by using the systems model outlined in Chapter 2.

In a similar vein, Blumer has emphasized that pain patients are often morally upright people who have difficulty acknowledging negative affects and so instead displace them onto somatic concerns. He has melded a profile consisting of Axis I and II features, as well as psychodynamic considerations. These patients typically have histories marked by personal and familial depression and alcoholism, physical abuse, and models for invalidism or pain. They tend to be workaholics, are so-called solid citizens in their premorbid state, and become depressed and somatically preoccupied (23). The clinical features are outlined in Table 3.

Blumer's work, as well as that of the investigators previously reviewed, represent a series of relatively consistent findings, thus suggesting their validity. However, this work also raises questions. Are Blumer's pain-prone patients primarily depressed? Do they have specific personality types? Are the characteristics of the solid citizen more common in chronic pain disorders than in the public at large, particularly if one controls for depression? Does the chronic pain patient, referred to either a pain center or to a psychiatrist, differ in personality characteristics or affective life from chronic pain patients not so referred? Psychological

Table 3. Clinical Features of the Pain-Prone Disorder*

Somatic complaint
  Continuous pain of obscure origin
  Hypochondriacal preoccupation
  Desire for surgery

Solid citizen
  Denial of conflicts
  Idealization of self and of family relations
  Ergomania (prepain): "workaholism," relentless activity

Depression
  Anergia (postpain): lack of initiative, inactivity, fatigue
  Anhedonia: inability to enjoy social life, leisure, and sex
  Depressive mood and despair

History
  Family and personal history of depression
  Past abuse by spouse
  Handicapped relative

---

* Reprinted from Blumer D, Heilbronn M: Chronic pain as a variant of depressive disease.
J Nerv Ment Dis 170:381–406, 1982. Reprinted by permission

conflicts and personality play roles at several points in the development of the chronic pain syndrome, and the picture that the patient presents is a blend of these components. The systems approach provides a framework for formulating hypotheses and for developing studies to validate them.

Psychogenic Pain and Depression

Blumer and Heilbronn have postulated that the pain-prone disorder represents a specific syndrome that they believe may be a variant of depressive disease, one that is distinctly different from well defined somatic disease (such as rheumatoid arthritis). He and Heilbronn contend that a factor in maintaining the chronicity of the disorder may be the continuous physical procedures aimed at correcting a "phantom peripheral source of pain" (23). They suggest that early recognition and diagnosis might avoid this costly and futile approach and lead to more effective treatment.

Pilowsky and Bassett (24) presented a study of 114 patients with chronic pain and compared them to 53 depressed inpatients. They noted numerous differences between the populations. Pain patients tended to be older (aged 45 versus 38), were more likely to be married, and more likely to have large families than were depressed patients. Patients with pain commonly attributed their problems of inactivity and insomnia to their pain and more often reported difficulties with motor function. Pain patients were less dysphoric than depressed patients and frequently were found to have a typical illness behavior profile suggestive of a conversion reaction. Pilowsky and Bassett observed that a salient feature of the chronic pain patient, which is also observed in the conversion patient, is the denial of emotional disturbance and life problems not related to pain. While depressed patients typically recalled stressful life events occurring in the year preceding the onset of their illness, pain patients seemed to focus on stressful events that occurred up to 9 or 10 years in the past. It was the authors' contention that the depressed population presented a more acute response to major stress, while the chronic pain population characteristically had longstanding unresolved problems without acute stressful events. They argued that the two groups could not be considered identical because chronic pain patients are distinguished from depressed patients by the presence of abnormal illness behavior. Finally, the authors noted that illness behavior typically is used by the chronic pain population as a coping mechanism. These two studies (23, 24) suggest that a characteristically vulnerable population may exist. Such a population may be susceptible to chronic maladaptive illness behavior as well as to depressive symptomatology.

It is of interest to note that prior to the publication in 1980 (by the American Psychiatric Association) of *The Diagnostic and Statistical Manual of Mental Disorders, Third Edition* (DSM-III), psychogenic pain had not been distinguished from conversion disorder and, in fact, had been diagnosed as conversion. Most of the studies on conversion prior to DSM-III included psychogenic pain, and there was no effort made to distinguish pain from other conversions. As psychogenic pain has acquired an important place in psychodynamic psychiatry, we will review the literature on conversion disorders with special reference to pain. A detailed account of the nosological criteria (DSM-III) for conversion disorder, psychogenic pain disorder, and somatization disorder are given in Chapter 9.

In a retrospective review of 285 patient charts in which diagnoses of hysterical conversion had been made, Bishop and Torch (25) attempted to distinguish conversion disorder from psychogenic pain (psychalgia). For comparison they randomly selected a control group of 94 patients having DSM-III nonpsychotic diagnoses other than conversion disorder or psychogenic pain disorder. They then attempted to rediagnose the 285 patients using DSM-III criteria, by which patients were defined as having either definite conversion disorder or psychogenic pain disorder when they met all the standards of DSM-III, and as probable cases when three or more of the DSM-III criteria were met. Of the 285 patients, 63 were thought to be definite and 28 probable conversion disordered while 9 were thought to be definite and 71 probable psychogenic pain disordered. Each of the four groups, as well as the controls, were then compared along a number of clinical variables and demographic features. It is of interest that no significant differences were found between definite and probable diagnostic groups, and no differences were found to discriminate psychogenic pain disorder from conversion disorder. In contrast, the control group varied significantly from both conversion disorder and psychogenic pain disorder groups in five areas: 1) symptoms possessing conflictual content; 2) symptoms having a psychological defensive function; 3) evidence of secondary pain; 4) presence of a history of trauma preceding onset of symptoms; and 5) past history of conversion phenomena. These data suggest that the DSM-III separation of psychogenic pain disorder from conversion disorder may be artificial.

DSM-III criteria for diagnosis of psychogenic pain disorder are as follows: 1) the predominant complaint is that of pain not medically explainable by a pathophysiological mechanism or by a physical disorder; 2) when organic findings are present, the severity of the pain complaint must be far in excess of observed pathology; 3) psychogenic pain is, by definition, mediated by an unconscious or involuntary mechanism; 4) at least one of the following qualifiers must be judged to be etiologically present: a) a temporal relationship between an affectively charged conflictual event with the onset or exacerbation of the pain; b) the pain in some way enables the individual to avoid noxious activity; and c) the pain enables the individual to get support from the environment. Finally, the pain cannot be symptomatic of another mental disorder.

The same criteria are applied to the diagnosis of conversion disorder, with the exception that the primary complaint is a loss or alteration of physical function, excluding pain or disturbance of sexual function. Unlike the diagnosis of psychogenic pain disorder, the diagnosis of conversion disorder does not allow for the severity of complaints to be far in excess of observed pathology (the overlay phenomenon). The rationale for this exclusion is obscure.

The term conversion was coined by Freud and Breuer (26) in *Studies on Hysteria* to define a psychic mechanism through which an unacceptable unconscious impulse may be kept from consciousness through the development of a physical symptom suggestive of illness. Thus, the forbidden unconscious impulse is kept from consciousness through the process of being "converted" to a physical complaint that is relatively less threatening. Consequently, with the sudden onset of a physical complaint, the conscious realization of an aggressive or sexual impulse may be avoided. Not uncommonly, the symptom may have symbolic significance in relation to the underlying conflict, as, for example, when a sudden pain in the neck disrupts a visit with a demanding relative.

The psychological defensive function of a conversion symptom is referred to as primary gain, whereby the unconscious conflict is kept from awareness through the substitution of the physical symptom. Where primary gain is central, the psychogenic pain or conversion symptom would most probably develop as an acute phenomenon occurring in an affectively charged situation. Here, the disabling effects of the symptom prevent the conscious recognition or expression of the psychologically conflicted and forbidden impulses. In this situation of apparent sudden physical distress, the person suffering the disorder at times appears strikingly calm and lacking concern. This observation has been referred to as *la belle indifference*, in which the indifferent attitude seems to be in striking contrast to the sudden onset of a possibly catastrophic medical situation. From the psychodynamic perspective, the indifference is understandable in terms of the defensive relief provided by the symptom, the primary gain. Acute conversion episodes will predictably be transient events in which the defensive primary gain occurs in an acutely stressful situation, with the symptom remitting once the stressful situation has passed. In general, such episodes would not come to medical attention.

Chronic psychogenic pain and conversion are quite different disorders. Here, the physical complaint may persist for extended periods up to a lifetime. Unlike the situation that exists in the acute presentation, the afflicted individual is often severely disabled by the complaint. Here, primary gain is of minimal to no significance compared to the alterations in lifestyle and interpersonal relationships necessitated by continued disabling physical symptoms. Thus, the underlying secondary gain becomes the central focus. By secondary gain we mean that the perpetuation of the symptom is either rewarded by special treatment and enhanced attention from others or by anticipation of such rewards. Self-esteem is maintained through the adoption of the sick role. This necessitates an investment in and perpetuation of the symptom as a complaint, and encourages the pursuit of medical relief essentially as a justification for the continuation of the secondary gain. With chronic conversion or pain, the perpetuation of the disability often leads to psychological regression with marked increased dependency.

In the population of chronic pain patients, one would expect to find a high incidence of developmentally primitive character pathology where issues of dependency are predominant areas of conflict. This has been borne out by the data (25, 27, 28, 30). Since the problem is one of chronicity or disability with characterologic incorporation of a maladaptive sick role, the prognosis for recovery is poor. Finally, the combination of increased dependency and fragile self-esteem predisposes the chronic pain patient to depressive affect, frequently observed in this population.

Engel and Schmale (27) took exception to the earlier psychoanalytic concepts of the conversion process enumerated by Alexander (28) and others (29, 30), who believed that psychic energy was transformed by the conversion process and channeled somatically by motor and sensory pathways. They suggested, rather, that the conversion occurs only as an intrapsychic process comparable to any other neurotic symptom in which no "mysterious leap from mind to body occurs" (27). They suggested that with conversion, memories of past physical symptoms are utilized as models. The memories may be of real or imagined physical experiences occurring in the recent or distant past, and may have involved either the patient directly or other significant individuals in the patient's life. In this manner, Engel and Schmale contend, the physical conversion symptom simply represents an unconscious reactivation or reexperiencing of previously experienced, observed, or fantasied somatic symptomatology. They believe that this accounts nicely for the often observed inconsistencies on careful physical examination distinguishing conversion symptoms from organic disorders, since the symptoms are, in fact, intrapsychic with no real peripheral components. Numerous recent studies have been designed to better define and characterize the conversion disorder. These studies can be divided into two categories: retrospective and cross-sectional studies (summarized in Table 4) and follow-up studies (summarized in Table 5).

Retrospective and Cross-Sectional Studies. Chodoff and Lyons (31) reviewed 17 military veteran patients (15 men and 2 women) diagnosed as having conversion reaction. They noted that only three (two women and one man) were diagnosed as having hysterical personalities, but noted that all were believed to have pathological personality types, including: seven passive-aggressive; three hysterical; two emotionally unstable; two inadequate; two schizoid; and one paranoid. They observed that no single personality pattern could be associated with conversion symptoms, suggesting that conversion could occur in a wide spectrum of personality types or psychiatric disorders.

Table 4. Retrospective and Cross-Sectional Study Data Conversion Disorder*

Studies	Number of Patients	Organic Finding (percent)	Depression (percent)	Schizophrenia (percent)	Personality Disorder (percent)
Ziegler (32)	134	—	30	14	50
McKegney (33)	144	50	22	—	30
Merskey (34, 35)	89	48	—	—	39
Stefansson (36)	64	56	50	8	48

* Adapted from Maltbie (43)

Table 5. Conversion Disorder: Summary of Follow-up Studies

Studies	Follow-up Period (years)	Number of Patients	Organic Finding at Follow-up	Organic Finding with Hysterical Overlay	No Organic Finding	Conversion Diagnosis — Associated Diagnosis		
						Depression	Schizophrenia	Other
Garfield (37)	3–10	24	5 (21%)	—	19 (79%)	—	—	—
Slater (38)	10	73	22 (30%)	19 (26%)	32 (44%)	9 (28%)	2 (6%)	21 (66%)
Raskin (39)	.5–1	50*	7 (14%)	3 (6%)	32 (64%)	0	7 (22%)	25 (78%)
Watson (40)	10	40	10 (25%)	—	30 (75%)	—	—	30 (100%)
Rada (41)	1–3	20	3 (15%)	2 (10%)	15 (75%)	3 (20%)	—	12 (80%)
Hafeiz (42)	1	57	—	—	57 (100%)	—	—	57 (100%)

* 8 patients undiagnosed

Ziegler and colleagues (32) reported on a review of 134 patients diagnosed with conversion, noting that 40 had diagnosable depression and 19 had schizophrenia. They suggested that the conversion symptom for these patients served the defensive function of avoiding the intolerable affect of depression, or of experiencing the psychotic disorganization of schizophrenia. Less than 50 percent of their patients met criteria for hysterical personality. They noted that the majority of the conversion patients rejected psychotherapy because they perceived themselves as physically ill.

McKegney (33) reviewed 1,052 psychiatric consultations on medical and surgical inpatients and found that of this number, 144, or 13.7 percent, carried the diagnosis of conversion reaction. He then compared this conversion patient population to the remainder of the 1,052 patient consultations as controls. He observed that for the conversion group, females outnumbered males three to one; while of the nonconversion group, females outnumbered males three to two. He noted overt depression in 22 percent of the conversion patients, with covert depression suspected in another 35 percent of the conversion group. In comparison, 43 percent of the controls were believed to be overtly depressed, and 18 percent were believed to be covertly depressed. Taken together, overt and covert depression was essentially the same, or 60 percent, in both groups. He noted that one-third of both groups had apparent character disorders, that organic deficit was apparent in 50 percent of the conversion patients and 70 percent of the others, and that patients referred for outpatient psychotherapy from both groups were unlikely to follow through with the treatment plan.

Merskey and Buhrich (34) reported on 89 patients diagnosed as having hysterical conversion with neurological symptomatology, in an effort to better define the association between conversion symptoms and organic cerebral disease. The patients included in this study met criteria on neurologic examination or observation for conversion. Of these 89 patients, 24 were selected and matched by age and sex, with 24 control patients chosen from psychiatric consultation seen in the same setting, where neither hysterical conversion nor pain were symptom complaints. Of the 89 patients, 48 percent had demonstrable organic cerebral disorder or systemic illness affecting the cerebral function. Fifty percent of the 24 matched subgroup of conversion patients had organic findings, as did 58 percent of the controls. Merskey and Buhrich noted that because their data reflected patients seen in a neurological hospital, a disproportionate number of patients with organic disease would be expected. In an additional report, Merskey and Trimble (35) further elaborated these data by evaluating the relationship of conversion symptoms to the presence of hysterical personality or sexual maladjustment in their patients. Hysterical personality occurred in 19 percent of 89 conversion patients,

21 percent of the conversion subgroup, and none of the controls. In addition, a diagnosis of passive-dependent personality was made in a further 20 percent of the conversion patients as compared to none of the controls. Forty-two percent of the conversion patients complained of symptomatic sexual adjustment problems, with only 16 percent of the controls having similar complaints. Merskey and Trimble noted that a disproportionate number of the conversion patients having sexual adjustment problems occurred in those diagnosed as having hysterical or passive-dependent personalities. The authors concluded from these two studies that personality disorder and sexual maladjustments seem to be important correlates of conversion symptoms. They suggest that conversion disorder is multifactoral in genesis and is likely to be associated with hysterical personality, sexual maladjustment, or chronic brain pathology.

An epidemiologic study done by Stefansson and colleagues (36) reviewed data on the registration rate for hysterical neurosis in Monroe County, New York, and in Iceland from 1960 to 1969. They noted a registration rate for hysterical neurosis in Monroe County to be 22 per 100,000 per year as compared to 11 per 100,000 per year in Iceland. They looked further at the psychiatric consultation records for the University Teaching Hospital in Monroe County over this time period and identified 64 cases diagnosed with conversion or probable conversion symptoms. Most patients had more than one conversion symptom, the majority had an accompanying organic illness or psychopathology, with 32 described as depressed, 22 as having "hysterical personality," 5 as schizophrenic, 9 as alcoholic, and 36 as physically ill. The authors made the additional observation that a disproportionate number of patients diagnosed with hysterical conversion died within a year of receiving the diagnosis. This observation lead them to suggest that there may have been a failure in making the proper diagnosis of organic illness.

Follow-up Studies. A follow-up study of 24 patients who had been diagnosed as having conversion reaction while they were patients on either a neurology or neurosurgery service was reported by Gatfield and Guze (37) (Table 5). They performed follow-up interviews 3 to 10 years after the original diagnosis was made. Of the 24 patients, 14 were found to have hysterical personality (Briquet's syndrome) and 4 had developed neurologic disorders. Nine were free of conversion symptomatology at the time of follow-up, while 15 continued to have their original complaints or had developed new complaints.

Perhaps the most comprehensive study of conversion was published by Slater and Glithero in 1965 (38). They reported data on 85 patients (32 males and 53 females) diagnosed as having "hysteria" at the British National Hospital during the early 1950s. Of the 85, 12 were deceased (4 from suicide and 8 from organic diseases). Two of those committing suicide had organic disorders at the time of their death. Of the 73 remaining patients, 19 (26 percent) were found to have diagnosed organic disorders with superimposed "hysterical overlay" complicating their symptom presentation. An additional 22 patients (30 percent) were felt to be misdiagnosed as hysterical when organic disorders accounted entirely for their symptoms. Only 32 patients (44 percent) had no established organic disease. Two of the 32 patients (6 percent) were found to be schizophrenic and 8 had recurrent symptomatic depressions, leaving 21 conversion patients (66 percent) without major psychiatric disorders or organic disturbance. Of these, eight patients had chronic disabling conversion symptomatology. The authors did not comment on the frequency of personality disorders.

A prospective study of 50 patients referred from an outpatient neurologic service for suspected conversion disorder was reported by Raskin and associates (39). The authors were blind to the actual neurologic data and rated each patient in terms of eight criteria that they believed would be useful in distinguishing conversion from organic disorders. Neurologically, 32 of the 50 patients were diagnosed as conversional, while 7 were eventually found to have organic neurologic pathology. Three had organic findings with hysterical overlay and the remainder were not diagnosed. They compared the 32 conversion patients to the 7 organic patients. They believed that of their eight diagnostic criteria, those most useful in distinguishing conversion disorder from organic pathology were: 1) a history of prior use of somatic symptoms as psychological defense; 2) demonstration of significant emotional stress at the time of onset of symptoms; and 3) evidence that the symptom served a defensive function in the solving of a conflict brought about by the precipitating stress. Raskin and colleagues suggested that when at least two of these criteria were met, a 93 percent correct prediction of diagnosis of conversion would occur. They noted a 29 percent false positive rate with the organic patients. The remaining five criteria were thought not to be diagnostically predictive. These included the positive demonstration of Briquet's syndrome or demonstration of a symptom model, either in the patients themselves or in significant others. The authors suggested that either of these two criteria may be useful in formulating the diagnosis of conversion reaction, but since they were absent in a substantial number of patients, they could not be considered diagnostically predictive. Finally, three criteria that the authors believed were not useful diagnostically included the presence of a hysterical personality, the presence of *la belle indifference*, and the expression of symbolism in a symptom.

In a 10-year follow-up study, Watson and Buranen (40) compared 40 male veteran patients having conversion diagnoses to 40 matched controls with neurotic disorders. They found a 25 percent rate for false positive conversion diagnosis, in which organic pathology had been misdiagnosed as conversion. They noted an inability to differentiate patients misdiagnosed as having conversion from those with true conversion symptoms, using Minnesota Multiphasic Personality Inventory (MMPI) scores as both groups demonstrated conversion patterns. Watson and Buranen cautioned that care be used in the medical evaluation of apparent conversion reactions in an effort to minimize false positive diagnosis. They noted that 57 percent of those diagnosed with conversion disorder presented with symptomatic complaints similar to actual symptoms of physical disorders that they had suffered in the past, a symptom model.

Rada and colleagues (41) reported data on 20 children aged 7 to 18 who were diagnosed as having visual conversion symptoms. It was noted that 9 were male and 11 female; 35 percent were diagnosed as having hysterical personality. Numerous other personality diagnoses were observed with only 10 percent, or 2 of the 20 children, considered to have healthy personalities. One- and three-year follow-up data on 18 of the 20 patients found that 3, or 17 percent, had bona fide organic eye disease. Four, or 27 percent, continued unimproved at follow-up with persistent chronic eye symptoms, although two were felt to have improved psychologically despite persistent symptomatology. The remaining 11 patients had improved on ophthalmologic exam but only 6 were believed to have improved psychologically as well. Three of the six reported transient recurrence of visual symptoms with stress (acute pattern without chronicity).

Hafeiz (42) reported a series of 61 conversion patients seen in an African population. He noted that patients were carefully evaluated to rule out organic pathology, with no organic disease occurring in a one-year follow-up of 57 of the patients. Treatment was aimed at symptom removal through suggestion utilizing various techniques, the combination of which eventually was successful in acute symptom improvement in the hospital situation. The patients were seen one year after discharge for follow-up: 21 percent, or 12 patients, had relapsed, 8 of whom complained of the same symptoms with which they had initially presented. Hafeiz noted that most of those who relapsed had their symptoms for extended periods of time prior to treatment and thus could be considered chronic when admitted for treatment. He suggested that the high recovery rate observed in his population (79 percent) might represent a high incidence of recent symptom onset in the majority of the patients, coupled with a follow-up interval of only one year.

Review of Studies on Conversion Disorder

Review of these data supports the observation that conversion symptoms and psychogenic pain are not specifically related to any particular personality type, but would be expected to be found in a wide variety of personality types. Conversion and psychogenic pain might also be found in association with other major psychiatric disorders and organic medical conditions. Common to most of these studies is a remarkably high incidence of organic disease being misdiagnosed as conversion disorder or psychogenic pain disorders. Follow-up reports range from a low of 14 percent to a high of 56 percent of patients being misdiagnosed as having conversion disorder (37–42). An additional, common observation is the conversional overlay that complicates organic medical disorders. Raskin and colleagues observed a 6 percent occurrence of conversional overlay, while Slater and colleagues (38) reported a 26 percent overlay. The perplexing problem of psychogenic overlay complicating organic pathology is frequently encountered clinically particularly in chronic pain patients, when a patient with known organic pathology has complaints that are markedly exaggerated from what would reasonably be expected. The overlay must be viewed as serving a psychological defensive function using the existing organic substrate as a symptom model. Both primary and secondary gain factors may be involved.

An additional characteristic of conversion disorder suggested by these studies is the distinction between its acute and chronic forms (43, 44) (Table 6). Patients with acute conversion, if seen medically at all, would be seen shortly after the sudden onset of their complaint, with the onset having occurred in a stressful situation. Primary gain would be the central feature when the psychological defensive nature of the symptom is clear. In addition, the symptom may seem to have symbolic meaning in terms of the stressful situation, and through its presence may allow the individual to avoid a conflicted activity. If defensively effective, *la belle indifference* would be observed. When not effective as a defense, anxiety would be expected.

Case Example

A 34-year-old married white male veteran presented to the emergency room complaining of crushing chest pain with a strikingly indifferent attitude to his problem. His cardiac work-up was unremarkable. His alcoholic father died the day before of a myocardial infarction. His conflicted feelings about his father's death and funeral were avoided by way of his own complaints.

PSYCHOLOGICAL TREATMENT

Traditionally, treatment has been focused on eliminating the cause of pain. There is now a great deal of interest developing in the treatment of depression in patients with chronic pain. Furthermore, considerable interest is developing on working with a patient's adaptive response to pain. Since the adaptive response to pain has both psychological and

Table 6. Acute and Chronic Forms of Conversion or Psychogenic Pain Disorders

Acute	Chronic
Onset recent	Onset distant
Precipitating stressful event apparent and affectively charged	Precipitating event not apparent, or vague and lacks effect
Primary gain is predominant where conversion symptom serves a clear defensive function	Secondary gain is predominant where conversion symptom serves as necessary requirement of sick role
La belle indifference more likely if conversion defense is effective; anxiety if defense is not effective	La belle indifference not apparent as secondary gain requires a focus on the conversion symptom as disabling
Anxiety is the predominant affect; the symptom may be warding off a psychotic decompensation	Depression is the predominant affect; secondary depression features are common
Single conversion symptom is common	Multiple conversion symptoms are likely, simultaneously or in a sequence
Acute form is not specific to any personality type or mental disorder	High incidence of occurrence with somatization disorder (Briquet's syndrome) or other dependent personality disorder
Prognosis is generally good for spontaneous lasting recovery, and for complete recovery with treatment if other major mental disorder is not present	Prognosis is generally poor for spontaneous lasting recovery and for complete recovery with treatment

Adapted from Maltbie (43, 44)

behavioral components (see Chapters 17 and 20), the treatment approaches have to be based on assessment of the patient's family, the individual's defensive mechanisms, personality structure, and interpersonal relationships. Any one of a wide variety of therapies may be indicated (such as supportive psychotherapy, cognitive psychotherapy, psychodynamic psychotherapy, family and marital therapy, and group therapy).

As we have already noted, chronic pain may result in an alteration of family dynamics which are often maladaptive (for example, the spouse and children may inadvertently reinforce the psychological need for denial of the loss). This, unfortunately, limits the rehabilitation of the individual, and family therapy may be indicated in such situations.

When pain appears to be the result primarily of a psychological process, the clinician must first evaluate whether the pain is an adaptive or maladaptive symptom, and whether it is a result of an acute or chronic process. Pain may be an adaptive symptom when it serves to provide structure to a chaotic, disorganized personality (such as the borderline personality disorder or other severe personality disorder such as narcissistic personality disorder). In such instances, considerable care must be exercised in formulating diagnosis and treatment. Since pain is serving as an adaptive mechanism in such cases, ablation of the symptoms without personality reorganization may be detrimental. However, when pain is maladaptive, it is necessary to formulate and treat the symptom with or without personality restructuring.

So far we have discussed pain as a result of unconscious conflicts; however, one must be aware that the experiencing of pain may sometimes be a deliberate or conscious process (for example, as in malingering).

Many chronic pain patients are fiercely resistant to any consideration of the emotional or psychological aspects of their illness. Nevertheless, these very same patients may, when allowed to, freely elaborate the impact of the pain on their lives and may develop a most useful and enriching descriptive view of themselves, their feelings, and their disorder so that the psychodynamic issues become clear.

If pain is a result of an organic process, the major aim of the psychological treatment is to help the patient face reality. It is essential to this process that the patient recognize an alteration in the integrity of self, an alteration that represents a permanent loss. This is generally experienced as a narcissistic injury and must be dealt with emotionally, much as any other major loss is dealt with.

FUTURE DIRECTIONS

Although a wealth of clinical material exists on the psychological and personality aspects of chronic pain, there are few empirical data. Furthermore, there is little literature on the psychodynamic assessment and management of chronic pain patients. Both empirical and theoretical studies are needed to clarify and extend our understanding of the psychological process in chronic pain patients. Psychotherapy outcome studies similar to the ones currently being conducted for depression need to be done in appropriately selected chronic pain patients with significant psychopathology.

REFERENCES

1. Cabot RC: Differential Diagnosis. Philadelphia, W. B. Saunders, 1911
2. Brown T, Nemiah JC, Barr JS, et al: Psychological factors in low back pain. N Engl J Med 251:123–128, 1954
3. Hanvik LJ: MMPI profiles in patients with low back pain. Journal of Consulting Psychology 15:350–353, 1951
4. Gentry WD, Shows WD, Thomas M: Chronic low back pain: a psychological profile. Psychosomatics 15:174–177, 1974
5. Philips EL: Some psychological characteristics associated with orthopedic complaints. Current Practices in Orthopedic Surgery 2:165–176, 1964
6. Sternbach RA: Psychological aspects of pain and the selection of patients. Clin Neurosurg 21:323–333, 1973
7. Wilfing FJ, Flonoff J, Kokan P: Psychological, demographic, and orthopedic factors associated with prediction of outcome of spinal fusion. Clin Orthop 90:153–160, 1973
8. Beals RK, Hickman NW: Industrial injuries of the back and extremities. J Bone Joint Surg 54-A(8):1593–1611, 1972
9. Pilowsky I: Abnormal illness behavior. Br J Med Psychol 42:347–351, 1968
10. Bond MR: Pain: Its Nature, Analgesics and Treatment. New York, Churchill Livingstone, 1984
11. Hendler HN: The four stages of pain, in Diagnosis and Treatment of Chronic Pain. Edited by Hendler NH, Long DM, Wise TN, et al. Littleton, MA, PSG Inc., 1982
12. Krishnan KRR, France RD, Pelton S, et al: Chronic pain and depression, I: classification of depression in chronic low back pain patients. Pain 22:279–287, 1985
13. Pilowsky I, Chapman CR, Bonica JJ: Pain, depression, and illness behavior in a pain clinic population. Pain 4:183–192, 1977
14. France RD, Houpt JL, Skott A, et al: Depression as a psychopathological disorder in chronic low back pain patients. J Psychosom Res 30:127–133, 1986
15. Pilowsky I: Pain and illness behavior assessment and management, in Textbook of Pain. Edited by Wall PD, Melzack R. London, Churchill Livingstone, 1984
16. Pilowsky I: Abnormal illness behavior and sociocultural aspects of pain, in Pain and Society. Edited by Kosterlitz AW, Terenius L. Weinhelm, Verlag Uremie, 1980
17. Pilowsky I, Spence ND: Manual for the Illness Behavior Questionnaire (IBQ). Adelaide, Australia, University of Adelaide, 1978
18. Pilowsky I, Bassett DL, Bassett R, et al: The illness behavior assessment schedule, reliability and validity. Int J Psychiatry Med 13:63–71, 1984
19. Freud S: Inhibitions, Symptoms, and Anxiety (1926), in Complete Psychological Works, Standard Edition, vol 20. Translated and edited by Strachey J. London, Hogarth Press, 1955
20. Rangell L: Psychiatric aspects of pain. Psychosom Med 15:22–37, 1953
21. Delaney JF: Atypical facial pain as a defense against psychosis. Am J Psychiatry 133:1151–1154, 1976

22. Engle GL: Psychogenic pain and the pain prone patient. Am J Med 26:899–918, 1959
23. Blumer D, Heilbronn M: Chronic pain as a variant of depressive disease. J Nerv Ment Dis 170:381–406, 1982
24. Pilowsky I, Bassett DL: Pain and depression. Pain 7:331–341, 1979
25. Bishop ER Jr, Torch EM: Dividing "hysteria": a preliminary investigation of conversion disorder and psychoalgia. J Nerv Ment Dis 167:348–356, 1979
26. Breuer J, Freud S: Studies on hysteria (1895), in Complete Psychological Works, Standard Edition, vol. 2. Translated and edited by Strachey J. London, Hogarth Press, 1955
27. Engle GL, Schmale AH: Psychoanalytic theory of somatic disorder: conversion, specificity, and the disease onset situation. J Am Psychoanal Assoc 15:344–365, 1967
28. Alexander F: Fundamental concepts of psychosomatic research: psychogenesis, conversion, specificity. Psychosom Med 5:205–210, 1943
29. Rangell L: The nature of conversion. J Am Psychoanal Assoc 7:632–662, 1959
30. Deutsch F: On the Mysterious Leap from the Mind to the Body. New York, International Universities Press, 1959
31. Chodoff P, Lyons H: Hysteria, the hysterical personality, and "hysterical" conversion. Am J Psychiatry 114:734–740, 1958
32. Ziegler FJ, Imboden JB, Meyer E: Contemporary conversion reactions: a clinical study. Am J Psychiatry 116:901–909, 1960
33. McKegney FP: The incidence and characteristics of patients with conversion reactions: a general hospital consultation service sample. Am J Psychiatry 124:542–545, 1967
34. Merskey H, Buhrich NA: Hysteria and organic brain disease. Br J Med Psychol 48:359–366, 1975
35. Merskey H, Trimble M: Personality, sexual adjustment and brain lesions in patients with conversion symptoms. Am J Psychiatry 136:179–182, 1979
36. Stefansson JG, Messina JA, Meyerowitz S: Hysterical neurosis, conversion type: clinical and epidemiological considerations. Acta Psychiatr Scand 53:119–138, 1976
37. Gatfield PD, Guze SB: Prognosis and differential diagnosis of conversion reactions. Diseases of the Nervous System 23:623–631, 1962
38. Slater ETO, Glithero E: A follow-up of patients diagnosed as suffering from "hysteria." J Psychosom Res 9:9–13, 1965
39. Raskin M, Talbott JA, Meyerson AT: Diagnosis of conversion reactions. JAMA 197:530–534, 1966
40. Watson CG, Buranen C: The frequency and identification of false positive conversion reactions. J Nerv Ment Dis 167:243–247, 1979
41. Rada RT, Krill AE, Meyer GG, et al: Visual conversion reaction in children, II: follow-up. Psychosomatics 10:23–28, 1969
42. Hafeiz HB: Hysterical conversion: a prognostic study. Br J Psychiatry 136:548–551, 1980
43. Maltbie AA: Conversion disorder, in Signs and Symptoms in Psychiatry. Edited by Cavenar JO Jr, Brodie HKH. Philadelphia, J.B. Lippincott, 1983
44. Maltbie AA: Chronic pain, in Biomedical Psychiatric Therapeutics. Edited by Sullivan JL, Sullivan PD. Boston, Butterworths, 1984

Chapter 8

Behavioral Concepts in the Analysis of Chronic Pain

Suzanne L. Ross, M.A.

Francis J. Keefe, Ph.D.

Karen M. Gil, Ph.D.

Preparation of this manuscript was supported by NIMH grant number 1 RO3 MH38407–01 (Behavioral Assessment of Chronic Low Back Pain), NIADDK grant number 1 RO1 AM35270–01 (Coping with Osteoarthritic Knee Pain), and a grant from the John D. and Catherine T. MacArthur Foundation.

There is a growing recognition that behavioral and psychological factors play an important role in determining how patients adapt to persistent pain. In this chapter, we review basic concepts that underly the behavioral approach to chronic pain and describe four theoretical models that help us understand the behavior of chronic pain patients.

BASIC BEHAVIORAL CONCEPTS

Behavioral approaches to the analysis of chronic pain differ in fundamental ways from traditional psychodynamic or psychological approaches. Psychodynamic theorists view the emotional distress of the chronic pain patient as resulting from underlying conflicts between inferred needs, drives, or motives. Psychological trait theorists maintain that a patient responds to chronic pain in a particular way because he has a particular trait or personality characteristic such as dependency, hostility, or anxiety. Both psychodynamic and psychological-trait theories view maladaptive behavior as simply a symptom or sign of the patient's underlying problem. To be properly understood the patient's behavior needs to be analyzed and interpreted. Unresolved problems such as conflicts over dependency, the expression of anger, or sexual feelings are viewed as root causes of maladaptive behavioral reactions to chronic pain. Traditional psychodynamic and psychological approaches, therefore, attempt to treat pain patients primarily by helping them to understand and change underlying psychological conflicts or problems.

Behavioral approaches, in contrast, focus their attention primarily on behavior—how the individual acts and responds in a variety of life situations. The hallmark of the behavioral approach is its insistence that behaviors are acquired and maintained through a process of conditioning and learning. While these behaviors may be labelled as "abnormal" or "normal" by society, they are nevertheless learned in the same fashion that all behavior is. A variety of types of learning can play roles in determining how a chronic pain patient behaviorally responds to pain. In the next section, we consider four conceptual models that describe somewhat different forms of learning that influence how patients respond to chronic pain.

A second major characteristic of the behavioral approach is its tendency to focus on *immediate* factors that may effect the patient's behavior. This is in contrast to traditional approaches that emphasize the importance of early childhood experiences or conflicts that occurred at times remote from the present. Behavioral treatment, therefore, is concerned with modifying the patient's current life situation and is not so much centered upon the patient's past history. While behavioral therapists view early experiences as important in the initial development of behavior, the maintenance of a behavior pattern is viewed as primarily under the control of *current* factors.

Two sets of variables are of great importance. These are the *antecedents* and *consequences* of behavior. The antecedents of behavior are those variables that immediately precede the occurrence of behavior. These might include stimuli such as being in a crowded room, walking up stairs, or talking with a spouse. In many patients, these stimuli elicit characteristic learned reactions that form an important part of how the patient copes with pain. For example, some patients adopt a very inactive and dependent lifestyle when their spouse is home; however, when the spouse leaves for work they become much more active and involved in tasks around the house. In this case, the presence of the spouse may be serving as a cue that elicits a maladaptive behavior pattern. Cognitive variables such as the patient's interpretation of stressful events or distortion of life experiences are also important stimuli that can elicit learned pain reactions.

The immediate consequences that the patient's behavior has are also important. Patients may learn, for example, that when they limp or cry, they get a sympathetic response from their spouse or family member. Alternatively, when they are doing well, they may get no noticeable response from those in their environment. In this case, differential attention from the spouse or family serves as a social reinforcement for pain behavior. We often find that significant progress can be made by redirecting family members to pay attention to positive coping behaviors elicited by the patient. Other important consequences may also follow the display of pain behavior. These include taking time to rest or ingesting narcotic medications. By pairing these powerful rewards repeatedly with high levels of pain and pain behavior, these pain responses may unwittingly become reinforced and strengthened. In some patients, of course, the financial contingenies for pain behavior are significant. Patients may actually lose their income if they stop engaging in pain behavior and return to a more effective lifestyle.

BEHAVIORAL MODELS

The Operant Model

The operant model focuses attention on the relationship between behavioral responses that are emitted by the individual and the consequences which subsequently occur. This model maintains that the best way to understand the behavior of certain chronic pain patients is to examine the consequences of their behavior (see Figure 1).

B. F. Skinner (1) was one of the first theorists to systematically examine the principles that underlie operant or instrumental conditioning. In his experiments, the behavior of animals was studied in a specialized laboratory setting (the Skinner box). Animals emitted simple motor behaviors such as key pecking or bar pressing, and the consequences of

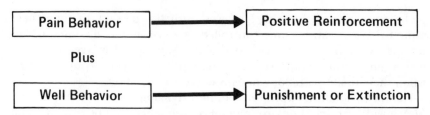

Figure 1. The operant model

these behaviors were manipulated. Skinner found that the type of consequence that was delivered altered the probability that behavior would be emitted in the future. The delivery of positive reinforcement (reward such as food) increased the likelihood that the animal would respond in a similar manner on subsequent occasions. Likewise, when a behavior was followed by an aversive stimulus (shock or punishment), the animal was less likely to respond similarly in the future. Skinner also found that the schedule of reinforcement was quite important. Animals given reinforcement each time they exhibited a response rapidly learned the behavior; but when the reinforcement was withheld, they also quickly extinguished or stopped engaging in the behavior. Animals trained using intermittent reinforcement (for example, delivery of food every third to fifth time they pressed a key) learned this response more slowly but this response was much more resistant to extinction (2). This observation is important because most behaviors acquired in the natural environments—such as responses to pain—have been reinforced on an intermittent basis and are therefore resistant to extinction.

Numerous studies have demonstrated that much of human behavior is acquired and maintained through operant conditioning. Applications of operant conditioning principles to clinical populations indicate that these simple learning principles are useful in understanding not only adaptive behavior but also maladaptive behavior patterns. Behaviorally oriented clinicians maintain that a wide variety of dysfunctional behaviors are acquired and maintained through the influence of operant conditioning (1). Moreover, the operant conditioning model can be used effectively to direct treatment efforts for psychiatric disorders such as depression, anxiety, phobias, anorexia nervosa, and marital and/or sexual problems (3–7).

Fordyce (8) was the first to argue that operant conditioning principles could explain the maladaptive behavior displayed by some chronic pain patients. Fordyce observed that pain patients exhibit overt behaviors that communicate to those around them the fact they are having pain. These behaviors include verbal complaints of pain, taking medication, body posturing, and certain facial expressions. Since these pain behaviors are quite overt, Fordyce maintained that they are easily subject to conditioning and learning influences. Pain behaviors initially may arise from pathological tissue changes. However, with the passage of time these same behaviors can become controlled by environmental consequences irrespective of their underlying pathology. Moreover, Fordyce found that in certain chronic pain patients, these pain behaviors continue even when their tissue pathology basis is decreased or absent.

Pain behaviors are expressed within a dynamic social system. Therefore, a wide variety of environmental consequences can be instrumental in the maintenance of these behaviors. The pain patient's spouse or family members may unwittingly reinforce pain behaviors by responding to them with reassurance or sympathy. Likewise, physicians and other medical professionals may inadvertently positively reinforce pain behaviors by responding with increased attention whenever they occur. Social reinforcement by family members or professionals is often frequently paired with additional potent reinforcers such as narcotics and other pain medications. The patient's financial security in the form of disability or workmen's compensation payments can also become contingent on the continued display of pain behavior. Patients, in fact, may lose their income if they continue to complain of pain but do not show pain behavior. Rewards may also take the form of an opportunity to rest, being provided with a back rub or massage, or being allowed to avoid unwanted responsibilities at home or work.

Several characteristics are evident in chronic pain patients whose pain behavior is influenced by operant conditioning. First, their behavioral patterns do not appear to be closely linked to nociception. These patients are likely to show pain behavior that is in excess of what might be expected on the basis of their underlying tissue damage. They may exhibit a great deal of pain behavior at times when one might not expect to see it, for example, while reclining. Second, the families of these patients are often quite anxious and hypervigilant to the patient's displays of pain. The patient's spouse, for example, may actively encourage the patient to take excess amounts of narcotics and may become angry if the patient attempts to become active or return to higher levels of functioning since past attempts at increased activity may have exacerbated the pain. Third, it is quite clear that the behavior of patients who are involved in pending litigation or disability decisions may be controlled by operant conditioning. Fourth, patients who have few vocational skills and limited formal education often develop an operantly maintained pain problem, as these patients may find that it is very difficult for them to return to their former occupations. In essence, these patients' efforts to engage in "well behaviors" can be very punishing. Finally, patients who have a long history of emotional problems may learn that persistent pain provides them with a legitimate excuse to avoid behaviors that they have found to be stressful and difficult in the past; for example, carrying out the responsibilities of a parent, spouse, or worker.

Behavioral treatment interventions based on the operant conditioning model attempt to change the behavior of the patient by systematically manipulating the consequences of pain and well behavior. Patients are often hospitalized on inpatient units where positive reinforcers such as staff attention and narcotic medication delivery can be carefully controlled. On these units, the staff selectively minimizes attention to pain behaviors while simultaneously attending to and positively reinforcing adaptive behaviors such as increased activity, socializing, and decreased medication intake. Family members are encouraged to visit the unit and become part of the program so that they can also positively reinforce well behaviors, thereby increasing the likelihood that the patient will continue to engage in these behaviors in the future. To reduce the reinforcing value of narcotics, these medications are delivered on a time-contingent schedule as opposed to an as needed schedule. The specifics of this treatment approach are discussed in subsequent chapters. Suffice it to say here that operant conditioning methods have been successful in helping many chronic pain patients who previously failed to respond to conventional medical and surgical approaches.

Conditioned-Fear Response Model

The conditioned-fear response plays a role in many psychiatric medical and psychophysiological conditions. The behavioral perspective maintains that fear is a learned response to anxiety that occurs in situations that the organism has learned will produce punishment or pain. Fear often has an adaptive function in that it motivates the individual to engage in behaviors that will minimize or reduce pain. For example, the symptom of pain may motivate the patient to seek out medical assistance. However, it is clear that fear can also become overwhelming and dysfunctional. Some patients become immobilized by fear and are unable to participate in daily activities they are capable of.

Watson (9) was an early behaviorist who investigated the principles underlying conditioned-fear responses in an experimental paradigm. In a landmark study, Watson and Rayner (10) exposed a child named Little Albert to repeated pairings of an unconditioned stimulus (loud noise) and a conditioned stimulus (white rat). After several pairings, the child routinely exhibited a fear response each time he was exposed to the white rat. It is now known that a similar process of conditioning plays a role in the development and maintenance of a wide variety of phobic and anxiety states (4). In phobic patients, anxiety or fear that is initially associated with a clearly aversive situation can, over time, occur in other situations in which similar cues or stimuli are present. For example, an individual who experiences a very rough airplane ride may subsequently feel quite anxious when approaching the airport to take a flight. The anxiety experienced is often quite salient because it is accompanied by autonomic arousal responses such as increased heart rate, blood pressure, and sweating.

The individual's behavioral response to anxiety is believed to be a key factor in the maintenance of a phobic response. For example, if the traveler cancels his airplane flight because of the anxiety experienced on the way to the airport, there will be an immediate decrease in anxiety and reinforcement of an avoidance response. Because the feared situation is not confronted, the individual never is able to experience a decrease in his anxiety in the presence of the feared stimulus (being on the plane). The avoidance response can become stronger and stronger, and the fear response perpetuated. Ultimately, avoidance behavior may continue and extend to other situations even when there is no indication that the situation is objectively dangerous or harmful. It is at this point that the conditioned-fear response has become a maladaptive habit.

Pain patients are predisposed to the development of conditioned-fear reactions because pain is often conceived of as a "warning signal" of impending danger. As a result, the link between pain and fear is central to the understanding of a wide variety of pain syndromes. Figure 2 illustrates the basic elements of this theoretical model. Patients having pain readily learn that specific activities (such as walking or standing) produce an exacerbation of pain. When pain persists, patients may believe that their pain will invariably increase if they attempt to engage in these activities. Often this avoidance response generalizes situations that would not objectively result in increased pain. The conditioned-fear response can become so strong that patients avoid a variety of simple daily activities that they can easily manage. Unfortunately, these activities often include pleasurable, social, recreational, or vocational pursuits. As patients' lives become more limited by fearful avoidance responses, they often become more preoccupied with pain and physical complaints. As

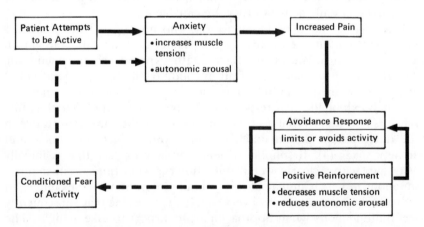

Figure 2. The conditioned fear model

the level of pleasant activities become quite low, depression also increases.

Thus, the conditioned-fear response model maintains that pain behaviors can be conceptualized as avoidance responses. By resting in bed or taking medication, patients may be avoiding increases in pain that they are certain will occur. Because pain behaviors reduce anxiety, they tend to be repeated again and again in the future.

As conditioned-fear reactions persist over time, the likelihood that social reinforcement may function to operantly condition these responses increases. Patients who are so overwhelmed by fear and anxiety that they spend only two to four hours a day out of bed demand a great deal of attention from the family. Spouse and family members take over many of the patient's former responsibilities and often become overly solicitous and responsive to pain behavior. The operant conditioning of pain behavior through social reinforcement serves to increase the strength of the conditioned-fear response. Over time, patient and family are plagued by anxiety and convinced that simple daily activities will invariably increase pain.

A number of behavioral interventions have been developed to alter conditioned-fear responses. The main assumption underlying these approaches is that patients need to be encouraged to confront, in a more adaptive manner, the activities and situations that they fear. Patients are typically trained to control the cognitive and psychophysiologic concomitants of the fear reaction, and then they are encouraged to gradually confront feared events. This process has been called *in vivo desensitization*. For example, patients who have learned to fear a simple activity such as being up and out of bed can benefit from training in relaxation techniques and then gradual exposure to higher levels of activity. A structured schedule of activity using an activity-rest cycle is often helpful. Initially, the activity period within this cycle is set at a very low level that allows the patient to be out of bed without experiencing any increase in pain. Since the pain does not increase, these patients learn that they need no longer fear the activity. By subsequently increasing activity in very small steps, patients can have similar positive experiences and become more confident that they can tolerate progressively longer periods of time out of bed. As patients progress through such a desensitization program, they are encouraged to replace negative self-statements that reinforce and exacerbate fear responses (for example, "I know this will make my pain worse and I can't deal with this") with positive coping self-statements (for example, "I know it is difficult, but I can do this"). They are also encouraged to minimize and control autonomic responses such as increased heart rate, respiration, and blood pressure by utilizing relaxation techniques.

In summary, behavioral treatments can minimize the impact of conditioned-fear reactions by reinforcing activity, promoting mastery experiences, and encouraging the use of a relaxation response that is incompatible with anxiety and fear. By incorporating these techniques in a comprehensive treatment package, patients are often able to return to a more active and fulfilling lifestyle.

The Psychophysiologic Model

The psychophysiologic model of chronic pain provides the conceptual foundation for many of the commonly employed behavior treatment procedures for chronic pain. The model is summarized in Figure 3. As can be seen, it emphasizes the importance of environmental events in eliciting psychological and physiological responses that cause pain. Pain problems that are stress related can best be conceptualized using this model. The basic assumption is that severe stress produces muscular or autonomic responses that result in increased nociception in the periphery. In many cases of muscular reactions, spasm, vasoconstriction, and the release of pain-producing substances appear to be responsible for the pain that patients experience. Emotional reactions to the pain in the form of increased anxiety, depression, or somatization in turn increase the patient's stress level and produce a vicious cycling phenomenon.

The psychophysiologic model is particularly applicable to the analysis of migraine headache. Current research indicates that migraine headache patients are predisposed to autonomic disturbances because of neurovascular instability. Stressful events can set off a series of reflex changes that produce unilateral cerebral vasoconstriction. The vasoconstriction is accompanied by a release of serotonin from platelets that in turn further decreases blood flow. Focal neurologic symptoms such as a visual aura or strange taste will often occur. These symptoms are believed to be due to decreased blood flow to the most effected areas of the brain. Marked vasoconstriction also reduces oxygen and leads to acidosis. Serotonin levels drop further in response to this and other metabolic

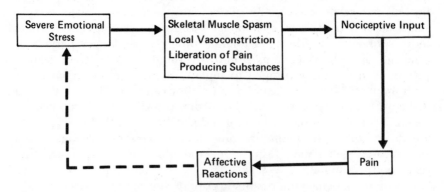

Figure 3. The psychophysiologic model

changes. At the same time that cerebral vasoconstriction is occurring, significant increases in blood flow in the extra and intracranial arteries take place. This pronounced vasodilatation, along with inflammation of the blood vessels and sensitization of pain receptors, produces much of the pain of migraine headaches. With the onset of severe pain, patients often become more anxious, emotionally distressed, and depressed. These affective reactions in turn increase pain. Medical approaches to migraine headache focus on both direct treatment and prevention. Analgesics are often used for mild headaches, and vasoconstrictors are often used in the treatment of severe headaches. Preventive therapy relies on the use of drugs that prevent dilatation of blood vessels such as propranolol, a beta blocker, or drugs such as antihistamines that block both histamines and serotonin receptors.

Behavioral approaches to psychophysiologic disorders such as migraine headaches have two major goals. First, patients are taught to become more aware of the influence of behavioral and psychological factors of their pain. Patients can be asked to keep a pain diary in which they record not only the frequency and severity of pain episodes, but also stressful life events that occur just before the onset of pain. Patients who deny that stress plays a role in pain onset often are better able to recognize the impact of stress after keeping such records. The second major goal in behavioral treatment is teaching patients to directly control the physiologic responses that create pain. The migraine patient, for example, can be taught to vasoconstrict extracranial arteries and to reduce muscle tension in the scalp and facial muscles using biofeedback or relaxation techniques.

Psychophysiologic mechanisms play a primary role in producing pain in patients who have peptic ulcer, colitis, coronary artery disease, temperomandibular joint pain, and muscle contraction headaches. It is clear, however, that psychophysiologic responses often play a secondary role in other chronic pain conditions such as chronic low back pain and arthritis.

Muscle Reeducation Model

In some patients, persistent pain is primarily related to muscle tension, spasm, or inappropriate use of musculature. The high levels of muscle activity that occur produce sustained nociceptive input that results in pain. Figure 4 displays the sequence of events that may result.

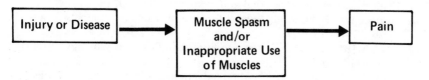

Figure 4. The muscle reeducation model

In many patients, musculoskeletal pain begins following an injury or accident. A typical example would be the patient who was hit from behind while driving a car and experienced a whiplash injury. Muscle spasm often ensues, producing a significant amount of pain. The patient may attempt to minimize additional pain by restricting movement of the head and neck. When this becomes a habit, shortening of the muscles may occur. When the muscles are not used as much, they fatigue more easily and are more likely to go into spasm. Patients compensate by using other muscles, thereby increasing the stress on other areas of the body.

The behavioral approach to musculoskeletal pain problems is designed to teach patients to reduce excess muscle activity in targeted muscles. Muscle activity is recorded from these muscles either directly, using psychophysiologic techniques, or through careful observation of the patient by a therapist. Patients are provided with feedback about muscle activity and are taught to produce a more normal pattern of activity under conditions of rest and during activity. Because inappropriate use of the musculature may be a long-standing habit, treatments to reverse these habits often need to be intensive and continued for some time. Patients, for example, are often unaware of their postural abnormalities and need to be reminded to use the muscles appropriately. We find that combining behavioral training with physical therapy often has synergistic effects for patients with musculoskeletal pain problems.

REFERENCES

1. Skinner BF: Science and Human Behavior. New York, Macmillan, 1953
2. Ferster CB, Skinner BF: Schedules of Reinforcement. New York, Appleton-Century-Crofts, 1957
3. Lewinsohn PM: The behavioral study and treatment of depression, in Progress in Behavior Modification. Edited by Hersen M, Eisler RM, Miller PM. New York, Academic Press, 1975
4. Marks IM: Fears and Phobias. New York, Academic Press, 1969
5. Agras S, Werne JH: Behavior modification of anorexia nervosa: research foundations, in Anorexia Nervousa. Edited by Vigersky R. New York, Raven Press, 1977
6. Patterson GR, Weiss RL, Hopps H: Training of marital skills: some problems and concepts, in Handbook of Application of Operant Techniques. Edited by Leitenberg M. New York, Appleton-Century-Crofts (in press)
7. Hartman WE, Fithian MA: Treatment of Sexual Dysfunction. Long Beach, California, Center for Marital and Sexual Studies, 1972
8. Fordyce WE: Behavioral Methods for Chronic Pain and Illness. St. Louis, CV Mosby, 1976
9. Watson JB: The place of the conditioned reflex in psychology. Psych Rev 23:89–116, 1916
10. Watson JB, Rayner R: Conditioned emotional reactions. J Exp Psychol 3:1–14, 1920

Clinical Concepts

Chapter 9

Pain in
Psychiatric Disorders

Randal D. France, M.D.
K. Ranga Rama Krishnan, M.D.

In this chapter we will review pain as a symptom in psychiatric disorders (Figure 1). While pain is a symptom commonly seen in psychiatric disorders, only in a few instances is pain the presenting complaint. In this section, we will review the psychiatric disorders in relation to the occurrence of pain symptoms.

Table 1 lists the occurrence of pain complaints (both acute and chronic pain) in various psychiatric disorders as defined by *The Diagnostic and Statistical Manual of Mental Disorders, Third Edition* (DSM-III) criteria (1). There are relatively few studies of pain complaints in psychiatric disorders despite the fact that pain is a common symptom in psychiatric patients (2). Most available studies do not use defined criteria for psychiatric disorders. Table 1 is based on clinical experience and extrapolation from the literature (3–7).

TYPES OF PAIN IN PSYCHIATRIC DISORDERS

Pain complaints commonly seen in psychiatric disorders are listed in Table 1. In many of these patients, pain complaints are transient. Table 2 lists some pain complaints and the frequency or infrequency with which they occur. From Table 2, we clearly can see that pain complaints are most often located in the cephalic and truncal areas (3, 8, 9). Pain in the limbs or other peripheral parts of the body is rare (except in central pain states such as thalamic syndrome).

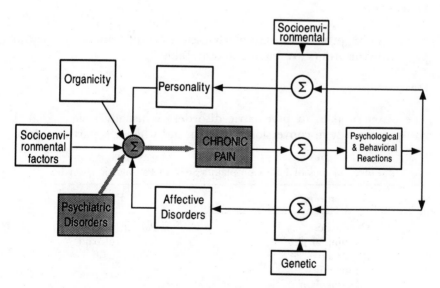

Figure 1. Systems model for chronic pain: chronic pain in psychiatric disorders

Table 1. Pain Complaints in Psychiatric Disorders

Psychiatric Syndrome	Frequency of Pain	Pain as Primary Complaint
Major depression	Common	Rare
Dysthymia	Common	Occasional
General anxiety disorder	Common	Rare
Somatoform disorder	Common	Common
Dementia	Occasional	Occasional
Schizophrenia	Rare	Rare
Alcohol dependence	Common	Rare
Opioid dependence	Common	Rare
Paranoid disorder	Rare	Rare
Bipolar disorder (manic phase)	Rare	Rare
Conversion disorder	Common	——
Psychogenic pain disorder	——	Always
Atypical somatoform disorder	Common	Common
Factious chronic disorder with physical symptoms	Common	Common
Personality disorder	Common	Rare
Hypochondriasis	Common	Common

CLINICAL CHARACTERISTICS OF PAIN IN PSYCHIATRIC DISORDERS

Some of the prominent clinical characteristics of pain secondary to psychiatric disorders are highlighted in Table 3.

Onset

The onset of pain in psychiatric disorders is usually insidious. It is abrupt primarily in conversion disorders and when it is part of a delu-

Table 2. Types of Pain Complaints Seen in Psychiatric Disorders

Common	Rare
Headaches	Pain in periphery
Abdominal pain	Unilateral pain
Back pain	Genital pain
Chest pain	
Cervical pain	
Pelvic pain	

sion. The psychological causes of pain usually affect the younger patient more than do organic causes (9).

Duration

When pain is part of the symptom complex of anxiety disorders or depression, the complaints are usually transient. In some cases of dysthymia, masked depression, generalized anxiety disorder, conversion disorder, hypochondriasis, and psychogenic pain disorder, it may become intermittent and chronic.

Character

Patients' verbal statements are used to gauge the qualitative nature of pain. The verbal description of pain has to be assessed from a multidimensional perspective. Generally, patients with pain from psychiatric disorders do not differ greatly from patients with organic pain on the basis of verbal description of pain (3) and severity (10). Patients with psychogenic pain often have difficulty describing the nature of the pain complaints and usually focus on describing the severity. Some authors contend that psychogenic pain does not awaken the patient at night (7, 8). However, this finding does not apply to pain in depressive illness, in which insomnia is a common symptom.

Site

The most common site of pain in psychiatric disorders is in the cephalic and truncal areas and rarely in peripheral areas (limbs and genitalia) (3, 11). Organic pain is usually recognized in its relation to its site of injury or nature of pathology. Some authors report pain in psychiatric disorders on the nondominant side (6, 12).

Table 3. Clinical Characteristics of Pain in Psychiatric Disorders

Characteristics	Common	Less Frequent
Onset	Insidious	Abrupt
Duration	Transient	Chronic
Site	Cephalic and threshold	Peripheral
Number of sites	Multiple	Single
Constancy of sites	Migraine	Continuous
Neuroanatomical correlation	Poor	Good
Exacerbating factors	Nonspecific	Specific
Alleviating factors	Nonspecific	Specific

Number of Sites

Pain is located in multiple sites in most psychiatric disorders (7). It usually occurs in a single site in delusional pain, psychogenic pain disorder, and conversion disorder.

Constancy of Sites

Pain in psychiatric disorders usually migrates from one location to another (13). Organic pain is stable in location. Psychologically based pain from conversion disorder, psychogenic pain disorder, and secondary to delusions may be more constant.

Neuroanatomical Correlation

There is lack of neuroanatomical and neurophysiological correlation in depression, generalized anxiety disorder, somatoform disorder, and most other psychiatric disorders. Good correlation can occur in medical professionals and medically sophisticated patients.

Exacerbating Factors

Organic pain is usually increased by specific physical factors such as directive movement, activity, palpation, and so on (13). Tenderness is usually not associated with pain of psychiatric origin. Exaggerated variable "tender points" may be seen in some patients with conversion, somatoform illness, and psychogenic pain (7). Similar points may be seen in patients with depression and myofascial pain syndromes.

Alleviating Factors

In patients with organic basis for pain, well defined alleviating factors are usually found. Patients with organic pain obtain some relief from analgesic drugs. Typically, patients with pain from psychiatric disorders report minimum relief from analgesic drugs.

Other Clinical Characteristics

Occasionally pain is described in bizarre, violent terms. Example: "Pain is like my insides are on fire; pain feels like someone is twisting a knife in my chest; and pain hurts so bad I feel like sticking an ice pick through my eyes." These verbal descriptions of pain are usually seen in patients suffering from severe depression with or without psychotic features, somatoform disorder, and generalized anxiety disorder. Devine and Mersky (9) discovered that patients presenting to a psychiatric clinic with pain complaints caused by psychiatric disorders have a more detailed complicated description of their pain than do pain patients presenting to a general medical clinic regardless of cause, psychological or physical. It is important to recognize the importance of selection in understanding this discrepancy. Usually in the case of pain patients presenting to a psychiatric clinic, pain will represent more psychological and social distress than it will in the case of patients presenting to a medical clinic.

Psychiatric patients with chronic pain complaints compared to those without pain have a tendency to have family members who have chronically painful illnesses (14). Most patients with persistent pain are married and come from large families.

Complications of Pain as a Symptom in Psychiatric Disorders

Patients with pain complaints secondary to psychiatric disorder often end up having multiple medical and surgical interventions. This leads to iatrogenic complications. The patient may then develop an organic pain syndrome.

Substance abuse is a frequent complication observed. These patients, in an attempt to alleviate the pain, initially abuse nonnarcotic analgesics. When no pain relief is obtained they gravitate toward narcotic analgesics. Tolerance soon develops and narcotic addiction becomes the major problem. Patients with organic pain rarely develop narcotic addiction (15). Patients, in an attempt to treat their pain, also begin to use alcohol. Alcohol dependency is a common problem in patients with depression and anxiety disorders. It is less common in conversion disorder. Depression is another frequent complication. This is discussed in Chapter 11.

DEPRESSION

Pain complaints are commonly seen in depressive disorders. Table 4 lists the occurrence of pain complaints in depressive illness in various studies (4, 5, 16–24). The incidence of pain complaints in depressed patients ranges from 30 to 84 percent. None of these studies used defined or structured interview to make the diagnosis of depression. Only three studies used a control group (22–24). Among patients admitted to the inpatient psychiatric service of Duke University Medical Center with a diagnosis of major depression using DSM-III criteria, 45 percent had pain complaints.

It should be noted that data on the occurrence of pain complaints in different, well defined subtypes of depression are not available. The study with the best defined criteria is that of von Knorring and colleagues (16). According to these researchers, approximately 57 percent of patients with unipolar depression (patients with major depression who have not had a manic episode) had pain. Forty-four percent of bipolar

Table 4. Depression: Pain as a Symptom

Author (Year)	Incidence of Pain Symptoms (percent)	Number of Subjects
Cassidy (1957)	40	100
von Knorring (1983)	57	161
Spear (1967)	48	85
von Knorring (1975)	60	40
Gallemore (1969)	30	300
von Knorring (1983)	46	140
Diamond (1964)	84	423
Delaplaine (1978)	52	29
Mathew (1981)	78	51
Lindsey (1981)	59	196

patients in the depressed phase had pain complaints. Sixty-nine percent of patients with reactive depression as defined by Perris (25) had pain complaints. Lesse reported that pain is characteristic of patients with agitated depression (26). Bond (6) and Delaplaine and colleagues (21) report that pain complaints are more common in neurotic depression than they are in endogenous depression.

Clinical Characteristics of Depressed Patients with Pain Complaints

Female depressed patients have a greater number of pain complaints than males (16, 26). Pain complaints are more common in older depressed patients than in younger ones (16). Several studies showed no difference in depression between patients with functional and those with organic pain (27, 28). However, others have showed that patients presenting with functional pain are more depressed than patients suffering from organic based pain (29–31). Anxiety and muscle tension are common in depressed patients with pain complaints (16, 26, 32). Autonomic disturbances are also prevalent (16). The backache and headache seen in patients may be related to the muscle tension. Chest and abdominal pain may be related to the autonomic disturbance.

As noted earlier (26), agitation is frequent. Table 5 profiles the common clinical characteristics of depressed patients with pain complaints. Depressed patients with pain complaints do not differ from depressed patients without pain complaints in neurovegetative symptoms, suicidal ideation, fatigue, or concentration difficulties (16). Bond states that hypochondriasis is common in depressed patients with pain complaints (6), but von Knorring and colleagues (16) found no difference in depressed patients with and without pain complaints.

Table 5. Profile of Clinical Characteristics of Depressed Patients with Pain Complaints

Age	Older
Sex	Female
Type	Agitated
Severity	Mild
Anxiety	Frequent
Muscular tension	Frequent
Autonomic Disturbance	Frequent
Site	Head > trunk > extremities

The head and neck appear to be the most common sites of pain complaints in depressed patients (19, 22, 23). Tension headache is the most common type of pain complaint (20). Pain in genitalia and upper and lower extremities are rare. Backache, abdominal, and thoracic pain occur in 10 to 15 percent of depressed patients.

Onset of Pain in Depressed Patients

Retrospective self-report studies (23, 33) suggest a majority of patients report that pain and depression develop at the same time (Table 6). In a few patients depression precedes pain. This suggests that pain, like insomnia, is an early symptom of depression. This is interesting in view of the clinical finding that antidepressants relieve pain prior to alleviating the depressive symptom complex.

Psychological Characteristics in Depressed Patients with Pain

Pain may serve to resolve unconscious conflicts (34). Several authors report a relationship between pain, aggression, hostility, and guilt (35–41). von Knorring and colleagues (18) showed interjected aggres-

Table 6. Temporal Relation Between Pain and Depression

Study	Onset of Pain Prior to Depression (percent)	Onset of Pain and Depression Together (percent)	Onset of Depression Preceding Pain (percent)
Bradley (1963)	46	54	0
Lindsay (1981)	38	50	12

sion in depressed patients with pain complaints. They did not find an association between guilt and the occurrence of pain in depressed patients. It is reported that elements of the depression precede the physical complaints in patients using pain as a defense (38, 42).

Pain Threshold in Depressed Patients

Since pain is a common complaint in depression, the question arises as to whether this is due to a change in the sensitivity to pain among depressed patients. Early studies have shown that depressed patients have a higher pain threshold (39, 43–47) than nondepressed patients. These authors have demonstrated that anxiety disorders are accompanied by a relative decrease in pain threshold as compared to endogenous depression. The altered perception to pain is related to the depressed state. This indicates that pain in depressive disorders probably *is not* due to nociceptive stimulation. The pain threshold is increased in depressed patients both with and without pain complaints (47). Davis and colleagues reported an increase in pain threshold in bipolar patients as in unipolar patients, and the increase is seen in both the depressed and manic phases (45). Ben-Tovim and Schwartz (46) demonstrated an elevation of pain threshold in two severely depressed patients. After recovery from depression, the pain threshold returned to a range seen in normal controls.

Masked Depression

Depression has myriad presentations. Among the various ways in which depression can be presented include hypochondriasis, alcoholism, behavior disorders, dementia, psychosomatic disorders, and specific pain syndromes. Chronic pain is a common presentation of depression (27, 48, 49). When patients with depression present with complaints other than depression, the underlying depression may not be recognized. On further questioning, these patients report vegetative and cognitive symptoms of depression. They may also appear overtly depressed. In rare cases some of these patients, especially those who are not psychologically minded, will deny their depressed mood. Even these patients will *appear* depressed and will admit to fatigue, altered sleep and appetite, weight change, irritability, and anhedonia. The term "masked depression" or "depressive equivalent" has been applied to describe these patients (27, 32, 48, 50). It must be clearly understood that the term describes both patients in whom depression is overtly present but misdiagnosed as a physical illness, and in patients in whom the depression is not clearly recognized and completely overshadowed by the presenting physical symptoms. The concept of considering all chronic pain as a masked depression is not only oversimplifying the issue, but may itself serve to mask the presence of other physical or psychiatric illness. The common types of pain syndromes that appear to be masked depression are angina, atypical facial pain (20, 32), cervical pain, chronic abdominal pain, headache, joint pain, low back pain (49, 51), myalgia, and pelvic pain.

PAIN PRONE PATIENT

Engel, in a study of headaches, showed that pain was associated with the experience of guilt from overt hostility (52). He later expanded this concept and described the "pain prone patient" (38). A detailed discussion of Engel's concept of the pain prone patient is described in Chapter 7.

SCHIZOPHRENIA

Perceptual dysfunction is commonly seen in schizophrenia. This has been well studied in relation to the senses; that is, visual, auditory, and olfactory. This involves an alteration in both the perception and integration of sensory information. Studies of pain thresholds in schizophrenia show their elevation (44, 53). This relative insensitivity to experimental pain is reflected by the reported denial of pain in schizophrenic patients (54–60). Schizophrenic patients with recent onset of their illness were less able to discriminate among the intensities of thermal stimulation than normals and patients with other psychiatric illnesses (58). Chronic schizophrenics have higher thresholds for experimentally induced pain (60). Even though the schizophrenic patients were less able to discriminate among various noxious stimuli or have elevated pain thresholds, the accompanying physiological reaction (muscle tension, heart rate, blood pressure) associated with such stimulation was marked and similar to that seen in anxious patients (58, 60). Similarly, Earle and Earle (61) demonstrated the reaction time of schizophrenics to a cold pressor test to be significantly lower than controls, but the autonomic response to the stress was similar. Process schizophrenics appear to have higher pain thresholds than reactive schizophrenics (59). Bender and Schilder (62) showed schizophrenics in a catatonic stupor to have little reactivity to pain, while other subtypes of schizophrenic patients have normal reactions. Stengel and colleagues (63) did not demonstrate pain insensitivity in a group of chronic schizophrenics using similar methodology. More recently, Davis and colleagues (64) demonstrated a greater degree of pain insensitivity in 17 drug-free schizophrenic patients as compared to 17 sex-matched normal controls. Naltrexone (opioid antagonist) increased the sensitivity to pain in five schizophrenic patients in a placebo controlled trial.

Clinically, this denial of pain can obscure the presentation of many major medical illnesses including peptic ulcer disease, myocardial infarction (65), fractures, and rupture of appendix (66). Marchand (67) reported that 82.5 percent of psychotic patients with myocardial infarction

present without complaints of pain. Physicians working with schizophrenic patients must be alert to the subtle clues and behaviors associated with pain that will aid in the diagnosis of undetected medical or
surgical emergencies in schizophrenic patients.

When pain occurs in patients with schizophrenia and is not related to
organic conditions, the pain may be part of the delusional or somatizing
process. If part of a delusional process, the pain is unusual and bizarre in
description and ill-defined. Behavior is not appropriate to the pain
complaint. Delusional pain is relatively uncommon in schizophrenic patients (8). It is usually seen in the hebephrenic or disorganized schizophrenic patients (6). The pain as part of a somatizing process is more
commonly seen in these patients than is delusional pain. Pain is rarely
the only symptom, and it is rare for it to be the presenting complaint in
patients with schizophrenia (14, 68). Headache is the most common pain
complaint, followed by back and leg pain (69). Watson and colleagues
(69) in a study of pain complaints in schizophrenic patients noted 29 out
of 78 patients with pain complaints. The pain complaints in 13 out of 29
complaining of pain had appropriate physical findings to explain the
pain. The overall incidence of pain complaints is low in schizophrenic
patients as compared to patients with depression or anxiety (8).

PAIN IN BIPOLAR DISORDER: MANIC PHASE

In manic patients decreased sensitivity to experimental pain is seen (53).
However, unlike the case in depressed patients, pain complaints are
rarely seen in the manic patients (21). Crompton-Smith reported a bipolar patient with anginal pain complaints in the depressed phase and
absence of pain complaints in the manic phase (70). Pain insensitivity in
the bipolar patient is seen in the manic and depressive phases of the
illness.

PAIN AND GENERALIZED ANXIETY DISORDER

Among the DSM-III criteria for generalized anxiety disorder are motor
tension and autonomic hyperactivity (1). The motor tension is often
manifested in the form of muscular aches that include both tension
headaches and backaches. The headaches are usually described as tight
bands or pressure. Patients with generalized anxiety disorder also complain of cervical pain. Palpation of the neck muscles often reveal tension
and spasm. Occasionally the neck muscles involved may be tender to
palpation. The autonomic symptoms may be part of cardiac neurosis
(DaCosta syndrome) and may include chest pain.

Spear reported that among psychiatric patients, pain was commonly
seen in anxiety disorders (5). Spear, in his studies of pain in psychiatric
disorders, reported that patients with depressive illness have a good

prognosis at follow-up, whereas patients with anxiety disorders/hysteria have a poor prognosis. Patients suffering from anxiety have lower pain thresholds than patients with major depression and other neurotic conditions (43). This suggests that the mechanism for the occurrence of pain complaints in anxiety disorder may not be the same as in depression.

SOMATIZATION DISORDER

Somatization disorder is defined by DSM-III criteria as a chronic but fluctuating disorder which begins early in life and is characterized by recurrent and multiple somatic complaints for which medical attention is sought, but which are not apparently due to physical illness (Table 7). Somatization disorder is believed to be more common in women and in female relatives of patients. This is based primarily upon findings from a single study (71). The incidence of somatization disorder is unknown. Among patients attending pain clinics the incidence is low, less than one percent in our experience. Reich and colleagues (71) reported that the incidence may be as high as 30 percent. Somatization disorder may be more frequent in patients with pelvic pain (72, 73) than other types of pain. Conversion symptoms are frequently found in patients with somatization disorder.

Clinical Features

The disorder usually manifests itself in the second or third decade of life, is usually lifelong, and has a highly variable course. It is generally characterized by vague, poorly defined, variable somatic complaints when pain occurs. The common sites for pain are back, head, and neck; often patients have pain in all three sites. Usually the pain, although chronic, waxes and wanes in response to attention and specific treatment directed toward the relief of pain. The patients' pain and attendant pain behaviors may lead to multiple medical and surgical interventions. The DSM-III diagnostic criteria for somatization disorder are given in Table 7. These criteria are useful as an aid in the diagnosis of somatization disorder but should not be taken as essential for its diagnosis. Some of the other important clues that aid in the diagnosis of these patients are:

1. The *dramatic, vivid, vague, and circumstantial, and tangential* description of the complaints.
2. As the clinician tries to focus on the description of the complaint, patients describe the reason for the complaint and tend to get angry when the questioning is persistent.
3. Pain complaints when present, never occur by themselves and are always accompanied by other symptoms (paralysis, for example).

4. As one complaint gets better, another takes its place (relief from all complaints is rarely seen except for brief periods).
5. Some patients, both male and female, tend to have histrionic and exhibitionistic characteristics.

Table 7. DSM-III Diagnostic Criteria for Somatization Disorder

---

A. A history of physical symptoms of several years' duration beginning before the age of 30.

B. Complaints of at least 14 symptoms for women and 12 for men, from the 37 symptoms lists below. To count a symptom as present the individual must report that the symptom caused him or her to take medicine (other than aspirin), alter his or her life pattern, or see a physician. The symptoms, in the judgment of the clinician, are not adequately explained by physical disorder or physical injury, and are not side effects of medication, drugs, or alcohol. The clinician need not be convinced that the symptom was actually present, e.g., that the individual actually vomited throughout her entire pregnancy; report of the symptom by the individual is sufficient.

> *Sickly:* Believes that he or she has been sickly for a good part of his or her life.
>
> *Conversion or pseudoneurological symptoms:* Difficulty swallowing, loss of voice, deafness, double vision, blurred vision, blindness, fainting or loss of consciousness, memory loss, seizures or convulsions, trouble walking, paralysis or muscle weakness, urinary retention or difficulty urinating.
>
> *Gastrointestinal symptoms:* Abdominal pain, nausea, vomiting spells (other than during pregnancy), bloating (gassy), intolerance (e.g., gets sick) of a variety of food, diarrhea.
>
> *Female reproductive symptoms:* Judged by the individual as occurring more frequently or severely than in most women: painful menstruation, menstrual irregularity, excessive bleeding, severe vomiting throughout pregnancy, or causing hospitalization during pregnancy.
>
> *Psychosexual symptoms:* For the major part of the individual's life after opportunities for sexual activity: sexual indifference, lack of pleasure during intercourse, pain during intercourse.
>
> *Pain:* Pain in back, joints, extremities, genital area (other than during intercourse); pain on urination; other pain (other than headaches).
>
> *Cardiopulmonary symptoms:* Shortness of breath, palpitations, chest pain, dizziness.

American Psychiatric Association, Diagnostic and Statistical Manual of Mental Disorders, Third Edition. Washington, DC, American Psychiatric Association, 1980. Used with permission.

6. Most patients tend to show a preoccupation with themselves, their complaints, and the attitudes of others toward their complaints.
7. Most patients with somatization disorder tend to go to multiple physicians ostensibly seeking help but often wanting something active intervention (that is, medications, surgery, and so on). They become angry and go to other doctors when told that medication or surgery is not necessary. In the course of doctor shopping, they become manipulative and skillful in obtaining what they want.

Another feature seen in these patients with pain complaints is the discrepancy between pain and pain behaviors. When patients are seen in naturalistic situations, pain behavior is often markedly less than the described intensity of pain. However, when patients know they are being observed, there is a *marked but often poorly correlated exaggeration of pain behavior* in relation to the pain complaint.

Complications

Due to the varied presentation and nature of the illness, a significant proportion of these patients, especially the ones with pain, become addicted to narcotics and benzodiazepines. Furthermore, a number of these patients in the later stages of illness become depressed and anxious. The depression seen is usually intermittent and related to the familial and environmental situation. Usually the patients become disabled either from the illness itself or from the complications. Many of these patients, especially those with back pain, often end up with multiple operations which might, in themselves, lead or contribute to the persistence of pain and disability. On occasion surgery might lead to relief of a symptom but another symptom usually takes its place. Suicidal complaints and behavior may be seen. Sometimes the behavior is manipulative and at other times it might be secondary to depression.

Treatment

The most important aspect of treatment of this disorder is *early diagnosis*. Thus, a patient presenting with multiple, poorly defined, variable complaints, a history of doctor shopping, dramatic presentation of symptoms with exaggeration of pain behavior in the case of pain complaints, should arouse suspicion of somatization disorder. At this point the diagnostic evaluation should be clearly defined and the diagnostic tests should be ordered in a specific manner, with attention paid to the diagnosis of treatable medical/surgical disorder rather than to try desperately to identify an abnormality. When no abnormality exists, the patient should be told that the physician believes that the pain and or other complaint is *real* and that a conservative treatment approach is warranted.

It will be important to emphasize several issues at this point to the patient and the family, including: a) that unnecessary treatment will make matters worse; b) that going to several doctors will not be of benefit; instead, staying with one physician will be the best course; c) that conservative management avoiding potentially harmful and addictive medications and surgery is best. From this point, a caring attitude—a willingness to listen both to the patient's complaint and to the patient's perception of the way people react to the complaint—will gradually bring about a rapport enabling the patient to stick with a single physician. It is essential that the physician recognize the chronic and lifelong nature of the illness, for failure to do so often leads to aggressive treatment, the failure of which makes the physician and the patient mutually angry. Concomitantly, an apathetic and defeatist attitude should not be adopted, as this will be interpreted by the patient as reflecting a lack of caring on the part of the physician. Furthermore, when new complaints are presented, physicians should be alert to the possibility of physical illness and should evaluate these complaints appropriately rather than dismissing them or evaluating them too aggressively. No specific therapeutic approaches have been shown to be of any benefit in the treatment of this disorder. The prognosis is, in general, poor.

CONVERSION DISORDER (HYSTERICAL NEUROSIS–CONVERSION TYPE)

In conversion disorder, psychological conflicts lead to the simulation of physical disease and loss of function. The disturbance is not under voluntary control and not limited to pain complaints.

Before the introduction of DSM-III, patients with multiple aches and pains of uncertain etiology were classified under conversion disorder. In DSM-III, patients with such complaints are primarily classified under somatization disorder. However, certain categories of pain are assigned to conversion disorder. As in the case of somatization disorder, pain in conversion disorders can be chronic. However, few patients with chronic pain syndromes seen in pain clinics have conversion disorder.

Clinical Features

The DSM-III diagnostic criteria for conversion disorder are given in Table 8. One of the criteria states that the symptoms should not be limited to pain. When symptoms are limited to pain a diagnosis of psychogenic pain disorder is considered. In both somatization disorder

Table 8. DSM-III Diagnostic Criteria for Conversion Disorder

A. The predominant disturbance is a loss of or alteration in physical functioning suggesting a physical disorder.
B. Psychological factors are judged to be etiologically involved in the symptom, as evidenced by one of the following:
   1. there is a temporal relationship between an environmental stimulus that is apparently related to a psychological conflict or need and the initiation or exacerbation of the symptom.
   2. the symptom enables the individual to avoid some activity that is noxious to him or her.
   3. the symptom enables the individual to get support from the environment that otherwise might not be forthcoming.
C. It has been determined that the symptom is *not* under voluntary control.
D. The symptom cannot, after appropriate investigation, be explained by a known physical disorder or pathophysiological mechanism.
E. The symptom is not limited to pain or to a disturbance in sexual functioning.
F. Not due to Somatization Disorder or Schizophrenia.

American Psychiatric Association, Diagnostic and Statistical Manual of Mental Disorders, Third Edition. Washington, DC, American Psychiatric Association, 1980. Used with permission.

and conversion disorder, pain is only one of a number of features that define the specific diagnosis. Conversion disorder frequently begins in adolescence or early adulthood. The clinical course is variable. In some patients the symptoms may be transient, and in others it may be unremitting. Pain when present is often accompanied by other symptoms; for example, patients complaining of chest pain may also describe other symptoms, sweating, fatigue, shortness of breath, and so on. Pain and weakness may be symbolic in other patients. For example, a man may develop pain and paralysis of his right arm as a symbolic somatic manifestation of his psychic desire to harm his father. The pain when present is often described in vivid terms (for instance, a headache may be described as a spike or nail being driven through the head). Although in DSM-III a distinction between conversion disorder and psychogenic pain disorder is made, such a distinction may not be warranted, as often the symptoms are variable and may change.

The symptoms of conversion disorder may stimulate bodily disease and/or complicate symptoms of physical illness. Conversion symptoms can occur in patients with organic problems even after the organic pathology is healed. For example, pain persists after successful treatment of local disease process secondary to psychological factors. When pain is the sole or predominant complaint, it is classified as psychogenic pain disorder. When it occurs with other symptoms and is secondary to psychological factors, it is called conversion disorder. Conversion symptoms may be symbolic in nature, may result in gratification of dependency needs, and may be a reaction to environmental stress. Although conversion symptoms can occur in patients with somatization disorder, they are not the predominant or sole feature. A diagnosis of conversion disorder is strongly considered when there is a past or current history of conversion symptoms, history of sexual disturbances, and recent stressful life events. Although *la belle indifference* has been considered as a pathogenic feature, this feature is not usually present, and patients often show anxiety in accordance with their clinical presentation.

Treatment

The choice of treatment depends upon the clinical characteristics, personality characteristics, motivation, family structure and relationship, interpersonal relationships, level of ego development, marital relationship, and work history. Medications, electroconvulsive therapy (ECT), and psychosurgery are not usually effective. Psychoanalysis or insight oriented psychotherapy are considered the treatments of choice only for a small proportion of patients. The criteria for insight oriented psychotherapy include: 1) stable work, family, and interpersonal relationships; 2) motivation to change behavior; 3) capacity for introspection; 4) capacity to feel, understand, and express emotions; 5) well circumscribed symptoms; 6) well defined conflicts; 7) no evidence of history or signs of psychosis or schizophrenia; 8) no evidence of severe personality disorder; 9) capacity to step aside and examine conditions, feelings, and thoughts without the development of severe anxiety, depression, or psychosis; and 10) no evidence of pregenital conflicts.

Most of the patients who are not suitable candidates for individual insight oriented psychotherapy may benefit from supportive therapy that can be individual, group, or a combination of the two. The focus of the supportive psychotherapy should be directed toward reemphasizing positive capabilities still present in patient, aim to return the patient to the premorbid state, encourage independence, and reduce emphasis on disability caused by symptoms. Hypnosis and direct suggestion are not usually helpful.

PSYCHOGENIC PAIN DISORDER

In psychogenic pain disorder, pain is the prominent symptom. The pain is related to significant psychological factors. Table 9 gives DSM-III diagnostic criteria for psychogenic pain disorder.

Table 9. DSM-III Diagnostic Criteria for Psychogenic Pain Disorder

---

A. Severe and prolonged pain is the predominant disturbance.

B. The pain presented as a symptom is inconsistent with the anatomic distribution of the nervous system; after extensive evaluation, no organic pathology or pathophysiological mechanism can be found to account for the pain; or, when there is some related organic pathology, the complaint of pain is grossly in excess of what would be expected from the physical findings.

C. Psychological factors are judged to be etiologically involved in the pain, as evidenced by at least one of the following:
   (1) a temporal relationship between an environmental stimulus that is apparently related to a psychological conflict or need and the initiation or exacerbation of the pain
   (2) the pain's enabling the individual to avoid some activity that is noxious to him or her
   (3) the pain's enabling the individual to get support from the environment that otherwise might not be forthcoming

D. Not due to another mental disorder.

American Psychiatric Association, Diagnostic and Statistical Manual of Mental Disorders, Third Edition. Washington, DC, American Psychiatric Association, 1980. Used with permission.

Incidence

Psychogenic pain disorder is relatively infrequent in pain clinic settings. It constitutes only a small number of patients suffering from chronic pain syndrome. In our experience the incidence of psychogenic pain disorder is less than one percent.

Etiology

The psychological mechanisms that produce or lead to psychogenic pain disorder are examined in Section Two of this volume, "Basic Concepts." As noted in the diagnostic criteria for psychogenic pain disorder, psychological factors can initiate and exacerbate the pain in these patients, and the pain may be a method of secondary gain, either by enabling the patient to avoid activity or by enabling the patient to receive support from the environment.

Clinical Characteristics

Psychogenic pain disorder is more often seen in female than in male patients. It can occur at any age. In children it often appears in the form of abdominal pain. In adults it can be any type of pain, most often in the form of a headache. The pain may be localized in one site, may be at multiple sites, and may vary from one site to another. The pain is unrelated to clearly defined organic processes. The pain is inconsistent with anatomical distribution of the nervous system and to referred pain. Many of these patients have alexithymia. It is believed that in these patients emotionally stressful events are translated into somatic symptoms without the psychic characteristics that commonly occur.

Management

Psychotherapy may be useful in treating these patients. However, it must be noted that many of these patients are not psychologically minded, and insight oriented psychotherapy is often difficult.

HYPOCHONDRIASIS

The DSM-III criteria for hypochondriasis are given in Table 10. As indicated, the predominant disturbance is an unrealistic interpretation of physical signs or sensations as abnormal, leading to preoccupation with the fear or belief of having a serious disease. It is important to realize that: 1) hypochondriacal complaints can occur in other psychiatric disorders, such as depression or schizophrenia; and 2) hypochondriacal concerns can occur in many chronic pain patients, sometimes as normal illness behavior and at other times as abnormal illness behavior. Hypochondriasis per se is relatively rare among chronic pain patients. Treatment for hypochondriasis is very difficult and is rarely successful. Medications and ECT are not useful. Insight oriented psychotherapy is usually impossible, as these patients have great difficulty in examining and dealing with emotions. Long-term supportive psychotherapy may offer the best solution. Prognosis is poor.

Table 10. DSM-III Diagnostic Criteria for Hypochondriasis

A. The predominant disturbance is an unrealistic interpretation of physical signs or sensations as abnormal, leading to preoccupation with the fear or belief of having a serious disease.

B. Thorough physical evaluation does not support the diagnosis of any physical disorder that can account for the physical signs or sensations or for the individual's unrealistic interpretation of them.

C. The unrealistic fear or belief of having a disease persists despite medical reassurance and causes impairment in social or occupational functioning.

D. Not due to any other mental disorder such as Schizophrenia, Affective Disorder, or Somatization Disorder.

American Psychiatric Association, Diagnostic and Statistical Manual of Mental Disorders, Third Edition. Washington, DC, American Psychiatric Association, 1980. Used with permission.

MALINGERING

Malingering is voluntary and conscious falsification of symptoms and signs in order to obtain clearly recognizable gain that goes beyond a need to be in a patient or a sick role. The possible gains could be financial, could be an avoidance of unpleasant obligations, or could be the access to addictive drugs, singly or in combination. As pain is one of the symptoms that can never be clearly verified, chronic pain is often one of the presentations of malingerers. Thus, a patient may complain of severe neck pain or back pain following an accident (either an automobile or a work related accident, for example). The pain might have been initially present but in order to obtain compensation and/or disability, the patient complains of pain, and pain related behaviors are continued even after the pain disappears. On occasion, the accident may be faked, the symptoms invented, or both. Sometimes pain might be used as a method of obtaining opioid drugs. Depending on the sophistication of the patient, it is often difficult to evaluate whether or not the symptom is due to malingering.

In addition, issues of secondary gain (including compensation) can affect the symptoms both in a conscious and unconscious fashion. Distinguishing the voluntary conscious element from the unconscious element is often very difficult. Thus, distinction between malingering and somatization disorder, conversion disorder, or psychogenic pain disorder may be difficult. However, unlike patients with conversion disorder, somatization disorder, or psychogenic pain disorder, these patients may tamper medical records, avoid treatment that is potentially risky—that is, they usually do not undergo surgery—and have clearly identifiable gains (financial, social, or the ability to obtain narcotic drugs). Many of these patients may also have a concomitant diagnosis of antisocial personality disorder. Furthermore, on obtaining a past history, a history of falsification of illness may be obtained. Malingerers usually stop their symptom production when it is no longer profitable, when the stakes get too high, or when there is risk or danger to themselves. Another condition that has to be distinguished from malingering is Munchausen syndrome. In Munchausen syndrome, no gain is clearly evident. Malingering is usually seen in association with low self-esteem and antisocial personality traits. An important and diagnostic characteristic is that the illness dramatically clears after the goal is reached. Sometimes, in the case of narcotic addicts, the purpose is self-perpetuating.

Treatment

Diagnosis and understanding that there is no effective treatment for malingering is essential. In understanding the reason for the falsification, countertransference and other issues have to be kept in mind. A high index of suspicion should be aroused when several of the characteristics of malingering are noted: 1) multiple vague complaints; 2) tampering with records; 3) poor corroboration of the patient's history; 4) clearly defined financial gain; 5) suspicion of narcotic addiction; 6) apparent avoidance of legal and social responsibility; 7) noncooperation in diagnostic evaluation; and 8) avoidance of painful treatment and/or diagnostic intervention.

It is important to keep several principles in mind while managing these patients:

1. Physicians and psychiatrists should be aware of the reason for the potential malingering (they will have to keep in mind that the behavior may not be malingering but may be unconscious).
2. Physicians should not get into a struggle to prove that the patient is malingering or fooling (furthermore, it may be difficult to prove conscious, willful falsification).
3. If antisocial personality disorder is diagnosed, treatment response and prognosis are poor, and psychiatric treatment should not be undertaken.
4. If there is a concomitant psychiatric disorder such as schizophrenia or affective disorder, it should be treated.
5. When a clear suspicion of opioid addiction exists, the physician should not fall into the trap of prescribing opioids.
6. On recognizing the existence of a clearly defined gain and lack of evidence for a physical or psychiatric disorder, the physician should not fall into the trap of nonspecific treatment.
7. Physicians should be constantly aware of countertransference issues.

PERSONALITY DISORDERS IN CHRONIC PAIN

Reich and colleagues (71), in their study of chronic pain patients, found that 47 percent of patients with chronic pain satisfied DSM-III criteria for a personality disorder. Fourteen percent had histrionic personality disorder, 12 percent dependent personality disorder, 7 percent borderline personality disorder, 5 percent schizotypal personality disorder, 5 percent mixed personality disorder, 2 percent schizoid personality disorder, and 2 percent narcissistic personality disorder. We are unaware of any other systematic study of personality disorders in chronic pain patients. Blazer (74) has reported that narcissistic personality traits are common among chronic pain patients. Others have reported an association between pelvic pain and borderline personality (75). In our clinical experience, personality disorders are not very common, but personality traits of various types are clearly seen in many chronic pain patients. Early studies of chronic pain patients assessed some dimensions of personality but did not examine the incidence and nature of personality disorders in chronic pain patients. Further study of this question is sorely needed.

When DSM-III is used to classify psychiatric diagnosis in chronic pain patients, a variety of diagnoses for one or all patients may be appropriately selected. As noted in this and other chapters of this book, chronic pain patients often have subjective symptoms and complaints that can either arise from the associated psychological distress they experience and/or a pathophysiological illness. If the clinician uses the DSM-III classification and does not fully appreciate the various etiological causes for these subjective complaints in chronic pain patients, then a disproportionate number of psychiatric diagnoses will occur in these patients. For example, the description of the psychogenic pain disorder can apply to many patients with chronic pain but it does not accurately define the multiple other causes and interactions leading to the chronic pain syndrome. Furthermore, the psychogenic pain disorder found in DSM-III is changed to somatoform pain disorder in DSM-III-R (76). As stated in the revision of DSM-III, somatoform pain disorder is present when the predominant disturbance is at least six months of preoccupation with pain and one of two of the following: 1) after extensive evaluation, no organic process accounts for the pain; and 2) when there is related organic pathology, the complaint of pain is in excess of the organic findings. Using these new guidelines, all patients with postherpetic neuralgia, for example, would be classified as having somatoform pain disorder since their pain complaints are usually chronic (> 6 months) and there are few physical changes to explain the severity of their pain complaints and the resulting disability. It should be noted that the DSM-III may be readily applied in classifying psychiatric disorders in chronic pain patients, but if the clinician fails to account for the other etiological causes for chronic pain and the clinical manifestation of chronic pain syndromes, then inappropriate diagnosis and treatment will occur.

In this chapter we have reviewed the occurrence and characteristics of pain complaints in various psychiatric disorders. Although pain complaints are frequently seen in various psychiatric disorders, chronic pain (that is, pain lasting more than six months) is only rarely seen. It is apparent from this review that there is a considerable dearth of information regarding pain in psychiatric disorders, pointing out the need for systematic studies aimed at exploring this question. Such studies, in addition to filling the gap in information, could also lead to a greater understanding of the nature of pain.

REFERENCES

1. American Psychiatric Association: Diagnostic and Statistical Manual of Mental Disorders, Third Edition, Washington, DC, American Psychiatric Association, 1980

2. Devine R, Merskey H: The description of pain in psychiatric and general medical patients. J Psychosom Res 9:311–316, 1965
3. Merskey H, Boyd D: Emotional adjustment and chronic pain. Pain 5:173–178, 1978
4. Paul L: Psychosomatic aspects of low back pain. Psychosomatics 12:116–124, 1950
5. Spear FG: Pain in psychiatric patients. J Psychosom Res 11:187–193, 1967
6. Bond MR: Pain: Its Nature, Analgesics, and Treatment. New York, Churchill Livingstone, 1984
7. Merskey H, Spear FG: Pain, psychological and psychiatric aspects. London, Bailliere, Tindall and Cassel, 1967
8. Merskey H: The characteristics of persistent pain in psychological illness. J Psychosom Res 9:191–198, 1965
9. Devine R, Merskey H: The description of pain in psychiatric and general medical patients. J Psychosom Res 9:311–316, 1965
10. Woodforde JM, Merskey H: Some relationships between subjective measures of pain. J Psychosom Res 16:173–178, 1972
11. Walters A: Psychogenic regional pain alias hysterical pain. Brain 84:1–18, 1961
12. Agnew DC, Merskey H: Words of chronic pain. Pain 2:73–81, 1976
13. Adler R: The differentiation of organic and psychogenic pain. Pain 10:249–252, 1981
14. Merskey H: Psychiatric patients with persistent pain. J Psychosom Res 9:299–309, 1965
15. France RD, Urban BJ, Keefe FJ: Long-term use of narcotic analgesics in chronic pain. Soc Sci Med 19:1379–1382, 1984
16. von Knorring L, Perris C, Eisemann M, et al: Pain as a symptom in depressive disorders, I: relationship to diagnostic subgroup and depressive symptomatology. Pain 15:19–26, 1983
17. von Knorring L: The experience of pain in depressed patients. Neuropsychobiology 1:155–165, 1975
18. von Knorring L, Perris C, Eisemann M, et al: Pain as a symptom in depressive disorders, II: relationship to personality traits as assessed by means of KSP. Pain 17:377–384, 1983
19. Gallemore JL, Wilson WP: The complaint of pain in the clinical setting of affective disorders. South Med J 62:551–555, 1969
20. Diamond S: Depressive headaches. Headache 4:255–258, 1964
21. Delaplaine R, Ifabumuyi OI, Merskey H, et al: Significance of pain in psychiatric hospital patients. Pain 4:361–366, 1978
22. Mathew R, Weinman M, Misales M: Physical symptoms of depression. Br J Psychiatry 139:293–296, 1981
23. Lindsey PG, Wyckoff M: The depression-pain syndrome and its response to antidepressants. Psychosomatics 22:571–577, 1981
24. Cassidy WL, Flanagan NB, Spellman M, et al: Clinical observation in manic-depressive disease. JAMA 164:1535–1546, 1957
25. Perris C: A study of bipolar (manic-depressive) and unipolar recurrent depressive psychoses. Acta Psychiatr Scand (Suppl) 42:194, 1966
26. Lesse S: Masked depression: diagnostic and therapeutic problems. Diseases of the Nervous System 29:169–173, 1968

27. McCreary C, Turner J, Dawson E: Differences between functional versus organic low back pain patients. Pain 4:73–78, 1977
28. Marback JH, Lund P: Depression, anhedonia, anxiety in temporomandibular joint and other pain syndromes. Pain 11:73–84, 1981
29. Kremer E, Atkinson J: Pain measurement: construct validity of the affective dimension of the McGill Pain Questionnaire with chronic benign pain patients. Pain 11:93–100, 1981
30. Hanvik LJ: MMPI profiles in patients with low back pain. Journal of Consulting Psychol 15:350–353, 1951
31. Freeman C, Colsyn D, Louks J: The use of MMPI with low back pain patients. J Clin Psychol 32:294–298, 1976
32. Lascelles RG: Atypical facial pain and depression. Br J Psychiatry 112:651–659, 1966
33. Bradley JJ: Severe localized pain associated with the depressive syndrome. Br J Psychiatry 109:741–745, 1963
34. Breuer J, Freud S: Studies on hysteria (1895), in Complete Psychological Works, Standard Edition, vol. 2. Translated and edited by Strachey J. London, Hogarth Press, 1955
35. Tinling DC, Klein RF: Psychogenic pain and aggression: the syndrome of the solitary hunter. Psychosom Med 28:738–748, 1966
36. Engel GL: Primary atypical facial neuralgia: a hysterical conversion symptom. Psychosom Med 13:375, 1951
37. Szasz TS: Pain and Pleasure: A Study of Bodily Feeling. New York, Basic Books, 1957
38. Engel GL: 'Psychogenic' pain and the pain-prone patient. Am J Med 26:899–918, 1959
39. Merskey H: The effects of chronic pain upon the response to noxious stimuli by psychiatric patients. J Psychiatr Res 8:405–419, 1965
40. Weiss E: Psychogenic rheumatism. Ann Intern Med 26:890–900, 1947
41. Eisenbud J: The psychology of headache. Psychiatr Q 2:592–619, 1937
42. Rangell L: Psychiatric aspects of pain. Psychosom Med 15:22–37, 1953
43. Hemphill RE, Hall KRL, Crookes TG: A preliminary report on fatigue and pain tolerance in depressive and psychoneurotic patients. Journal of Mental Science 98:433–440, 1952
44. Hall KRL, Stride E: The varying response to pain in psychiatric disorders: a study in abnormal psychology. Br J Med Psychol 27:48–60, 1954
45. Davis GC, Buchsbaum MS, Bunney WE: Analgesia to painful stimuli in affective illness. Am J Psychiatry 136:1148–1151, 1979
46. Ben-Tovin DI, Schwartz MS: Hypoalgesia in depressive illness. Br J Psychiatry 138:37–39, 1981
47. von Knorring L: The Experience of Pain in Patients with Depressive Disorders: Clinical and Experimental Study. Umea Sweden, Umea University Medical Dissertations, 1975
48. Lopez-Ibor JJ: Masked depression. Br J Psychiatry 120:245–258, 1972
49. Forrest AJ, Wolkind SN: Masked depression in men with low back pain. Rheumatology Rehabilitation 13:148–153, 1974
50. Lesse S: Masked Depression. New York, Jason Aronson, 1974
51. Sternbach RA, Murphy RW, Akeson WH, et al: Chronic low back pain, "the low-back loser." Postgrad Med 53:135–138, 1973

52. Engel GL: Studies of ulcerative colitis, IV: the significance of headaches. Psychosom Med 13:375, 1951
53. Davis GC, Buchsbaum MS, Bunney WE: Pain and psychiatric illness, in Pain, Discomfort, and Humanitarian Care. Edited by Ng LKY, Bonica JJ. New York, Elsevier North Holland, 1980
54. Marchand WE, Shrota B, Marble HC: Occurrence of painless acute surgical disorder in psychotic patients. N Engl J Med 260:580–585, 1959
55. Geschwind N: Insensitivity to pain in psychotic patients. N Engl J Med 296:1480, 1977
56. Fishbain DA: Pain insensitivity in psychosis. Ann Emerg Med 11:630–632, 1982
57. Torrey EF: Headaches after lumbar puncture and insensitivity to pain in psychiatric patients. N Engl J Med 301:110, 1979
58. Malmo RB, Shagass C: Physiologic studies of reaction to stress in anxiety and early schizophrenia. Psychosom Med 11:9, 1949
59. Sappington J: Thresholds of shock-induced discomfort in process and reactive schizophrenics. Percept Mot Skills 37:489, 1973
60. Malmo RB, Shagass C, Smith AA: Responsiveness in chronic schizophrenia. J Pers 19:359–375, 1951
61. Earle A, Earle BV: The blood pressure response to pain and emotion in schizophrenia. J Nerv Ment Dis 121:132–139, 1955
62. Bender L, Schilder P: Unconditioned and conditioned reactions to pain in schizophrenia. Am J Psychiatry 10:365–384, 1930
63. Stengel E, Oldham AJ, Ehrenberg ASC: Reactions to pain in various abnormal states. Journal of Mental Science 101:52–69, 1955
64. Davis GC, Buchsbaum MS, von Kammen DP, et al: Analgesia to pain stimuli in schizophrenia and its reversal by naltrexone. Psychiatry Res 1:61–69, 1979
65. Jetter WW, White PD: Rupture of heart in patients in mental institutions. Ann Intern Med 21:783–802, 1944
66. Hackett TP: The pain patient: evaluation and treatment, in MGH Handbook of General Hospital Psychiatry. Edited by Hackett TP, Cassem NH. Saint Louis, C.V. Mosby, 1978
67. Marchand WE: Occurrence of painless myocardial infarction in psychotic patients. N Engl J Med 253:51–55, 1955
68. Chapman K: The early symptoms of schizophrenia. Br J Psychiatry 112:225–251, 1966
69. Watson GD, Chandarana PC, Merskey H: Relationship between pain and schizophrenia. Br J Psychiatry 138:33–36, 1981
70. Compton-Smith RN: Psychological factors in pain. Br Med J 2:535, 1965
71. Reich J, Tupin JP, Abramovitz SI: DSM-III diagnosis of chronic pain patients. Am J Psychiatry 140:1495–1498, 1983
72. Benson RC, Hansen KH, Matarazzo JD: Atypical pelvic pain in women: gynaecologic-psychiatric consideration. Am J Obstet Gynecol 77:806–825, 1959
73. Gidro L, Gorden T, Taylor HC: Pelvic pain and female identity: a survey of emotional factors in 40 patients. Am J Obstet Gynecol 79:1184–1202, 1960
74. Blazer DG: Narcissism and the development of chronic pain. Int J Psychiatry Med 10:69–79, 1980

75. Gross RJ, Doerr H, Goldiorla D, et al: Borderline syndrome and incest in chronic pelvic pain patients. Int J Psychiatry Med 10:79–96, 1981
76. American Psychiatric Association: Diagnostic and Statistical Manual of Mental Disorders, Third Edition, Revised.Washington, DC, American Psychiatric Association, 1987

Chapter 10

Chronic Pain Syndromes of Idiopathic and Organic Origin

K. Ranga Rama Krishnan, M.D.

Randal D. France, M.D.

In this chapter, we will focus on chronic pain syndromes of both organic (Figure 1) and idiopathic (Figure 2) origin; that is, headache, cervical and low back pain, pelvic pain, atypical facial pain, abdominal pain, arthritis, cancer, neuropathies, postherpetic neuralgia, trigeminal neuralgia, phantom limb pain, myofascial pain syndrome, causalgia, and central pain syndromes. Specific management and assessment of some of these conditions are briefly described. For a more complete discussion of the general methods of assessment and management of chronic pain syndromes, please see the sections on Assessment and Management, respectively.

HEADACHE

Headache is not a condition that is commonly seen by psychiatrists. When a psychiatrist is asked to evaluate a patient with headache, it is often as a last resort. The psychiatrist evaluates patients in cases where the headache is chronic and often resistant to standard methods of treatment.

CLASSIFICATION OF HEADACHE

There are several methods of classifying a headache. It is important to have a simple classification, one which is both heuristic and practical, such as that shown in Table 1. The classification is not exhaustive.

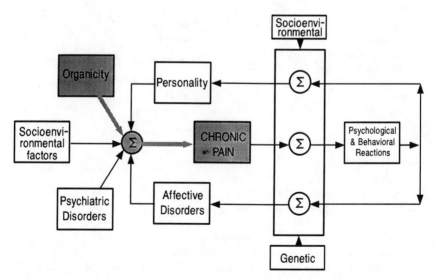

Figure 1. Systems model for chronic pain: chronic pain of organic etiology

143

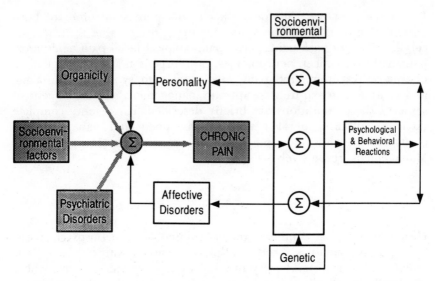

Figure 2. Systems model for chronic pain: chronic pain of idiopathic etiology

Table 1. Classification of Headache

Vascular

    Migraine
      classic
      common
      hemiplegic
      ophthalmoplegic

    Cluster
      episodic
      chronic

    Toxic
      pyrexia
      drugs

    Hypertension

    Psychiatric disorders
      anxiety
      depression

    Posttraumatic

Musculoskeletal

    Temporomandibular joint syndrome
    Cervical spondylosis/arthritis
    Psychogenic: depression and anxiety

Headache Secondary to Specific Causes

    Intracranial: trauma, edema, hemorrhage, etc.
    Extracranial: disease of eye, ear, nose, throat; inflammation of cranial
      arteries, etc.

Headache is classified into three major groups: vascular, musculoskeletal, and headache secondary to specific causes. Vascular headache includes migraine, cluster headache, headache secondary to toxic factors in which the headache is evoked by vascular dilation, and hypertensive headache. The most common cause of headache is the tension headache, which is a form of musculoskeletal headache. This is the type of headache commonly seen secondary to anxiety disorders, depression, and other psychiatric disorders. The other causes of musculoskeletal headache include cervical osteoarthritis, myositis, temporomandibular joint syndrome, and, occasionally, trauma.

Vascular Headache

Migraine

Migraine can be defined as a recurrent disorder of the cranial vasculature in which the headache is usually bilateral, periodic, and is often associated with irritability, nausea, photophobia, vomiting, constipation, and diarrhea (1, 2). The attacks are often preceded by aura such as hemianopia, speech disorders, and unilateral, or occasionally bilateral, sensory disturbance. On occasion, in some patients, there may be transient neurological defects such as difficulty speaking, dysarthria, dysphagia, vertigo, hemiparesis, hemianesthesia, memory problems, impairment of consciousness, confusion, and so on. Migraine can be precipitated by medications, chemical substances such as reserpine, monosodium glutamate, exertion, and psychological factors such as anxiety and depression. Migraine can be classified into classic, common, hemiplegic, and ophthalmoplegic types. In classic migraine, preheadache experiences usually occur. In common migraine such experiences are not readily evident.

Management. *Treatment of the acute attack:* The drug of choice is ergotamine tartrate. It can be given orally, sublingually, subcutaneously, or rectally. Oral preparations commonly used are Migral or Cafergot. The other drugs that are used include dihydroergotamine mesylate, which is administered subcutaneously (3).

Prophylaxis: Prophylactic management includes identification of trigger factors and/or avoidance where possible. This might include dietary restrictions if dietary factors are found to precipitate migraine attacks. Similarly, if some medications are found to increase the periodicity of migraine attacks, then these medications should be discontinued. Among the drugs that are commonly used in the prophylaxis of migraine include propranolol and other beta blockers. Tricyclic antidepressants and other nontricyclic antidepressants have been used in some patients with migraine, both in patients with and without depression (4).

Serotonin antagonists such as cypropheptadine or methysergide are also used for prophylactic purposes (5). Biofeedback, on occasion, may be useful (6).

Cluster Headache

Cluster headaches are also known as migrainous neuralgia (7). In this condition the pain usually occurs in attacks of high intensity localized to the orbital, facial, and temporal regions. On occasion it may extend into the cervical and into the shoulder region. This condition is usually seen in middle-aged people. Each attack usually affects the same site. Unlike migraine, males are more commonly affected than females.

Management. The treatment of cluster headaches is symptomatic. The drugs used include ergot alkaloids. Other drugs include salicylates. As there are usually no prodromal symptoms, the ergot preparations used are better given subcutaneously. Prophylactic therapy is also similar to that for migraine. Ergot alkaloids can be used for short-term prophylaxis.

Other Causes of Vascular Headache

Hypertension. Hypertension, especially when malignant, can cause severe headaches that are often throbbing in nature. Moderate hypertension can aggravate migraine but it is unlikely to produce severe headache of its own.

Toxic vascular causes. Among the toxic causes of headaches, alcohol, vasodilator drugs such as nitrites, and caffeine are important. Other conditions include fever and disturbances of fluid and electrolyte balance.

MUSCULOSKELETAL HEADACHE

The most common causes of musculoskeletal headaches are psychiatric disorders. Thus, musculoskeletal headaches, much more commonly known as tension headaches, are often a symptom of depression and anxiety. Musculoskeletal headache is steady, nonpulsatile, and is often characterized as a feeling of tightness or a band-like sensation about the head. It is usually seen around the forehead and temporal regions and occasionally in the back of the head and neck regions. It is commonly bilateral and on occasion it may be unilateral. The duration can vary from a few minutes to hours, days, and, on occasion, years. In the chronic types of tension headaches, tender areas may be found over the muscles involved.

Other causes of musculoskeletal headache include temporomandibular syndrome, cervical spondylosis, and myositis.

Management.   Management depends upon the condition causing the tension headache. Where the headache is chronic, is not alleviated by nonspecific analgesic treatment, and there is no evidence of cervical spondylosis, myositis, or temporomandibular joint syndrome, the headache may be a manifestation of depression and/or anxiety. Psychiatric assessment is clearly indicated for these types of patients. Appropriate treatment, including the use of tricyclic antidepressants, is often needed. Benzodiazepines such as alprazolam may be useful on occasion. Biofeedback and relaxation training may also be useful.

HEADACHE SECONDARY TO SPECIFIC CAUSES

In the assessment of headache, especially when it is persistent, evaluation for organic etiology is of primary importance. The headache may be a symptom of an underlying intracranial pathology and a careful neurological exam for the presence of intracranial pathology should be done. Sometimes computerized tomograms, EEG, and other laboratory techniques are useful. Occasionally, the headache may be a symptom of diseases of other cranial structures such as the eye, ear, nose, throat, teeth, and so on. Evaluation of these sites should also be done. One of the other conditions associated with severe headache is cranial arteritis.

Giant Cell Arteritis.   In this condition the temporal artery is commonly affected. The first symptom is usually a severe headache, throbbing in character, localized to that vessel. The scalp adjacent to the vessel is usually tender. There is usually reddening over the affected arteries. In later stages of the illness the arteries do not pulsate. The dangerous complications of this condition include occlusion of the retina and, on occasion, cerebral arteritis. Laboratory examination usually reveals an elevated sedimentation rate.

Treatment.   Corticosteroids are the drugs of choice. Prednisolone is usually used. Treatment response is usually dramatic. Maintenance steroid treatment is often required.

SUMMARY

Headache may not only be a symptom of other conditions, it may also be the sole condition. Chronic headache is often a manifestation of underlying psychiatric disorders and/or psychological difficulties. Careful evaluation of patients, paying particular attention to a detailed history, physical examination, neurological evaluation, and, where necessary, use of ancillary aids such as a computerized tomographic (CT) scan and electroencephalogram (EEG) are necessary to arrive at the correct diagnosis. Treatment of chronic headache without attempts to arrive at a diagnosis may lead to drug abuse problems in these patients. Narcotic drugs should be used with extreme caution. Psychiatrists, when asked to evaluate patients with chronic headaches, should not assume that organic factors have been ruled out and should evaluate the patient carefully.

TRIGEMINAL NEURALGIA

Trigeminal neuralgia is a syndrome of rapid onset characterized by brief, severe, paroxysmal episodes of acute pain occurring in the area of distribution of the trigeminal nerve (8). Synonyms for this syndrome are tic douloureux, dolor facei Fothergillii, facii morbus nervorum Crucians, LaGrande neuralgie, and epileptiform neuralgia (9).

ETIOLOGY

Most cases of trigeminal neuralgia are believed to be idiopathic in origin. In a few cases, clearly identifiable causes of the pain may be found, such as: vascular anomaly (aneurism, meningioama of the base of the skull); tumor of the fifth and eighth nerves; metastases of the base of the skull; and multiple sclerosis.

CLINICAL FEATURES

Women are affected slightly more often than men (10). Trigeminal neuralgia can occur at any age, but is most commonly seen between the ages of 50 and 70 (10).

Characteristics of Pain

Onset, while usually rapid and often reaches maximum intensity in minutes, is brief in duration and rarely lasts longer than a few minutes. The pain is usually very severe and is described as sharp or stabbing. The pain is usually unilateral; in rare cases, however, it may be bilateral. Trigger areas are quite common and, when present, they clinch the diagnosis. The trigger areas do not necessarily bear a relation to the area of pain (11). Some of the common trigger areas include the lower lip, upper lip, eyebrow, scalp, and the nasal region (12). The pain can often be triggered by the slightest contact and even a sudden draft of air. Another important characteristic of trigeminal neuralgia is that most patients will be absolutely pain free between the paroxysmal episodes of pain. Only a few patients will describe a dull ache between episodes.

The maxillary and mandibular divisions of the trigeminal nerve are affected about equally. The ophthalmic division is affected in less than two to five percent of patients (9). Radiation of the pain into an adjacent division is uncommon. When it occurs it is often an overflow phenomenon.

Remission

Sometimes spontaneous remission of the paroxysmal episode, which has never been clearly related to any physical or psychological factors, is seen. Sometimes several years can elapse between episodes. When the episodes recur they usually recur in the same area.

Other Characteristics

Usually no sensory loss is evident. Autonomic phenomena and local tenderness are rare. The manner in which the patient describes the pain is pathognomonic. The patient, especially after a recent episode, will hold the affected side of the face relatively immobile and will point to the involved area without touching it. He will also usually prevent the examiner from touching it.

Idiopathic trigeminal neuralgia is difficult to differentiate from trigeminal neuralgia secondary to other diseases. However, in the later stages it may be possible to differentiate. Some patients with trigeminal neuralgia secondary to other conditions usually show some degree of neurological deficit, especially sensory loss. They rarely have pain-free intervals between episodes. Occasionally, they may show involvement of other cranial nerves.

MANAGEMENT

Carbamazepine (Tegretol) is the drug of choice for the treatment of trigeminal neuralgia. Approximately 60 to 70 percent of patients will have complete pain relief. The mechanism of action of carbamazepine in the relief of pain is unclear (12).

Other drugs that have been reported to be of benefit in the management of these patients include diphenylhydantoin, baclofen, and sodium valproate (13–15). Psychotropic drugs are generally not useful.

Surgery is tried only after medical treatment fails or when there is a clear, identifiable surgical indication. A description of the surgical approaches are beyond the scope of this book. The interested reader should refer to references 16–18.

ATYPICAL FACIAL PAIN

Atypical facial pain is a term used to describe many conditions (19). Some of these conditions may be properly included in this chapter, others under pain in psychiatric disorders. The term was first used by Frazier (20). Atypical facial pain refers, in general, to pain in the facial region other than secondary to trigeminal neuralgia. Some of the differences between atypical facial pain and trigeminal neuralgia are given in Table 2. Since Frazier first used this term it has been used in a number of ways, often with the entities described having little relation to one another. Several classifications of atypical facial neuralgia have been proposed but are, in general, unsatisfactory (21). A simple classification of the conditions that can lead to atypical facial pain is given in Table 3.

A discussion of the organic causes of atypical facial pain is beyond the scope of this book. A brief description of a) psychological factors in development of atypical facial pain; b) atypical facial pain as a conversion symptom; and c) atypical facial pain as a form of masked depression follows.

PSYCHOLOGICAL FACTORS IN THE DEVELOPMENT OF IDIOPATHIC ATYPICAL FACIAL PAIN

At the current time very little is known about the development of atypical facial pain. Glaser suggested that atypical facial pain could occur as part of a psychoneuroses (21). Moulton suggested that the etiology of atypical facial pain is multifactorial (22). She suggested that personality factors may be involved. Weddington and Blazer (23) noted that many of their patients had psychiatric problems, although they were uncertain as to whether the psychiatric problems preceded the onset of atypical facial pain (23). It has been suggested that, as in the case of other chronic pain syndromes of idiopathic origin, personality factors may play a role. However, the nature and influence of personality has not been elucidated.

ATYPICAL FACIAL PAIN AS A CONVERSION SYMPTOM

Engel (24), in a study of atypical facial neuralgia, has emphasized the "masochistic" character structure seen in many of these patients. He describes the character disorder in these patients as marked by "many varieties of self-punitive behavior" (24). Engel conceptualized the occurrence of pain in these patients as a form of guilt displacement. In many of his patients, pain was a conversion symptom. Facial pain was a conversion symptom either by itself or, more commonly, as part of multiple somatic "conversion" symptoms. Weddington and Blazer (23) found that

Table 2. Differences Between Trigeminal Neuralgia and Atypical Facial Pain

Course Pain Free Intervals	Episodic present	Constant absent
Character	stabbing, sharp	aching, burning
Laterality	unilateral	can be either unilateral or bilateral
Trigger zones	present	absent
Sensory changes	none	may be present

Table 3. Causes of Atypical Facial Pain

Organic

  Dental—impacted teeth
          peridontal abscess
          unerupted teeth

  Mandibular/Maxillary—infection
                      acromegaly
                      tumors

  Sinus—mastoiditis
        sinusitis
        tumors

  Other soft tissues of the face—facial abscess
  Ocular
  Atypical neuralgia—glossopharyngeal
                    sphenopalatine ganglion neuralgia
                    geniculate ganglion neuralgia

  Vascular—temporal arteritis
          migrainous neuralgia

  Arthritis—temporomandibular joint

  Referred Pain—cardiovascular disease (angina)

Psychological

  Depression ("masked depression")
  Conversion disorder
  Somatization disorder
  Hypochondriasis
  Psychoses

Idiopathic

  Temporomandibular joint syndrome
  "Idiopathic" atypical facial pain

pain was a conversion symptom in only 17 percent of their patients. The difference in methodology and conceptualization probably accounts for this discrepancy.

ATYPICAL FACIAL PAIN AS A MASKED DEPRESSION

Lascelles (25, 26), in two interesting studies of atypical facial pain, reported that many of these patients had features similar to those found in atypical depression. Some of these features are listed in Table 4, which also lists the features of depression rarely seen in atypical facial pain. These features are similar to those described by West and Dally (27) as the characteristics of atypical depression. Hysterical traits were uncommon, as was a family history of depression.

Treatment with phenelzine was found to be effective in both controlled and uncontrolled studies.

COMMON PAIN STATES OF THE TRUNK

This section will describe common conditions giving rise to chronic pain states of the trunk. Correct diagnosis between chest or abdominal pain from referred pain of visceral organs and that of the chest or abdominal walls is often difficult. Chronic pain of the chest will be discussed initially, followed by chronic abdominal pain. For a more detailed discussion on the causes for chest and abdominal pain, one should refer to a standard text on medicine or surgery.

CHRONIC CHEST PAIN

One of the most common causes of chronic chest pain is angina pectoris. While the pain is typically brief, it can recur intermittently over the course of years (see Table 5). The pain is described as constricting, dull,

Table 4. Common Features of Depression in Atypical Facial Pain

Common	Rare
Sleep disturbance	Guilt, self reproach
Irritability	Suicidial ideation/gestures
Tenseness	Loss of libido
Fatigue	Weight loss
Crying spells	Psychomotor retardation

and as a heavy feeling in the chest with possible radiation to the arms, back, or neck. Duration of pain is several minutes and is usually relieved by rest or nitroglycerine. Pain typically is precipitated by exertion or stress. Electrocardiographic changes such as ST segment depression may occur. When the angina is brought on by minimal stress or exertion, the patient reacts by limiting lifestyle and activity.

Pericarditis may produce a sharp severe pain in a similar distribution as angina pectoris. The associated symptoms depend on the underlying cause of pericarditis, which can include infection, collagen vascular disease, drugs postmyocardial injury, and cancer.

Aneurysm of the aorta may produce a deep diffused central chest pain with radiation to the midscapular region. If there is dissection of the aneurysm, the pain is sudden and severe. Pain from the diaphragm may be present in the shoulders or midthoracic area. The pain is deep and poorly localized. The most significant causes for pain in the diaphragm are cancer and infection.

Compression fracture of a thoracic vertebrae can produce both thoracic pain and dermatomal pain. The fracture can lead to nerve root compression. A hypermobile rib cartilage can produce irritation of an intercostal nerve, causing the slipping rib syndrome. Pain is located at the costal margin and may be mistaken for visceral pain. Pain may be intermittent or constant and is reproduced with manipulation of the hypermobile rib.

Following mastectomy, phantom sensation of the amputated breast may be present and in some cases the sensations are painful. After extensive breast surgery with trauma to the intercostal or brachial nerves, paresthesia or burning pain may be reported in the axilla or upper chest and arm. This type of pain usually subsides with time. Chronic postmastectomy pain without any associated findings may occur.

Table 5. Causes of Chronic Chest Pain

Visceral origin	Referred pain from abdomen
angina pectoris	subphrenic abscess
pericarditis	esophageal dysmotility
aneurysm of the aorta	gastric and duodenal ulcer
esophagitis	cholelithiasis
diaphragm	
	Psychological origin
Chest wall	depression
postherpetic neuralgia	anxiety
compression fracture of thoracic vertebrae	conversion
slipping rib syndrome	
postmastectomy	
postthoracotomy	

The patient may describe the inability to wear a prosthesis or clothing, or the inability to tolerate touch. Psychological distress and impairment of sexual activities are present. Etiology is unknown. Recurrent cancer may produce pain one to three years following a mastectomy. Local metastasis may produce secondary physical changes to adjacent tissue.

Pain may develop in the chest wall following thoracotomy. The pain is described as aching or burning in nature. Any movement of the chest will increase the pain. Sensory loss and tenderness occur along the surgical scar. The pain may be caused by traumatic neuromatosis or local metastasis if the thoracotomy was performed for tumor resection. A deafferentation syndrome may occur following a thoracotomy. The pain is severe and a demonstrable sensory loss is present. The pain can be either intermittent or constant, and may be hyperpathic.

Subphrenic abscess produces referred pain to the shoulder. Esophageal dysmobility causes midline chest pain, often behind the sternum. Esophagitis produces a similar pain, but certain foods aggravate the pain.

Chest pain may also be caused by depression or anxiety. The conditions produce muscle tension leading to chest wall pain. Not infrequently, chest pain may be conversional, especially anginas. For a discussion on the psychiatric aspects of pain, see Chapter 9.

CHRONIC ABDOMINAL PAIN

The causes of chronic abdominal pain include gastric ulcer, gastric cancer, hiatal hernia, pancreatitis, carcinoma of the pancreas, and irritable bowel syndrome. These causes are listed in Table 6. A brief discussion of peptic ulcer and intractable bowel syndrome with special relevance to pain is presented below.

Peptic Ulcer

The term "peptic ulcer" describes an erosion of the gastric or duodenal mucosa that penetrates through the musculans. Peptic ulcers are, in general, believed to result from excessive vagal drive or excessive activity of gastrin-producing cells, or from defective mucous protection of the lining epithelium.

Chronic abdominal pain in peptic ulcer patients is fairly common. Patients with gastric ulcer generally complain of upper abdominal pain covering a fairly wide area. The pain starts soon after eating, is periodic, and is relieved by antacids. Patients with duodenal ulcer, however, have sharply localized pain in the epigastric region. The pain occurs in the fasting states and is often relieved by food. It is usually periodic at first but, when left untreated, may become chronic. Unlike gastric ulcer, which, by itself, has few associated symptoms, duodenal ulcer is associ-

Table 6. Causes of Chronic Abdominal Pain

Visceral Origin	gall bladder
stomach	chronic cholecystitis
ulcer	post cholecystectomy
carcinoma	
aerophagy	Generalized Diseases
	abdominal migraine
duodenum	porphyria
carcinoma (rare)	
	Abdominal Wall
pancreas	postherpetic neuralgia
chronic pancreatitis	segmental neuralgia
carcinoma	twelfth rib syndrome
	cutaneous nerve entrapment
small intestine	syndrome
malabsorption syndrome	
Crohn's disease	Psychological Origin
irritable bowel syndrome	depression
	anxiety
colon	conversion
diverticular disease	
cancer	

ated with frequent nausea, vomiting, and abdominal distension. Wolf has noted that many of the patients with peptic ulcer may have failed to achieve mature emotional development (28). Others, including Alexander, have pointed out that the occurrence of ulcers in these patients may be related to frustration of intense dependency needs (29). However, the specific role of psychological factors in the development of peptic ulcer remains controversial.

It is important to note that peptic ulcer disease may often be an important differential diagnosis for psychogenic abdominal pain.

Irritable Bowel Syndrome

Irritable bowel syndrome is a syndrome characterized by abdominal pain and other abdominal symptoms lasting either continuously or intermittently for three months or more, and is not due to clearly identifiable organic causes. This is a very common disorder seen most often in young adults, especially females. Pain is usually poorly localized and may occur anywhere in the abdominal region. The pain may vary in intensity from mild to excruciating. It may be intermittent and colicky, or dull and aching in character. It may occasionally last for days.

In addition to abdominal pain, alteration of bowel habits may occur. Constipation and diarrhea can occur interchangeably. Other symptoms including bloating, flatulence, and mucus in stools; nausea and vomiting may occur. In addition to abdominal symptoms, headache, urinary symptoms, dysmenorrhea, and palpitation may occur (30, 31).

Patients who suffer from irritable bowel syndrome generally are described as obsessive, compulsive, dependent, overconscientious, and sensitive individuals who score higher on anxiety, neuroticism, and introversion than do normal controls on formal testing (32). Furthermore, many of these patients may have a past or recent history of depression.

The abdomen is the third most common site of pain in psychiatric disorders (see Chapter 9, references 1–3). The characteristics of chronic abdominal pain of psychiatric origin has been described previously. Table 7 shows some of the characteristics that distinguish psychogenic abdominal pain, irritable bowel syndrome, and peptic ulcer.

LOW BACK AND CERVICAL PAIN

Low back pain may arise from several different causes. Table 8 shows a simple classification of the etiological conditions that cause chronic low back pain.

Table 7. Differences Between Abdominal Pain Secondary to Irritable Bowel Syndrome, Gastric Ulcer, Duodenal Ulcer, and Psychogenic Abdominal Pain

	Gastric Ulcer	Duodenal Ulcer	Irritable Bowel Syndrome	Psychogenic Abdominal Pain
Site	left upper quadrant or epigastric	epigastric	flanks, but may occur elsewhere	variable
Character	burning	burning	variable	variable
Onset	brought on by food	fasting	variable	variable
Relief	antacid	food	variable	variable
Stress	may be related	may be related	often related	often related
Associated GI Problems	rare	occasional	often	highly variable
Diarrhea/ Constipation	none	none	common	rare

EPIDEMIOLOGY OF LOW BACK PAIN

Approximately 70 percent of the population will have low back pain at some time in their lives (33, 34). Low back pain is usually characterized by a likelihood of recurrence. However, only one in seven have pain lasting more than two months (35, 36). Men are more likely to experience low back pain than women. Age of onset is usually in the fourth and fifth decade of life (37, 38). Fifty percent of the population show signs of degenerative changes in the spine by the end of the fourth decade, though not all patients with degenerative disc disease develop chronic low back pain. In fact, this is not a significant determinant of back pain in

Table 8.   Causes of Chronic Low Back Pain

Causes of Pain	Manifestations of Pain
Trauma	fracture dislocation
Infection	tuberculosis Pott's disease syphilis
Degenerative diseases	degenerative disc disease herniated disc Facet's syndrome
Neoplasms	multiple myeloma metastatic cancer
Referred pain	from abdomen and pelvis (pancreas—female reproductive system)
Psychiatric disorder	depression conversion disorder somatization disorder
Arthritic disorder	ankylosing spondylitis lumbar spondylosis osteophyte
Idiopathic	secondary to scoliosis poor posture, and other causes lumbar stenosis coccydynia
Neurological	archnoiditis demyelinating disease cauda equine lesion

Table 9. Risk Factors For Low Back Pain

Age—greater for individuals over 40 years of age

Physical fitness—greater for individuals in poor physical health

Posture—lordosis

Stress at work

Poor behavioral coping pattern

Poor support system

Psychological factor—poor ability to adapt to stressors

an individual subject. Disc degeneration does show a weak correlation with previous episodes of pain (39). Among the etiological factors listed above, idiopathic back disorder is probably the most common cause of low back pain. Several factors appear to be associated with the development of this type of low back pain. People who do light work seem to have a lower incidence of low back pain than those who do heavy work (40). Table 9 gives a history of some of the risk factors that are associated with the development of the low back pain syndrome.

NATURAL HISTORY OF LOW BACK PAIN

Low back pain is usually a self-limited condition. Ninety percent of all patients having episodes of back pain recover without a physician ever seeing them (41). Among those who attend a clinic for back pain, 50 percent improve within eight weeks (42). Only four percent have pain lasting more than six months (34).

DIAGNOSIS AND DIFFERENTIAL DIAGNOSIS

Only in a small number of patients can a clear-cut pathology be identified. In this section we will briefly describe some of the common specific conditions that produce back pain, many of which have been listed in Table 8, and describe some clinical manifestations that will aid in their diagnosis.

ANKYLOSING SPONDYLITIS

Etiology

The etiology of ankylosing spondylitis is uncertain. A high frequency of these patients have HLA-B27 antigen. It is usually seen in young men. It is characterized by inflammation of the sacroiliac joints and the apophyseal joints in the vertebrae.

Clinical Characteristics

Low back pain is often a presenting symptom. Several clinical tests such as the finger-to-floor test and direct compression over the sacroiliac joints assist in diagnosing this condition.

Radiological Evaluation

The typical radiological picture of an advanced case of ankylosing spondylitis is the bamboo spine. The bamboo spine is marked by paraspinal ligamentous calcification. The early signs usually are sclerosis around the sacroiliac joints and subchondral erosions. Another condition resembling ankylosing spondylitis may be seen in men over the age of 50; it is called Forestiers disease.

JUVENILE ANKYLOSING SPONDYLITIS

Ankylosing spondylitis can occur in boys and involve joints prior to spondylitis. The sacroilitis is usually seen later. HLA typing is a useful adjunct in the diagnosis of juvenile ankylosing spondylitis (43–45). A related condition is Reiter's syndrome, which is a triad of specific urethritis, conjunctivitis, and arthritis. HLA-B2 also is found commonly in this condition; sedimentation rate is usually elevated but unlike ankylosing spondylitis; and the sacroiliac joint inflammation is usually unilateral.

HERNIATED DISC

Another specific condition that can produce low back pain is herniated disc.

Incidence

The incidence is not known; it can occur at any age but usually occurs in males over the age of 40 more often than it does in females.

Etiology

The etiology of herniated disc is unknown. It can be caused by a number of factors, including trauma, heredity, and biochemical alterations (46). Disc herniations are usually classified into three groups: sequestered, extruded, and protruded (47). Prognosis is poor in patients with protruded disc herniations.

Clinical Characteristics

Herniated disc usually occurs in males between the ages of 40 and 50. The pain is usually present in onset and can be insidious. On close questioning, a history of low back pain preceding the onset of acute pain is usually found. The initial episode of pain is severe. The pain is described as occurring in the lower back radiating down the back or both legs. The most common site is the L4, L5, L5-S1 region. When herniation occurs in this region pain is reported to radiate into the legs (sciatic). When the herniation occurs at a little higher level—L3, L4 or L2, L3 region—the pain is usually reported as radiating into the thigh. On examination, a sciatic tension sign is usually seen. Depending upon the site of involvement, or depending upon the site of herniation, weakness of specific muscles and a decrease in different reflexes will be seen. If it is a large disc herniation, urinary and anal incontinence may be seen.

Management

Many cases can be conservatively managed, although surgical management is necessary in some patients. Surgical management is definitely indicated in those conditions in which there is a neurological deficit.

LUMBAR DISC DEGENERATION

Lumbar disc degeneration is a common finding in older people. However, very few report symptoms. It is uncertain to what extent this degeneration plays a role in symptom formation.

Etiology

Etiology is probably multifactorial (48). Degenerative changes occur both in the disc as well as in the facet joints.

Clinical Presentation

As noted earlier, the extent to which degenerative disc disease causes back pain is uncertain. When the degeneration is severe and extends to involve the neural foramina or the vertebral canal, then neurological symptoms as well as vascular symptoms may be seen. Otherwise, low back pain may be the only presenting symptom. Examination usually reveals no involvement of the sciatic nerve. There is limited motion or mobility of the lumbar spine. Management is again conservative with physical therapy and analgesic use.

TRAUMA

Minor trauma as well as major trauma can lead to chronic low back pain. Often the onset of chronic low back pain is related to a trivial traumatic episode. The extent to which these types of trauma contribute to the pathogenesis of low back pain is uncertain. Chronic pain that persists after major injury to the spine is common.

INFECTIONS OF THE INTERVERTEBRAL DISC

Among infections of the intervertebral disc, pseudomonas is often the most common. In other countries, tuberculosis is very common; fungal infections can also produce intervertebral disc disease. Radiological and bone evaluations aid in the diagnosis. A definitive diagnosis should be based upon disc biopsy and microbial analysis.

NEOPLASMS

Neoplasms rarely involve the spine. The most common condition that involves the spine is multiple myeloma; the second most common is metastatic disease. Other malignancies that can involve the spine and produce back pain include osteoid osteomata and giant cell tumors. Radiological evaluation usually aids in the diagnosis of these conditions. Congenital abnormalities occur in 5 to 10 percent of the population; the extent and role they play in the development of low back pain is uncertain.

METABOLIC DISEASES

Among the metabolic diseases, hyperparathyroidism and hyperthyroidism can play a role in the development of back pain. Paget's disease is another condition characterized by excessive bone turnover, usually in the lower spinal and pelvic region, which can cause pain.

DEMYELINATING NEUROLOGICAL DISORDERS

Demyelinating process of the spinal cord can lead to low back pain. Referred pain to the lower back in female patients can be secondary to pelvic inflammatory disease, ovarian tumors, endometriosis, uterine tumors, urinary infections, and the like. In males, the most common conditions include prostatic and urinary infections. Other causes of referred pain include peptic ulcer disease, gastric distress, heartburn, pancreatitis, and aneurysms of the major blood vessels (49).

ASSESSMENT OF LOW BACK PAIN

History

The following information should be obtained:

1. The nature of the pain complaint
2. the onset of the pain—whether it is acute, insidious, and so on
3. the factors that aggravate the pain
4. the factors that diminish the pain
5. any trauma that could have started the pain—either minor or major
6. the description and characteristics of the pain complaint
7. the radiation of the pain
8. whether the radiation occurs at all times
9. whether the radiation occurs in certain postures, certain movements, and so on

In asking questions about the radiation, it is necessary to find out whether the pain radiates beyond the knee or not. Other questions should include intensity of pain and the presence of other associated symptoms, such as abdominal pain, nausea, vomiting, pelvic infection in women, urinary infection in men, and so forth.

History of prior back pain should be obtained, as should history of any prior injuries or surgeries, careful employment history, history of psychiatric disorders, alcohol dependence, and psychosocial history. Characteristics of pain-prone personality should be sought. A careful review of other systems, especially the gastrointestinal and the genitourinary system, should be conducted.

Physical Examination

Details of the various procedures used in the physical examination of back pain patients can be found in several textbooks (50, 51).

Laboratory Evaluations

A complete blood count, urinalysis, and radiological evaluation (including myelogram when indicated) are some of the useful laboratory and radiological techniques used in the assessment of low back pain. Other assessment methodologies used include electromyogram and evoked sensory nerve potential (49, 50).

CERVICAL PAIN

The etiology of cervical pain includes trauma, infections, degenerative diseases, and other causes, including myeloma, metastatic tumors, spondylosis, cervical myelopathy, referred pain, and psychiatric disorders.

Cervical Spondylosis

This disorder is most commonly seen in C5-C6 region. It usually leads to radiculopathy secondary to irritation of the nerve root. Both sensory and muscle involvement can be elicited easily on physical examination. The pain is usually radicular. Tenderness of the involved segment is usually seen.

Cervical Myelopathy

Cervical myelopathy is secondary to a decrease in the size of the spinal canal. This occurs when osteophytes protrude into the spinal canal from the vertebral bodies. In addition to pain, other signs of spinal cord involvement are usually seen.

Rupture of the Cervical Disc

Rupture of the cervical disc is less common than is rupture of the lumbar disc (52). This can occur secondary to both minor injuries (whiplash) and severe trauma. Fractures of the cervical spine are also quite common causes of cervical pain. Referred pain to the cervical region can occur from myocardial infarction, hiatal hernia, esophagitis, and from other diseases in the neck, dental, and chest regions. Predisposing factors to pain in the vertebral region are listed in Table 10 (53).

Table 10.   Predisposing Factors to Pain in Vertebral Region

Congenital anomalies
   spondylosis
   spondylolisthesis
   spina bifida

Occupation
   those requiring repeated lifting, bending, and twisting
   those where there is prolonged vibration to the disc

Pregnancy

Pain-prone personality

Degeneration of the intervertebral disc

CHRONIC PELVIC PAIN IN WOMEN

Pelvic pain is one of the most common complaints in gynecological practice (54, 55). When pelvic pain is acute, it is usually caused by one of the following: 1) complications of pregnancy (abortion, ectopic pregnancy); 2) infection (pelvic inflammatory disease, hemorrhage of cyst, torsion of ovarian tumor, rupture of corpus luteum cyst); or 3) nongynecological causes (appendicitis, intestinal obstruction, urethral colic). Treatment is directed at the etiological cause, and the interested reader should refer to the gynecological literature. Chronic pelvic pain can result from metabolic or endocrine disturbances, structured abnormalities, tumor, infection, or menstrual dysfunction.

Gynecological pain is localized to two areas: ventral and dorsal zones (56). A pathological process occurring in the pelvic region refers pain to either or both of these zones. The ventral zone is in the lower abdominal region and does not extend above the level of the anterior superior iliac spines. The dorsal zone is located over the upper half of the sacrum and extends laterally over the gluteal area (56). Pain outside these zones is either not of gynecological origin or is caused by other factors complicating the pelvic abnormalities (tumor extending out of the pelvic cavity). Pelvic pain may occasionally radiate to the lower extremities, especially if the sacral nerve is involved. The innervation of the pelvic organs is not fully understood. This limits the understanding, to some degree, of the mechanism for pelvic pain (54). The external genitalia of the woman is acutely sensitive to injury, lesions, or inflammatory reaction (54). The vagina, except for the introitus, is relatively insensitive. Painful intercourse (dyspareunia) occurs when organs or tissue other than the vagina is the source of the pathology (54). The uterus is the source of painful sensation only if distended or during contractions (change in tissue tension). Stimulation of the internal os does produce pain. Fallopian

Table 11.　Causes of Chronic Pelvic Pain

Recurrent pain:	Dysmenorrhea
	Premenstrual syndrome
Continuous pain:	Endometriosis
	Chronic pelvic inflammatory disease
	Displacement of uterus
	Urinary tract pain
	Ovarian pain
	Gastrointestinal pain
	Chronic pelvic pain without organic pathology

tubes are also sensitive to mild pressure. The ovaries are insensitive to external pressure, but if there is a rapid increase in tissue tension, pain may develop. Fluid from ruptured cysts may be a local irritant to the peritoneal tissue. In the assessment of the patient with pelvic pain, attention to menstruation and pregnancy is important, since most pelvic pain states are either caused or associated with these conditions.

In most chronic pelvic pain conditions, the pain varies during the menstrual cycle. Pain that increases toward the end of the menstrual period is characteristic of endometriosis. Pain of musculoskeletal origin can also increase during the premenstrual period (55). Chronic pelvic pain can be episodic (dysmenorrhea) or continuous (chronic pelvic in-flammatory disease) (Table 11).

CLINICAL SYNDROMES

Dysmenorrhea

This condition refers to cyclic pelvic pain during the period of menstrual blood flow. It occurs mainly in women under the age of 30. Primary dysmenorrhea is pain not associated with a structural abnormality. The pain is colicky and located over the lower abdominal area, and may radiate to the sacral area and anterior surface of the thighs. Severe cases of dysmenorrhea may be associated with nausea, vomiting, and diarrhea. The cause of dysmenorrhea is unknown, but elevated levels of pros-taglandins are found in endometrial and menstrual fluids (55). In most cases, primary dysmenorrhea disappears after the first delivery. Second-ary dysmenorrhea is pain produced by structural abnormality. The most common causes for secondary dysmenorrhea are endometriosis, ade-nomyocystis, and fibroids. There is little evidence for psychological etiology for dysmenorrhea (55).

Premenstrual Syndrome

This syndrome comprises various symptoms occurring from 7 to 10 days prior to menses and disappears at the beginning of a period. Symptoms include distention of breast and abdomen, nervousness, emotional la-bility, depression, insomnia, and dizziness. Symptoms vary from one cycle to the next. Premenstrual syndrome is most frequently seen around the age of 30. The incidence of the syndrome affects between 25 and 75 percent of women in their reproductive years. The variation in incidence is due to the variation in definition of premenstrual syndrome required for diagnosis (55). The cause of premenstrual syndrome is unknown, but it is reported that some patients may have impaired progesterone secre-tion (55).

Endometriosis

Pain occurs in areas of ectopic foci of endometrial tissue. The most common locations are in the peritoneum of the pelvis (54, 55). The pain location is dependent upon the site of ectopic foci of endometrial tissue. As stated earlier, pain occurs during menses. Infertility and dyspareunia also may be present. Bleeding midcycle is a frequent symptom. Diagnosis is confirmed by laparoscopic examination. Pain due to endometriosis is relieved by pregnancy, hormonal therapy, or drug treatment with Danazol.

Chronic Pelvic Inflammatory Disease

After the acute infection of the pelvic area subsides, pain complaints may persist. Patients may, in addition, complain of dyspareunia, infertility, and abnormal menstrual periods.

Displacement of the Uterus

Retroversion of the uterus may give rise to pelvic pain. Genital prolapse is not associated with pain (55).

Ovarian Pain

Pain from the ovaries is usually caused by follicular, luteal, or endometrial cysts. Benign and malignant ovarian tumors usually do not cause pain, except when there is a rupture of a cyst or torsion of the ovarian tumor.

Chronic Pelvic Pain Without Organic Pathology

The previously mentioned causes of pelvic pain are typically diagnosed on the basis of specific pain complaints and findings on physical and laparoscopic examination. However, there are women who present with chronic pelvic pain where there is no discernible organic pathological process. This syndrome has been named by Renaer as chronic pelvic pain without obvious pathology (CPPWOP) (55). This syndrome occurs in women between the ages of 20 and 40, with the mean age around 30 years (57–61). The pain symptoms usually start during or after the first pregnancy (58, 61, 62). The possible causes of this syndrome include: 1) pelvic congestion secondary to circulatory factors (63); 2) traumatic laceration of the supporting structures of the uterus (64); 3) structural modification of the sacral-uterine ligament (56); and 4) psychological factors (57, 59, 62). A detailed review and discussion of the etiological causes of chronic pelvic pain without organic pathology is presented by Renaer and colleagues (61).

Allen and Master (64) stated that in certain women with this syndrome, there is a traumatic laceration of the sacro-uterine ligament or of a posterior leaf of the broad ligament. This observation has not been supportive by the findings of other investigators (61). Taylor (63) and Taylor and Duncan (62) described circulatory dysfunction leading to chronic pelvic congestion in women undergoing emotional distress. Recent studies have failed to support this cause in all cases (61). A common finding in these patients is that pressure on the internal pelvic organs usually produces pain; however, the mechanism for the tenderness or pain is unknown and does not explain the other multiple organic complaints associated with this syndrome. Several authors (57, 60, 65, 66) have described a significant degree of psychopathology in these women. Gidro-Frank and colleagues (60) found more psychiatric disturbance than in a controlled group of pregnant women. Murphy (65), in a study of 100 consecutive chronic pelvic pain patients without organic pathology, found 40 percent of the women with severe character disorders and 30 percent of women with depression. All patients studied in this series had a significant degree of psychopathology. Benson and colleagues (59), in a study of 35 women with chronic pelvic pain (with few or no physical findings to explain the pain), all had a psychiatric diagnosis (psychoneurosis, schizophrenia, hysteria).

Renaer and colleagues (67) compared the results of Minnesota Multiphasic Personality Inventory (MMPI) testing among three groups: Group I—women with pelvic pain and no organic cause; Group II—women with chronic pain secondary to endometriosis; and Group III—women who were pain free. The mean scale scores of the MMPI were not significantly different between Groups I and II, but Groups I and II were significantly different from Group III. In this study, no psychiatric diagnosis was made. Rosenthal and colleagues (68) compared the MMPI results in women complaining of chronic pelvic pain who had either a positive or negative laparoscopic examination for organic pathology. There was no significant difference between the MMPI scores in the group of women with pathology on laparoscopic examination versus those with a negative examination. Given these findings of a significant degree of psychopathology in women with chronic pelvic pain without organic pathology and results of the two studies described above, there appears to be a marked discrepancy. However, this difference has also been observed by Sternbach (69) in a study of low back pain patients, Bond (70) in a study of cancer pain patients, and Woodforde and Merskey (71) in a study of chronic pain patients secondary to physical problems. In summary, psychometric testing of personality traits does not distinguish whether a patient's pain is organic or psychogenic in nature. Pain, whatever the cause, does induce personality disturbances or changes that can be measured by psychological testing. In order to clarify the role of psychological factors in chronic pelvic pain, further studies are needed. Future studies should include control groups of women with and without chronic pelvic pain, psychometric testing, standardized assessment for psychiatric diagnosis, and longitudinal follow-up.

Clinical Description. The most frequent symptom is lower abdominal pain in the suprapubic region, and pain in either or both lower quadrants (Table 12). Pain can be referred to the sacral and anterior parts of the upper thighs. The pain is described as dull, heavy, burning, aching, and stabbing or cramp-like. Pain can increase with movement. Pain increases in the premenstrual period (59–61). The pain is often described in vague terms and accompanied by other multiple physical complaints (59, 61, 66). Many of the patients have had multiple abdominal or pelvic operations (59). Dyspareunia is a frequent finding (55, 57, 59, 61), and sexual dysfunction is apparent in most patients (55, 57, 59, 60). The ability to conceive a child is not a problem (59). There is the lack

Table 12.   Characteristics of Chronic Pelvic Pain Without Organic Pathology in Women

Demographic
  married
  age range—20–40 years

Pain Complaints
  lower abdomen or sacral area
  starts during or after first pregnancy
  poor description of pain
  varies with menstrual period
  dyspareunia
  presence of other physical complaints

Past History
  history of sexual abuse
  presence of psychological distress
  early marriage
  ability to conceive a child
  neglectful parents
  history of abdominal or pelvic operations

Psychological Functions
  frequent diagnosis of borderline or personality disorders
  poor interpersonal relationships
  dependency conflicts
  poor feminine identity

of organic findings on physical or laparoscopic examination (57). There is an increased incidence of psychological disturbance in these patients. Common psychiatric diagnoses found in women with chronic pelvic pain without organic pathology include borderline personality disorder, character disorder, depression, and adolescent adjustment disorder. No study reported in the literature notes little psychological disturbance or infrequent diagnosis of pyschiatric disorder.

Past history of these patients reveals childhoods characterized by neglectful parents, and early marriages on the part of these patients to escape from the family environment (59, 62). The parents of these patients are described as having problems with alcohol, promiscuity, and aggression control. The patients' relationship to the mothers is described as marked by hostility, the relationship to the fathers as cold and distant (59). There is the frequent finding of sexual abuse, especially incest, in these women (57, 65). Despite the frequent occurrence of marital conflicts, most of these patients are married (59, 60, 62, 67). The women are described as being immature and dependent, and see their marriages as a means to relieve their problems. Their pattern of psychological defenses includes repression, denial, phobic avoidance, and projection (60). They have a poor feminine identity (59–61). They have limited interpersonal skills, and relationships are characterized by dependency and lack of trust.

With the frequent finding of psychological disturbances, multiple symptoms, and lack of definite organic pathology, surgical treatment is often nonproductive (61). The personality profile of these patients also limits the type of psychological intervention that can be used. The defensive style and interpersonal skills seen most commonly in these patients do not make them candidates for psychotherapy aimed at personality alteration or conflict resolution. However, crisis intervention, short term psychotherapy, or supportive psychotherapy is often beneficial for these patients.

PERIPHERAL NEUROPATHIES

CLASSIFICATION

Peripheral neuropathies can be classified into two major groups: polyneuropathies and mononeuropathies. Table 13 gives a simple listing of the various etiological conditions that can produce polyneuropathies and mononeuropathies. The classification is limited primarily to neuropathies that are associated with chronic pain. Polyneuropathies can also be classified on the basis of the type of fiber loss. Larger fiber loss is associated with isoniazid toxicity and pellagra; small fiber loss is associ-

Table 13. Etiological Conditions for Mononeuropathies and Polyneuropathies

Mononeuropathies

    diabetes mellitus
    herpes zoster
    polyarteritis nodosa
    rheumatoid arthritis
    systemic lupus erythematosus
    nonmetastatic complications of malignant disease
    brachial plexus neuropathy

Polyneuropathies

    diabetes mellitus
    Guillain-Barre syndrome
    amyloid neuropathy
    myeloma neuropathy
    neuropathy related to nutritional deficiencies
    pellagra
    beriberi
    burning feet syndrome
    toxic drug-induced neuropathy
    INH (Isoniazid)
    alcohol
    arsenic

ated with diabetes and amyloid neuropathy. In neuropathy secondary to alcohol and to myeloma, the type of fiber loss can be quite variable, with both small and large fibers being affected. In the large number of neuropathies, the etiological factors are usually difficult to identify (72).

A comprehensive description of the various conditions mentioned above is beyond the scope of this book. We briefly describe one of the most common neuropathies and one which psychiatrists are sometimes asked to help manage in patients, postherpetic neuralgia. A brief mention of the use of psychotropics in the management of these conditions is presented in the final section of this book.

POSTHERPETIC NEURALGIA

Postherpetic neuralgia is a mononeuropathy characterized by painful, localized vesicular eruptions of the skin along the distribution of the involved nerves.

Etiology

The disease is caused by a virus, the varicella-zoster virus.

Pathogenesis

The virus initially infects the respiratory tract. This is followed by secondary involvement of the skin. The virus then ascends from the skin by way of peripheral nerves to the dorsal root ganglia (73). Here it becomes latent. Later, it can become reactivated. When it is reactivated, there is replication of the virus, followed by the virus traveling along the sensory nerves to the dermatome where it produces skin vesicles. Reactivation tends to occur more often in the elderly, immune compromised, and debilitated individuals.

Clinical Features

Pain. Pain is described as sharp, burning, and severe in intensity. It is localized to the dermatome involved. The pain precedes the development of the rash and pain may continue long after the rash has disappeared. The involved area is very sensitive to touch.

Skin lesions. Vesicles form over the region of the involved dermatome within a week after the onset of pain. The vesicles then evolve into pustules before disappearing.

The disease can lead to complications if it involves certain nerves; for example, uveitis and keratitis can occur when it involves the ophthalmic division of the trigeminal nerve.

MANAGEMENT

Management of postherpetic neuralgia is very difficult. Transcutaneous electrical stimulation, acupuncture, carbamazepine, antidepressants, and nerve blocks are sometimes useful. A brief discussion regarding the use of psychotropics is given in the Management section of the book.

CAUSALGIA

Causalgia is a relatively uncommon type of pain that follows injury to a nerve. The term causalgia means "burning pain"; and while most of the patients do complain of burning pain, some describe the pain in other ways.

CLINICAL CHARACTERISTICS

The pain, as just mentioned, is usually described as burning. The pain starts within a few hours after the injury and it usually spreads. The area of involvement is usually sensitive to touch, movement, and other stimulation. Pain can also be increased by anxiety, and even sometimes by any emotion. The pain is usually severe in intensity.

On examination of the affected area, vascular changes are usually observed. Later, trophic changes, including muscular atrophy, osteoperosis, dryness of the skin, stiffening of joints, changes in the hair covering the area, and altered sweating patterns are usually seen. The affected area is usually hyperpathic and hyperesthetic; that is, usually sensitive to any stimulation. Some of the conditions in which the pain is less severe goes under the name of minor causalgia, or Sudeck's atrophy. The characteristic common to both major and minor causalgia is the good response to sympathetic blockade. It is believed that both conditions are related to altered sympathetic nervous system activity in the region. It is also noted that hypersensitivity to norepinephrine secreted at the peripheral sympathetic terminals may be responsible for the pain.

Management

Sympathetic block is the treatment of choice. The type of sympathetic block or the site for the sympathetic block depends upon the site of the pain and causalgia. Regional sympathetic block with guanethidine sulfate is often useful. In the initial assessment of patients with causalgia it is important to note that on rare occasions it can be simulated by psychogenic mechanisms. Psychotherapy may be useful in these patients.

PHANTOM LIMB PAIN

Phantom limb sensation, which refers to the painful sensation that occurs in the amputated portion of the body, occurs almost universally in patients who have experienced the loss of a limb. Phantom limb pain has been estimated in 5 to 10 percent of patients (74), but recent reports indicate the incidence to be as high as 78 to 85 percent (75).

Phantom limb sensation varies from the exact duplication of the amputated body part to the mild sensation of the missing limb. Most amputees experience the phantom sensation twenty-four hours after the amputation, and only 10 percent of patients report the initiation of the sensation more than a month after the amputation (76). Phantom limb is rarely seen in the congenital absence of a limb (77) or in children whose body parts were amputated before the age of six (78). Amputees experience the sensation of position, length, volume, and movement of the amputated limb. They may also describe various cutaneous sensations such as cold, heat, itching, and so on. The phantom limb sensation may be altered by weather, emotional stress, ejaculation, defecation, micturition, and attention focused on the phantom. Usually the phantom sensation diminishes over the course of the year following the amputation, but may remain for years. The fading of the phantom limb has been termed "telescoping" where the distal part of the amputated limb approaches the stump. Phantom sensations can also be experienced with loss of nose, eye, tongue, teeth, penis, scrotum, and breast. Stump pain occurs in the distal end of the remaining limb. Stump pain is reported to be present in at least 50 percent of amputees and usually wanes in the first year after amputation (79). This pain is described as painful spots, stabbing sensations, or electrical shocks located in the stump. The causes of stump pain include skin breakdown, neuromas, bone spurs, infections, or circulatory disturbances.

ETIOLOGY OF PHANTOM LIMB PAIN

The exact cause of phantom limb pain is unknown. One possible mechanism is the loss of normal sensory input into the central biasing mechanism. It is this central biasing mechanism that exerts a tonic inhibitory influence on the transmission of nociceptive impulses (74, 80).

CLINICAL CHARACTERISTICS OF PHANTOM LIMB PAIN

The phantom limb pain is described as severe cramping, shooting, burning, crushing, or squeezing sensations. Some patients report distorted positions of the phantom limb or plantar flexion of the amputated hand or foot. The development of the phantom limb pain usually occurs within the first month following amputation. Parkes (79) reported 63 percent of amputees have severe phantom pain immediately postoperatively; 13 months later, 30 percent of the patients report this intensity of pain.

Factors intensifying the phantom pain include attention to the phantom limb, trauma to the stump, emotional distress, weather, wearing a prosthesis, and autonomic activity. Factors diminishing the phantom pain include rest, distraction, relaxation, cold or heat, using a prosthesis, elevation of the stump, massage, and movement of the stump (81). It has been noted that pain in the phantom prior to amputation is common in patients with postoperative pain in the phantom (79).

Phantom sensation of the breast (82, 83) is occasionally experienced by mastectomized women. Jamison and colleagues (82) found that 54 percent of women undergoing mastectomy had phantom breast sensation, and found that 80 percent of the women experienced this sensation as painful. It should be noted that most of the women did not report their sensations to their physician. Phantom anal pain is reported to occur in approximately 10 percent of patients who have undergone abdominoperineal surgical resection (84). Bladder phantom sensations and pain occasionally occur in patients who have undergone cystectomy (85).

PSYCHOLOGICAL AND BEHAVIORAL FACTORS IN PHANTOM LIMB PAIN

It has been shown that emotional stress can trigger phantom limb pain and that psychological intervention can lessen the intensity of the pain (74). Parkes (79), in a study of phantom limb pain, found a significant correlation between complaints of persistent pain in the phantom and a rigid, compulsive, and self-reliant personality. Sherman and colleagues (86) noted a strong correlation between severity of the phantom limb pain and anxiety in these patients. Despite the psychological contributions to phantom limb pain, there is no greater incidence of psychopathology in patients with phantom limb pain than those amputees without pain in the phantom limb (74).

SPECIAL TREATMENT FOR PHANTOM LIMB PAIN

There is no recognized successful method for the treatment of phantom limb pain. Sherman and colleagues (87) concluded that there are no treatments for phantom limb pain that produce positive long-term results. He also reported that surgical intervention was the least successful. However, Nashold and colleagues (88) reported pain relief occurring in patients with phantom pain following nerve root avulsion by focal destruction in the dorsal root entry zone of the spinal cord. Progressive muscle relaxation with biofeedback of stump and forehead muscle tension, control of anxiety and depression, and reassurance have been successful in the management of phantom limb pain (84). The use of fixed dose (81) or time contingent administered narcotics in combination with antidepressants (89) has been effective in controlling phantom limb pain.

CENTRAL PAIN

THALAMIC PAIN

Etiology

The etiological factors that can cause thalamic pain are listed in Table 14. The most common cause of thalamic pain is vascular disease.

Clinical Characteristics

Pain is usually described as "shooting, boring, gnawing, crushing, burning, or aching." It is usually associated with dysesthesia and the intensity of pain is usually severe. The trunk is often the site of the pain, but limbs

Table 14.   Conditions Which Cause Thalamic Pain

Trauma

Cardiovascular diseases
  thrombosis
  embolism
  hemorrhage
  arteriovenous malformation

Tumors

Other
  surgical lesions

---

may be involved. Autonomic and vasomotor dysfunctions are associated with the pain. Upon painful stimulation, the sensation is referred to a wide area around the area of stimulation. Heat, cold, touch, or pain produces a more unpleasant sensation than is usually associated with the same sensation in the unaffected area. The pain sensation produced by certain stimulation may persist and outlast duration of the stimulation. Sensory loss is highly variable and can vary from severe analgesia to minimal sensory loss. Table 15 lists some of the clinical characteristics of thalamic pain.

Management

A comprehensive discussion of the management of this condition is beyond the scope of this book. Carbamazepine, phenothiazine, and diphenylhydantoin are the drugs that have been reported to be successful in central pain (90). Central pain is refractory to narcotic analgesics.

Table 15.   Clinical Characteristics of Thalamic Pain

Character	shooting, burning, aching
Site	variable—contralateral to side of lesion usually peripheral
Factors increasing pain	any stimulation of the affected area
Sensory loss	variable
Other associated factors	unpleasant sensations

Other Mechanics of Central Pain

Besides thalamic pain, diseases of the central nervous system (CNS) that destroy parts of the brain and spinal cord can lead to central pain. After onset of the pain, the pain is persistent. A list of the conditions that can produce central pain is given in Table 16.

PAIN SECONDARY TO SPINAL CORD LESIONS

Lesions of the spinal cord produce a central pain phenomenon, just as injury or disease of the thalamus produces the thalamic pain syndrome. The mechanism of central pain is unknown, but evidence suggests a loss of descending inhibitory influences and/or loss of sensory inputs (91). Three kinds of pain in patients with spinal cord lesions have been reported (92). Phantom body pain is felt in the area of complete sensory loss. Visceral pain is the sensation of abdominal fullness, cramps, or painful sensations in the hypogastric area. The visceral pain is precipitated by distention of the bladder or rectum and can be associated with autonomic disturbance such as nausea, flushing, headache, and sweating. Root or girdle pain is located near the level of the spinal cord lesion.

Occurrence

It has been reported that 27 percent of paraplegic patients with partial or total spinal cord lesions complain of some type of pain in body areas below the level of the lesion (91). The onset of pain may occur at the time of the injury or be delayed for years (93). It has been estimated that 5 to

Table 16. Other Causes of Central Pain

Spinal Cord	Bulbar
Traumatic injury:	Vascular
concussion	inferior/posterior cerebellar
hemisection	artery thrombosis
complete transection	
	Tumor
Vascular	
ischemia	Other
hematomyelia	syringobulbia
	spinothalamic tractotomy
Tumor	
	Corticol-Subcorticol:
Other	Traumatic lesions
syringomyelia	Vascular
toxic myelopathy	Tumor

10 percent of paraplegic patients have severe central pain (91). The causes of central pain secondary to spinal cord lesions include: 1) spinal cord trauma with partial or complete transection; 2) spinal cord concussion; 3) vascular lesions; 4) tumor; 5) myelopathies; and 6) disseminated sclerosis (94).

Clinical Description

Patients complaining of phantom body pain describe the pain as spontaneously aching, burning, or shooting. They also complain of dysesthesias, hyperalgesia, formications, and other unusual sensations. In some patients these unusual sensations can be more unpleasant than the pain itself. There is excessive reaction to peripheral stimuli, so there is often very little relationship between the intensity of the stimulus and the degree of sensation produced. This sensation usually continues long after the stimulation ends. The dysthetic pain can occur in totally anesthetic or hypoasthetic areas (95). Nonpainful stimuli can give rise to pain sensations. The onset of pain can be immediate or delayed for months or years after the injury (95). The pain is persistent and lasts for many years (94). The pain is exaggerated by cold, damp weather (96), smoking (96), and bladder or bowel distention (92). Psychological distress increases the level of pain in these patients (92). Both anxiety and depression have been shown to increase the level of central pain in paraplegics (96). However, there is little evidence to support a psychological cause for central pain. It appears that the emotional disturbance exaggerates the chronic pain in patients with spinal cord lesions.

Treatment

Neurosurgical ablative procedures to interrupt pain tracts in the spinal cord or thalamus have failed to produce lasting benefit (94). Electrical stimulation of peripheral nerves or dorsal columns and deep brain stimulation have not produced lasting results (94). Narcotic analgesics are generally of no benefit. Carbamazepine has been reported to be effective in the shooting pain of paraplegics (94).

MYOFASCIAL PAIN SYNDROME

Myofascial syndrome is used to describe pain arising from muscle and fascia. Pain from myofascial syndrome is associated with fatigue, sleep disturbance (97), stiffness of involved muscles, limited range of motion in affected muscles, irritability, and depression (98, 99). Myofascial syndromes occur in many other conditions, including backache, headache, soft tissue injury, whiplash, osteoarthritis, and hypothyroidism. Myofascial syndrome is also characterized by trigger points, which are local, sensitive, tender areas identified by palpation. The trigger point can be identified when pressure on it produces local pain. Trigger points are usually seen in palpable bands in muscle groups.

Other terms used to define the myofascial syndrome include: interstitial myofibrositis (100), myalagia (101), myofascial pain dysfunction syndrome (102), and fibrositis syndrome (103).

ETIOLOGY

The hyperirritable spot is believed to be initiated by muscle strain. This neuromuscular dysfunction produces pain and autonomic phenomena (99). The trigger points are associated with lowering of the pain threshold and are vulnerable to stress (104). When the trigger point fires in response to a stimulus, the impulses are relayed to the CNS. Impulses from the CNS cause autonomic changes, including muscle tension and vasoconstriction. These changes alter the extracellular environment near the trigger point and increase the sensitivity of nociceptors in the area. This further increases autonomic activity leading to pain. Fatigue can cause additional trigger points (105).

PATHOLOGY

Earlier studies did not show any pathological change in muscle. A recent study (106) has shown that muscle tension from trigger point areas have a moth-eaten appearance and show reduction of adenosine triphosphate and phosphocreatinine.

CLINICAL CHARACTERISTICS

Myofascial pain may begin either abruptly or gradually. When the pain begins suddenly, it is useful to pinpoint which muscles have been strained at the time. When the pain is gradual, muscles that have been repeatedly stressed are likely to be involved. Over a period of time, several muscle groups become involved. Patients complain of subjective swelling in the affected muscle groups and numbness (nonradicular). Pain is usually described as aching, swelling, or numb. On examination, the muscles that are involved show trigger points, palpable muscle bands, and restricted range of movement. Light pressure on active trigger points can reproduce the patient's pain. Most patients have more than four trigger points (107). Articular examination in these patients is normal. When the trigger point is subjected to rapid changing pressure, the local twitching phenomenon is seen.

The common sites of trigger points include masticatory muscles, neck muscles, muscles of shoulder girdle, paraspinal muscle groups, quadratus lumborium, and muscle groups of lower extremities. Myofascial pain syndromes become chronic when perpetuating factors are present, such as mechanical stress, viral and bacterial disease, and nutritional, endocrine, and metabolic disorders (Table 17) (108).

In the absence of perpetuating factors, the pain will resolve spontaneously. In the presence of perpetuating factors, symptoms can be exaggerated by cold or humid weather, fatigue, a sedentary state, anxiety, and overactivity (107). Symptoms may be relieved by hot showers, activity, warm, dry weather, and massage. When the pain and disability become chronic, this can lead to depression, which can intensify the process.

The lifetime rate of major affective disorder in these patients is higher as compared to normals. They also have a higher familial incidence of affective disorders (109).

Table 17. Perpetuating Factors for Chronicity of Myofascial Pain

GROUP I —Mechanical Stressors
           trauma
           short leg
           foot disorder
           small heavy pelvis
           poor posture
           prolonged immobility

GROUP II —Infections
           viral (flu)
           herpes simplex, Type I
           bacterial
           chronic sensitivity
           chronic urinary tract infection
           parasitosis (fish tapeworm, giardiasis, amebiasis)

GROUP III—Endocrine
           hypothyroidism
           estrogen deficiency

GROUP IV —Metabolic
           hypoglycemia
           hyperuricemia

GROUP V —Nutritional
           vitamin C/B-complex deficiency
           low serum calcium and potassium
           iron deficiency
           magnesium and zinc deficiency

Myofascial pain syndrome is infrequently diagnosed and poorly managed (107). When the condition arises from a compensated injury or injury involving litigation, the treatment becomes difficult as the potential for secondary gain is enhanced. The syndrome in its chronic form can lead to an extended period of absenteeism from work.

Myofascial pain syndrome has been differentiated from psychogenic rheumatism by various authors (110–113). In psychogenic rheumatism, the pain symptoms are described in a bizarre, exaggerated quality (cutting, burning) with changing sites and no clearly defined trigger points. The complaints are vague and emotional distress is usually a modulating factor. The response to physical treatment (trigger point injections, physical therapy) is poor. Psychogenic rheumatism is clearly related to a psychological etiology.

TREATMENT

Some of the specific treatment modalities include trigger point injections with local anesthetics (114), spray-stretch (fluoromethane spray mixture) (115, 116), and ischemic compression. Other treatment modalities are those applicable for chronic pain syndromes of multifactoral etiologies. They are described in the Management section of this volume.

ARTHRITIS

Chronic arthritis can be secondary to multiple diseases. These include rheumatoid arthritis, osteoarthritis, and infectious conditions leading to arthritis.

RHEUMATOID ARTHRITIS

The exact etiology is unknown. It is associated with histocompatability antigens DR4 and D4. The association is strongest for the most severe forms of rheumatoid arthritis. Slow viruses have also been suspected to be of importance in the development of rheumatoid arthritis. Clinical features include both articular and extra-articular symptoms. The extra-articular symptoms are primarily general malaise, lassitude, weight loss, low grade fever, rheumatoid nodules, vasculitis, anemia; in rare cases, Sjogren's syndrome, ophthalmic manifestations, kerato conjunctivitis, and scleritis; respiratory manifestations such as pleurisy; cardiovascular manifestations, peripheral neuropathies, myelopathy (especially of the cervical region), and renal and hepatic dysfunctions. The articular manifestations are usually symmetrical, peripheral, with involvement of the hands and feet, and in rare cases, the hip. The cervical spine may be involved occasionally.

Laboratory evaluation includes elevated sedimentation rate, decrease in serum albumin, alpha-2 and gamma globulin, increase in IGA, IGG, and IGM presence of rheumatoid factors in approximately 75 percent of patients, presence of antinuclear antibodies, and an increased frequency of association with DR4 and D4 antigens.

The mechanism of pain in rheumatoid arthritis is mainly peripheral. The complications of chronic pain including substance abuse and depression may be seen in rheumatoid arthritis. Psychological factors do not play a major role in the development of rheumatoid arthritis. The management includes the use of analgesics, immunosuppressive drugs, corticosteroids, and surgery, where indicated, for improvement of function.

OSTEOARTHRITIS

The etiology of osteoarthritis is also uncertain. Osteoarthritis is a very severe, disabling illness. It is defined as a disease of the articular cartilage, characterized by destruction of the articular cartilage with secondary destruction of the subchondral bone. Symptomatic osteoarthritis is predominantly a disease of middle-aged women and it is usually polyarticular. The joints affected are the knees, hands, and, in rare cases, the hip. The pain is related to use of the joint, is worse at the end of the day, and is associated with stiffness. On examination there is a reduction of joint movement, and some evidence of inflammation and tenderness of the joint. Pain is considered in these diseases to be caused by a mechanical and chemical stimuli. The pain can arise from the cartilage, the synovium, periosteum bone, and the periarticular structures, rarely from the cartilage itself. Psychogenic factors may play a role in the development of pain in osteroarthritis.

The management of these patients is often symptomatic and directed primarily toward the relief of pain. In addition, physiotherapy for maintenance of the strength of muscles, and sometimes surgery for providing relief from pain as well as for improvement in function, is indicated.

CANCER

Cancer is one of the most frequent forms of chronic pain (117). Chronic cancer pain, unlike other forms of chronic pain, is unrelenting, progressive, and often part of the terminal process (118). We have included cancer pain in this section because most forms of cancer pain are secondary to the tumor or to the treatment of the tumor. In this section, we give a brief overview of the incidence, etiology, psychophysiology, and the psychological and physical sequelae of pain in malignant disease. Some of these specific modalities for cancer pain will be covered in Chapter 25.

EPIDEMIOLOGY

It is estimated that 700,000 cases of cancer are diagnosed in the U.S. each year (119) and that one-half of cancer patients die each year (119). Cancer is often not painful in the initial phases, but pain increases as the illness progresses. The pain increases and exacerbates the psychological and, probably the physiological process involved in the disease (120). Twenty to 50 percent of cancer patients experience pain at the time the cancer is diagnosed (121) (Table 18). Forty percent of patients in the intermediate stage of the illness have moderate to severe pain (121). Sixty to 80 percent of patients with advanced cancer experience pain (120, 122–125). McKegney and colleagues (126) reported that 80 percent of terminally ill cancer patients had experienced pain. Severity and frequency of pain complaints increased as death approached. Similarily, Cartwright and associates (127) reported that 87 percent of patients dying from cancer experienced pain, and the pain prior to death was poorly controlled. Inadequate control of cancer pain has been reported by other authors (127–129), and Twycross and Lack (130) estimated that 25 percent of cancer patients die without relief from pain, regardless of whether care was provided in the home or hospital. Twycross and Fairfield (123) found that 80 percent of patients with advanced cancer had more than one site of pain, and that 34 percent of patients had four sites of pain.

Pain complaints are most frequently reported by patients having cancer affecting bone (85 percent), cervix (80 percent) stomach (85 percent), lungs (70 precent), and pancreas (70 percent) (Table 19) (120). Pain is less frequently reported in patients having breast cancer, cancer of the kidney, colon, and rectal cancer. Pain is infrequent in patients with leukemia (120, 121).

Table 18. Frequency of Pain at Various Phases of Cancer

Phase of Illness	Frequency of Pain (%)
At time of diagnosis	20 to 50
Intermediate	40
Advanced	60 to 80
Terminal	80 to 87

Table 19. Types of Cancer Associated with Pain

Type of Cancer	Frequency of Pain (%)
Bone	85
Cervix	85
Stomach	85
Lung	70
Pancreas	70
Prostate	73
Oral	80
Liver	73
Urinary organs	68
Central nervous system	68
Lymphoma	20
Leukemia	5

Adapted from: Benedetti C, Bonica JJ: Cancer pain: basic considerations, in Advances in Pain Research and Therapy, vol. 1. Edited by Benedetti C, Chapman CR, Moricca G. New York, Raven Press, 1984; and Foley KM: Pain syndromes and patients with cancer, in Advances in Pain Research and Therapy, vol. 2. Edited by Bonica JJ, Ventafridda V. New York, Raven Press, 1979

ETIOLOGY AND CLASSIFICATION

The etiology of cancer pain can be classified into one of four categories (Table 20). Direct tumor involvement is the most common cause of cancer pain (121, 131). Between 62 and 78 percent of cancer pain is due to direct tumor involvement. Nineteen to 30 percent of cancer pain is due to cancer treatment. Three percent of pain in cancer patients is unrelated to cancer. Degenerative disc disease, myofascial pain syndromes, migraine headaches, and osteopenia are the common nonmalignant pain syndromes in cancer patients (121).

MECHANISM OF CHRONIC CANCER PAIN

Bonica (120) has classified the mechanisms of cancer into four categories: peripheral, peripheral-central, central, and psychological. The systems approach is an ideal way to conceptualize the various forms of cancer pain. Cancer pain secondary to direct tumor involvement is primarily due to peripheral or peripheral-central mechanisms with psychological and sociocultural factors modulating the pain. Central mechanisms are operative in pain as a result of damage to or compression of the spinal cord, brain stem, or parts of the brain following treatment, or directly due to the tumor itself. Again, psychological factors modulate the pain. Psychiatric disorders are seen in 40 to 50 percent of cancer patients. Thirteen percent of patients with psychological disorders have a major affective disorder, eight percent have an organic mental disorder, seven percent have a personality disorder, and four percent have anxiety disorder (132). Depression and anxiety are seen in 70 to 80 percent of patients with cancer (132). It is uncertain whether the pain

Table 20. Classification of Etiology of Cancer Pain

Cancer Pain by Causes
  Tumor infiltration of bone
    primary
    metastatic
  Tumor infiltration and compression of nerves
    peripheral neuropathy
    brachial plexus neuropathy
    sacral neuropathy
    lumbar neuropathy
  Tumor infiltration of blood vessels and lymphatics
    primary
    metastatic
  Tumor infiltration of hollow viscus and ducts
    primary
    metastatic
  Necrosis and infections secondary to tumor of pain sensitivity structures

Pain Syndromes Associated with Treatment of Malignant Disease
  Postsurgical pain (damage to nerves during surgery)
  Postchemotherapy/immunosuppressive therapy pain
    steroid-induced arthralgia, myalgia, osteopenia
    postherpetic neuralgia
    peripheral neuropathy
  Postradiation therapy pain
    neuropathy
    obstruction of hollow viscus
    radiation myelopathy
    postherpetic neuralgia
    fibrositis
  Pain unrelated to cancer
    arthritis
    low back pain
    migraine headache
    myofascial pain syndrome
  Psychological pain

Adapted from Ng LKY, Bonica JJ (Eds): Pain, Discomfort, and Humanitarian Care. New York, Elsevier/North Holland, 1980 these patients experience is associated with these disorders. Further study is needed.

PSYCHOLOGICAL AND PHYSICAL SEQUELAE IN CANCER PAIN

As we have noted in earlier sections, chronic pain can lead to several emotional and psychological reactions. These include anxiety, depression, somatization, hypochondriasis, denial, and regression. Similar changes are seen in patients with cancer. It is difficult to separate the psychological sequelae caused by pain from that caused by other factors in these patients. However, the above disturbances are seen commonly. Cancer patients have greater emotional distress resulting from pain than do patients with nonmalignant disease (133–137). The greater impact of cancer pain is related to the physical deterioration from the cancer as well as the treatment of the cancer, often fatal nature of the illness and perception of the illness.

Woodforde and Fielding (138) showed that cancer patients with pain had an increased incidence of depression, somatization, and hypochondriasis as compared to cancer patients without pain. Kissen (139) showed a reduction in the elevated level of emotional distress with successful treatment of the cancer pain. Bond (134) studied the levels of neuroticism in cancer pain patients before and after percutaneous cervical cordotomy and found that low preoperative values in some patients rose postoperatively when the pain was relieved. In patients with high preoperative values of neuroticism, the score fell postoperatively. Bond postulated that personality factors may be altered by the presence of the cancer pain, and relief of only the pain may restore a more normal state in the patient. Depression was the most common psychological disturbance. The combination of depression and intractable pain represent a state of helplessness and inability to cope with the cancer (136). In addition, cancer patients with pain tend to respond less well to chemotherapy and die sooner than cancer patients without pain. Bond (134) found that cancer patients with pain were more hypochondriacal than pain-free cancer patients.

From these studies it appears cancer patients with pain have significantly greater emotional distress than cancer patients who are pain-free. Therefore, treatment of the pain in these patients should also include reduction of the emotional tension as well as the symptomatic treatment of the pain itself. What is unclear from these studies is whether the greater emotional distress in cancer patients with pain is dependent upon the coping abilities of the patient or progression of the cancer. This clinical dilemma emphasizes the need to evaluate the following: 1) the patient's coping style before and after the development of the cancer; 2) the phase of the cancer, 3) the patient's accompanying psychiatric illness, 4) the patient's coping skill for pain control, and 5) the patient's social support system.

Cancer pain tends to intensify the interpersonal and social problems that often are seen in these patients. The emotional turmoil in cancer patients intensifies as the treatment aimed at the cancer itself fails. Feelings of depression develop in cancer patients with pain as they learn that the factors causing the pain cannot be eliminated. The ensuing depression can produce an escalation of the pain complaints in the cancer pain patients.

When suicide occurs in cancer patients, Holland (140) observed that it occurs in the late stages of the disease and in patients with limited psychological defenses and inability to adjust to the cancer. Suicide potential in cancer pain patients should be considered when the patient has a low tolerance for pain and discomfort (141).

Nehemkis and colleagues (142) demonstrated that cancer patients with an external locus of control (patients who ascribed their illness to fate) rated their pain as less severe than patients with an internal locus of control. The less the patients feel self-direction and control, the less they perceive any pain.

As pain occurs in the cancer patients, fear and anxiety develops over several issues: anticipation of further pain, progression of the cancer, physical disability, disfigurement, and death. In some patients the anxiety level becomes so high as to produce anxiety disorder. As stated in an earlier section, anxiety produces pain intolerance and increases pain behaviors.

Physical deterioration is most severe in cancer pain patients; they have greater sleep disturbance and a greater number of physical symptoms including nausea, vomiting, and appetite and weight loss. Cancer patients with moderate to severe pain report significant interference with their activity and enjoyment of life (122). The use of multiple medications to symptomatically treat the cancer pain—narcotics and antiemetics—exacerbate the above problems. Often, pain relief with narcotic medications is obtained at the expense of mental alertness if the medications are not properly adjusted.

REFERENCES

1. Friedman AP: Overview of migraine, in Advances in Neurology, vol. 33. Edited by Critchley M, Friedman AP, Gorini S, et al. New York, Raven Press, 1982
2. Connor RCR: Complicated migraine: a study of permanent neurological and visual defects caused by migraine. Lancet 2:1072–1075, 1962
3. Friedman AP: Medicine for migraine. Modern Medicine 48:36–49, 1980
4. Couch JR, Zeigler Dk, Hassarein R: Amitriptyline in the prophylaxis of migraine. Neurology 26:121–127, 1976

5. Graham JR: Methysergide for prevention of headache: experience in 500 patients over 3 years. N Engl J Med 270:67–72, 1964
6. Sargant JD, Green EE, Walters ED: Preliminary report on the use of autogenic feedback training in the treatment of migraine and tension headache. Psychosom Med 35:129–135, 1973
7. Kunkle EC: Clues in the tempos of cluster headaches. Headache 22:158–162, 1982
8. Fothergill J: Of a painful affection of the face. Medical Observations and Inquiries by a Society of Physicians (London) 5:129–142, 1773
9. Stookey B, Ranshoff J: Trigeminal Neuralgia. Springfield, Ill., Charles C Thomas, 1959
10. Loeser JD: Tic douloureux and atypical facial pain, in Textbook of Pain. Edited by Wall PD, Melzack R. New York, Churchill Livingstone, 1984
11. Kugeberg E, Lindblom U: The mechanism of pain in trigeminal neuralgia. J Neurol Neurosurg Psychiatry 22:36–43, 1959
12. Crill W: Carbamazepine. Ann Intern Med 79:79–80, 1983
13. Chimitz A, Seelinger DF, Greenhouse AH: Anticonvulsant therapy in trigeminal neuralgia. Am J Med Sci 252:62–67, 1966
14. Peiris JB, Perera GLS, Devendra SV, et al: Sodium valproate in trigeminal neuralgia. Med J Aust 2:278, 1980
15. King KR: The medical control of tic douloureux. J Neurosurg 26:175–180, 1967
16. Miles J: Trigeminal neuralgia, in Persistent Pain: Modern Methods of Treatment, vol. II. Edited by Lipton S. New York, Grune and Stratton, 1980
17. Janetta PJ: Microsurgical approach to the trigeminal nerve for tic douloureux. Progress in Neurological Surgery 7:180–200, 1975
18. Loeser JD: The management of tic douloureux. Pain 3:155–162, 1977
19. Munsford JM: Atypical facial pain, in Persistent Pain: Modern Methods of Treatment, vol. 2. Edited by Lipton S. New York, Grune and Stratton, 1980
20. Frazier CH: Neuralgia of the trigeminal tract and facial neuralgia of other origins. Ann Otol Rhin and Laryngol 30:855–869, 1921
21. Glazer MA: Atypical facial neuralgia: diagnosis, cause and treatment. Arch Intern Med 65:340–367, 1940
22. Moulton RE: Psychiatric considerations in maxillofacial pain. J Am Dent Assoc 51:409–415, 1955
23. Weddington W, Blazer DG: Atypical facial pain and trigminal neuralgia: a comparative study. Psychosomatics 20:348–353, 1979
24. Engel GL: Primary atypical facial neuralgia. Psychosom Med 13:375–396, 1951
25. Webb HE, Lascelles RG: Atypical facial pain. Lancet 1:355–357, 1962
26. Lascelles RG: Atypical facial pain and depresssion. Br J Psychiatry 112:651–659, 1966
27. West ED, Dally PJ: Anxiety, depression. Br Med J 1:1491–1499, 1959
28. Wolf S: Peptic ulcer. Psychosomatics 23:1101–1105, 1982
29. Alexander F: Psychosomatic Medicine. New York, W. W. Norton, 1950
30. Latimer PR: Irritable bowel syndrome. Psychosomatics 24:205–217, 1983
31. Blendis LM: Abdominal pain, in Textbook of Pain, Edited by Wall PD, Melzack R. New York, Churchill Livingstone, 1984

32. Esler MD, Goulston K: Levels of anxiety in colonic disorders. N Engl J Med 288:16–20, 1973

33. Hult L: The Munkfors investigation: a study of the frequency of stiff neck brachalgia and lumbago–sciatica syndrome, as well as observations on certain signs and symptoms from the dorsal spine. Acta Orthop Scand (Suppl 16):1–76, 1954

34. Horal J: The clinical appearance of low back disorders in the city of Gothenburg, Sweden. Acta Orthop Scand (Suppl 118):1–109, 1969

35. Rowe ML: Low back pain in industry: a position paper. J Occup Med 11:161–169, 1969

36. Troup JDG, Martin JW, Lloyd DCEF: Back pain in industry. Spine 6:61-68, 1981

37. Curry HLF, Greenwood RM, Lloyd GG, et al: A prospective of low back pain. Rheumatology Rehabilitation 18:94–104, 1979

38. Hult L: Cervical dorsal and lumbar spinal syndromes. Acta Orthop Scand (Suppl 17):1–102, 1954

39. Lawrence JS: Disc degeneration—its frequency and relationship to symptoms. Annals of Rheumatoid Disease 28:121–136, 1969

40. Schaepe JL: Low back pain: an occupational perspective, in Chronic Low Back Pain. Edited by Hicks S, Bocus R. New York, Raven Press, 1982

41. Dixon ASJ: Diagnosis of low back pain—sorting the complaints, in The Lumbar Spine and Back Pain. Edited by Tayson M. New York, Grune and Stratton, 1976

42. Fry J: Back pain and soft tissue rheumatism. London, Advisory Services Colloquium Proceedings (Advisory Services, Clinical and General Ltd), 1972

43. Ansell BM: Ankylosing Spondylitis. Arthritis Rheum 20(Suppl):414–415, 1977

44. Calabro JJ: Early diagnosis and management of ankylosing spondylitis. Med Times 105:80–96, 1977

45. Calvin A, Porta J, Fries JF, et al: Clinical history as a screening test for ankylosing spondylitis. JAMA 237:2613–2623, 1977

46. White AA, Panjabi MM: Clinical biomechanics of the spine, in Kimematics of the Spine. Edited by White AA, Panjabi MM. Philadelphia, JB Lippincott, 1978

47. Spangfort EW: Lumbar disc herniation: a computer aided analysis of 2504 operations. Acta Orthop Scand (Suppl) 142:1–95, 1972

48. Nachemson A: The lumbar spone, an orthopaedic challenge. Spine 1:59–71, 1976

49. Spengler DM: Low back pain assessment and management. New York, Grune & Stratton, 1982

50. Hicks MS, Bocus RA: Chronic low back pain. New York, Raven Press, 1982

51. Hoppenfelds S: Physical examination of the lumbar spine, in Physical Examination of the Spine and Extremities. Edited by Hoppenfeld S. New York, Appleton-Century-Crofts, 1976

52. Crock HV: Traumatic disc injury, in Injuries of the Spine and Spinal Cord. Edited by Vinken PJ, Bruyn GW. Amsterdam, Elsevier North Holland, 1976

53. Frymoler JW, Pole MH, Lostranga MC: Epidemiologic studies of low back pain. Spine 5:419–423, 1980
54. Jeffcoate TNA: Pelvic pain. Br Med J 3:431–435, 1969
55. Renaer M: Gynecological pain, in Textbook of Pain. Edited by Wall PD, Melzack R. London, Churchill Livingstone, 1984
56. Renaer M, Guzinski GM: Pain in gyneocologic practice. Pain 5:305–331, 1978
57. Gross RJ, Doerr H, Caldirola D, et al: Borderline syndrome and incest in chronic pelvic pain patients. Int J Psychiatry Med 10:79–96, 1980
58. Friederick MA: Psychological aspects of chronic pelvic pain. Clin Obstet Gynecol 19:399–406, 1976
59. Benson RC, Hanson KH, Matarazzo JD: Atypical pelvic pain in women: gynecologic-psychiatric consideration. Am J Obstet Gynecol 77:806–825, 1959
60. Gidro-Frank L, Gordon T, Taylor HC: Pelvic pain and female identity. Am J Obstet Gynecol 79:1184–1202, 1960
61. Renaer M: Chronic pelvic pain without obvious pathology in women. Eur J Obstet Gynecol Reprod Biol 10:415–463, 1980
62. Duncan CH, Taylor HC: A psychosomatic study of pelvic congestion. Am J Obstet Gynecol 64:1–12, 1952
63. Taylor HC: Pelvic pain based on vascular and autonomic nervous system disorder. Am J Obstet Gynecol 66:1177–2296, 1954
64. Allen WM, Masters WH: Traumatic laceration of uterine support. Am J Obstet Gynecol 70:500–513, 1955
65. Murphy TM: Profiles of pain patients, including chronic pelvic pain, in New Approaches to Treatment of Chronic Pain. University of Washington Clinical Pain Services. National Institute on Drug Abuse Monograph 36:122–129, 1981
66. Castelnuovo-Tedesco P, Krout BM: Psychosomatic Aspects of Chronic Pelvic Pain. Int J Psychiatry Med 1:109–126, 1970
67. Renaer M, Vertommen H, Nys P, et al: Psychological Aspects of Chronic Pelvic Pain in Women. Am J Obstet Gynecol 134:75–80, 1979
68. Rosenthal RH, Ling FW, Rosenthal TL, et al: Chronic pelvic pain: psychiatric and laparoscopic findings. Psychosomatics 25:833–841, 1984
69. Sternbach RA, Wolf SR, Murphy RW, et al: Aspects of chronic low back pain. Psychosomatics 14:52–56, 1973
70. Bond MR: Pain and Personality in Cancer Patients, in Advances in Pain Research and Therapy, vol 1. Edited by Bonica JJ, Albe-Fessard D. New York, Raven Press, 1976
71. Woodforde J, Merskey H: Personality traits of patients with chronic pain. J Psychosom Res 16:156–172, 1972
72. Scadding JW: Peripheral neuropathies, in Textbook of Pain. Edited by Wall PD, Melzack R. New York, Churchill Livingstone, 1984
73. Lhermitte J, Nicolas M: Les lesions spinales du zana: la myelite zosterienne. Revue Neurologigue 1:361–364, 1924
74. Melzack R: Central mechanisms in phantom limb pain, in Advances in Neurology, vol. 4. New York, Raven Press, 1974
75. Sherman RA, Sherman CT, Parker L: Chronic phantom and stump pain

among American veterans: results of survey. Pain 18:83–95, 1984

76. Carlen PL, Wall PD, Nodvorna H, et al: Phantom limbs and related phenomena in recent traumatic amputations. Neurology 28:211–217, 1978

77. Weinstein S, Sersen EA: Phantoms in cases of congenital absence of limbs. Neurology 11:905–911, 1961

78. Simmel ML: Phantom experiences following amputation in childhood. J Neurol Neurosurg Psychiatry 25:69–78, 1962

79. Parkes CM: Factors determining the persistence of phantom pain in the amputee. J Psychosom Res 17:97–108, 1973

80. Melzack R: Phantom limb pain; implications of treatment of pathologic pain. Anesthesiology 35:409–419, 1971

81. Jensen TS, Rasmussen P: Amputation, in Textbook of Pain. Edited by Wall PD, Melzack R. London, Churchill Livingstone, 1984

82. Jamison K, Wellisch DK, Koty RL, et al: Phantom breast syndrome. Arch Surg 114:93–95, 1979

83. Weinstein S, Vetter RJ, Sersen EA: Phantoms following breast amputation. Neuropsychologia 8:185–197, 1970

84. Boas RA: Phantom anus pain syndrome, in Advances in Pain Research and Therapy, vol. 5. Edited by Bonica JJ, Lindblom U, Iggo A. New York, Raven Press, 1983

85. Breno SF, Sammons EE: Phantom urinary bladder pain—case report. Pain 7:197–201, 1979

86. Sherman RA, Gall N, Gosmby J: Treatment of phantom limb pain with muscular relaxation training to disrupt the pain-anxiety-tension cycle. Pain 6:47–55, 1979

87. Sherman RA, Sherman CJ, Gall NG: A survery of current phantom limb pain treatment in the United States. Pain 8:85–99, 1980

88. Nashold BS, Urban B, Zorub DS: Phantom pain relief by focal destruction of the substantia gelatinosa of Rolando, in Advances in Pain Research and Therapy, vol 1. Edited by Bonica JJ, Albe-Fessard D. New York, Raven Press, 1976

89. Urban BJ, France RD, Steinberger EK, et al: Long term use of narcotic/antidepressant medication in the management of phantom limb pain. Pain 24:191–196, 1986

90. Smith TR: The thalamic pain syndrome. Minn Med 55:257–261, 1972

91. Melzack R, Loeser JD: Phantom body pain in paraplegics: evidence for a central "pattern generating mechanism" for pain. Pain 4:195–210, 1978

92. Gutterman L: Spinal Injuries: Comprehensive Management and Research. Oxford, Blackwell, 1973

93. Botterell EH, Callaghan JC, Jousse AT: Pain in paraplegia: clinical management and surgical treatment. Proceedings of the Royal Society of Medicine 47:281–282, 1954

94. Pagni CA: Central pain due to spinal cord and brain stem damage, in Textbook of Pain. Edited by Wall PD, Melzack R. London, Churchill Livingstone, 1984

95. Pagni CA: Pain due to central nervous system lesion: physiopathological considerations and therapeutical implications. Adv Neurol 4:339–348, 1974

96. Davis L, Martin J: Studies upon spinal cord injuries, II: the nature and

treatment of pain. J Neurosurg 4:483–491, 1947

97. Moldofsky H, Lue FA: The relationship of alpha and delta EEG frequencies to pain and mood in fibrositis patients treated with chlorpromazine and L-tryptophan. Electro-encephalogr Clin Neurophysiol 50:73–80, 1980

98. Simons DG: Muscle pain syndromes, part I. Am J Phys Med 54:289–311, 1975

99. Simons DG: Muscle pain syndromes, part II. Am J Phys Med 55:15–42, 1976

100. Award EA: Interstitial myofibrositis. Arch Phys Med Rehabil 54:440–453, 1973

101. Hunter C: Myalagia of the abdominal wall. Can Med Assoc J 28:157–161, 1933

102. Mikhail M, Rosen H: History and aetiology of MPD syndrome. J Prosthet Dent 44:438–44, 1980

103. Moldofsky H: Psychogenic Rheumatism or the fibrositis syndrome, in Modern Trends in Psychosomatic Medicine, vol. 3. Edited by Hill O. Boston, Butterworths, 1976

104. Lamo T: The role of activity in the control of membrane and contractile properties of skeletal muscle, in Motor Innervation of Muscle. Edited by Thesleff S. London, Academic Press, 1976

105. Edagawa N, Friedman LW: The Treatment of Disordered Function. Smithtown, New York, Exposition Press, 1981

106. Henrikkson KD, Bengtsson A, Larson J, et al: Muscle biopsy findings of possible diagnostic importance in primary fibromyalgia. Lancet 2:1395, 1982

107. Yunus M, Mori AT, Calabro JJ, et al: Primary fibromyalgia (fibrositis): clinical study of 50 patients with matched normal controls. Semin Arthritis Rheum 11:151–171, 1981

108. Travell JC, Simons DG: Myofascial pain and dysfunction: The Trigger Point Manual. Baltimore, Williams & Wilkins, 1983

109. Hudson JI, Hudson MS, Plines LF, et al: Fibrositis related to major affective disorder by phenomenology and family history. Am J Psychiatry 142:441-446, 1985

110. Smythe HA: Non-articular rheumatism and the fibrositis syndrome, in Arthritis and Allied Conditions. Edited by Hollander JL, McCarty DJ Jr. Philadelphia, Lea and Febiger, 1972

111. Beetham WP: Diagnosis and management of fibrositis syndrome and psychogenic rheumatism. Med Clin North Am 63:433–439, 1979

112. Klinefelter HF: Primary fibrositis and its treatment with the pyrazolane derivatives, butazolidin and tandearil. John Hopkins Medical Journal 130:300–307, 1972

113. Boland EW: Psychogenic rheumatism: the musculoskeletal expression of psychoneurosis. Am Rheum Dis 6:195–203, 1947.

114. Sola AE: Treatment of myofascial pain syndrome, in Advances in Pain Research and Therapy, vol. 7. Edited by Benedetti C, Chapman CR, Moricca G. New York, Raven Press, 1984

115. Travell J: Ethyl chloride spray for painful muscle spasm. Arch Phys Med 33:291–298, 1952

116. Travell J: Myofascial trigger points: clinical view, in Advances in Pain

Research and Therapy, vol. 1. Edited by Bonica JJ, Albe-Fessard D. New York, Raven Press, 1976

117. Report on the Panel on Pain to the National Advisory Neurological and Communicative Disorders and Stoke Council. National Institute of Health Publication No 81-1912. Washington, DC, U.S. Government Printing Office, 1979

118. Holden C: Pain, dying, and the health care system. Science 203:984–985, 1979

119. American Cancer Society: Cancer Facts and Figures. New York, American Cancer Society, 1978

120. Ng LKY, Bonica JJ (EJS): Pain, Discomfort and Humanitarian Care. New York, Elsevier/North Holland, 1980

121. Foley KM: Pain syndromes in patients with cancer, in Advances in Pain Research and Therapy, vol. 2. Edited by Bonica JJ, Ventafridda V. New York, Raven Press, 1979

122. Daut RL, Cleeland CS: The prevalence and severity of pain in cancer. Cancer 50:1913–1918, 1982

123. Twycross RG, Fairfield S: Pain in far-advanced cancer. Pain 14:303–310, 1982

124. Pannuti E, Martoni A, Rossi AP, et al: The role of endocrine therapy for relief of pain due to advanced cancer, in Advances in Pain Research and Therapy, vol. 2, Proceedings of the International Symposium on Pain of Advanced Cancer. Edited by Bonica JJ, Ventafridda V. New York, Raven Press, 1979

125. Parkes CM: Home or hospital? Terminal care as seen by surviving spouse. J R Coll Gen Pract 28:19–30, 1978

126. McKegney FP, Bailey LR, Yates YW: Prediction and management of pain in patients with advanced cancer. Gen Hosp Psychiatry 3:95–101, 1981

127. Cartwright A, Hockey L, Anderson ABM: Treatment of pain in patients with advanced cancer, in Life Before Death. Edited by Gybels J, Andreaesen H, Cosyns P. London, Routledge and Kegan Paul, 1973

128. McGivney WT, Crooks GM: The care of patients with severe chronic pain in terminal illness. JAMA 251:1182–1188, 1984

129. Marks RD, Sachs EJ: Undertreatment of medical inpatients with narcotic analgesics. Ann Intern Med 78:173–181, 1973

130. Twycross RG, Lack SA: Symptom Control in Far Advanced Cancer: Pain Relief. London, Pitman, 1983

131. Benedetti C, Bonica JJ: Cancer pain: basic considerations in Advances in Pain Research and Therapy, vol. 7. Edited by Benedetti C, Chapman CR, Moricca G. New York, Raven Press, 1984.

132. Derogatis LR, Morrow GR, Getting J, et al: The prevalence of psychiatric disorders among cancer patients. JAMA 249:751–757, 1983

133. Bond MR: The relationship of pain to the Eysenck Personality Inventory, Cornell Medical Index, and Whitely Index of Hypochrondriasis. Br J Psychiatry 119:671–678, 1971

134. Bond MR: Psychologic and emotional aspects of cancer pain, in Advances in Pain Research and Therapy, vol. 2. Edited by Bonica JJ, Ventafridda V. New York, Raven Press, 1979

135. Bond MR, Pearson IB: Psychologic aspects of pain in woman with advanced cancer of the cervix. J Psychosom Res 13:13–19, 1969

136. Bonica JJ: Cancer pain: importance of the problem, in Advances in Pain Research and Therapy, vol. 2. Edited by Bonica JJ, Ventafridda V. New York, Raven Press, 1979

137. Bonica JJ: The Management of Pain. Philadelphia, Lea and Febiger, 1953

138. Woodforde JM, Fielding JR: Pain and cancer, in Pain, Clinical and Experimental Perspectives. Edited by Weisenburg M. St. Louis, Mosby, 1975

139. Kissen DM: The influence of some environmental factors on personality inventory scores in psychosomatic research. J Psychosom Res 8:145–152, 1964

140. Holland J: Psychological aspects of cancer, in Cancer Medicine. Edited by Holland JF, Frei E. Philadelphia, Lea and Febiger, 1973

141. Forman BF: Cancer and suicide. Gen Hosp Psychiatry 20:108–114, 1979

142. Nehemkis AM, Chester RA, Stampp M, et al: The meaning of pain to the cancer patient: the role of attribution theory. Pain (Suppl 1):570, 1981

Chapter 11

Depression as a Psychopathological Disorder in Chronic Pain

K. Ranga Rama Krishnan, M.D.

Randal D. France, M.D.

Jonathan Davidson, M.D.

In Chapter 10 we mentioned that depression is a complication or se-quelae of chronic pain syndromes. In this chapter we will expand our discussion of depression as a psychopathological disorder occurring secondary to chronic pain. Figure 1 highlights the development and occurrence of depression in chronic pain patients.

In evaluating chronic pain patients, it should be kept in mind that there may be at least four possible relationships between pain and de-pression: 1) pain may be a symptom of depression; 2) depression may be a complication of chronic pain; 3) pain and depression are linked inex-tricably; and 4) pain and depression coexist but are not related. In some syndromes, such as idiopathic atypical facial pain, the pain and depres-sion are so closely linked that it is often difficult to say exactly what the relationship is. Conceptually, in most such instances, pain is thought of as part of the symptom complex of depression. In others, depression and other organic/sociocultural/personality factors are believed to lead to the occurrence of pain.

In this chapter we will examine the following aspects of depression as a complication in chronic pain patients:

1. depression as a normal illness behavior
2. the prevalence of depression in chronic pain patients
3. the different subtypes of depression in chronic pain patients
4. the clinical characteristics of depression in chronic pain patients
5. neuroendocrine markers for depression in chronic pain patients

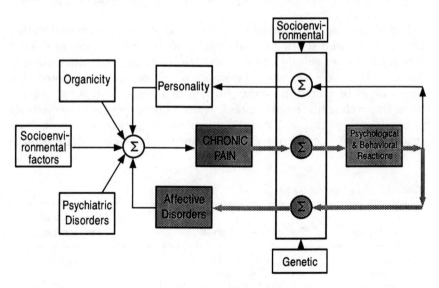

Figure 1. Systems model for chronic pain: pathogenesis of affective disorders in chronic pain

6. genetic factors in the development of depression in these patients
7. socioenvironmental factors
8. theories behind the development of depression in these patients

Depression as a Normal Illness Behavior

Nelson Hendler considers depression to be a normal illness behavior in patients with chronic pain (1, 2). He states that almost all chronic pain patients will pass through a period of depression (2). He describes conceptually a four-stage response to pain akin to the stages of dying described by Kubler-Ross. The four stages, listed in Table 1, are described below:

Stage I (Acute). This is the initial stage following pain. During this time both the patient and physician are hopeful that the pain will get better. Little or no depression is seen during this stage.
Stage II (Subacute). In the second stage the patient grows more worried about the pain and seeks further help for it. Again, depression is rare during this stage.
Stage III (Chronic). In this stage the patient begins to believe that the pain will be permanent and thus feels hopeless, helpless, and depressed.
Stage IV (Subchronic). During this stage the patient moves toward accepting the reality of pain and starts to make changes to cope with the physical, social, and psychological aspects of the condition. During this stage patients become less depressed if they cope well. (1, pp. 2–8)

It must be noted that these are stages based on clinical experiences that have not yet been studied or validated. They should not be considered rigidly but rather should be taken as a useful method of understanding the ways in which patients cope with pain. It must also be noted that these stages of pain apply more to pain that has at least some organic basis. In psychogenic pain, depression also may be seen, but the methods of coping are often poor, and the subchronic stage is seldom seen. The relationship between depression as an illness behavior and depression as

Table 1. Pain Response Stages

Stage	Period	Presence of Depression
Acute	0–2 months	(−)
Subacute	2–6 months	(−)
Chronic	6 months – 8 years	(+)
Subchronic	3–12 years	(+)

a psychopathological disorder is unclear, as is the difference between the two. Just as grief following a loss can precipitate depression as a psychopathological disorder, so too can loss secondary to chronic pain precipitate depression. It is therefore not uncommon to see depression as a psychopathological disorder in the chronic stage.

Prevalence of Depression in Chronic Pain Patients

Despite several studies of depression in chronic pain syndromes, the data concerning its prevalence can best be described as unreliable. Depression in chronic pain patients has been reported to vary from less than 10 percent up to 100 percent. Table 2 lists the major studies in which the prevalence of depression was assessed, and notes the methods used in making the assessment. The wide variance in the prevalence of depression is probably due to any one or more of the following factors:

1. the definition of depression: that is, symptom, mood or syndrome (and, if syndrome, the criteria used, if any)

Table 2.   Prevalence of Depression in Chronic Pain Patients

Study	Criteria	Assessment	Number	Percent of Depression
Blumer and Heilbronn (3)	none	psychological tests, Rorschach, TAT*	89	83
Hill and Blendis (4)	unclear	? interview	27	22
Large (5)	unclear	? interview	127	31
Lascelles (6)	unclear, ?	interview	53	100
Lindsay and Wyckoff (7)	RDC**	unstructured interview	300	87
Maruta et al. (8)	unclear	chart review	31	16
France et al. (9)	RDC	unstructured	80	21†
Krishnan et al. (10)	RDC	semistructured (SADS-L)***	71	43†
Kramlinger et al. (11)	RDC	? interview	100	25†
Pilowsky et al. (12)	unclear	LPDQ****	100	10
Turkington (13)	Kupfer-Detre system	interview	59	100
Wilson et al. (14)	unclear	interview	36	78

   * TAT = Thematic Apperception Test
  ** RDC = Research Diagnostic Criteria
 *** SADS-L = Schedule of Affective Disorders and Schizophrenia—Lifetime Version
**** LPDQ = Levine-Pilowsky Depression Questionnaire
† = Major depression
? = not specified; probably clinical interview

2. the nature of the chronic pain: that is, the site, presence or absence of organic finding, duration of pain, and so on (in previous chapters we have emphasized the importance of assessing these qualities of chronic pain and not considering them as single entities)

3. the setting: whether the study was carried out in an outpatient clinic, private practice, family practice, mental health center, tertiary care center, or pain clinic

4. variability in the assessment procedures: self-report, psychological testing, clinical interview, semistructured interview, or structured interview

Only four studies used Research Diagnostic Criteria (RDC) for assessing depression. Kramlinger and colleagues noted that 25 percent of chronic pain patients also satisfied RDC criteria for major depression (11). Lindsey and Wyckoff (7) reported that 31 percent of 300 patients were depressed by RDC criteria. The other two studies were done by Krishnan and France, the details of which are noted in the next subsection.

SUBTYPES OF DEPRESSION

As noted earlier, most of the studies did not define the type of depression they were trying to identify. Pilowsky and colleagues noted that the incidence of endogenous depression was low in chronic pain patients, but did not state the criteria used for diagnosing endogenous depression (12). The incidence of major depression as defined by RDC was found to vary from 20 to 43 percent (7, 9–11). The lowest figure (20 percent) was found at a point of first entry into the pain program (9). The highest incidence was found on an inpatient pain management unit (10). This indicates that the setting influences the rate of occurrence of major depression. Almost all patients with major depression have primary depression as defined by RDC criteria. The depression may be classified as endogenous in a small percentage of these patients; that is, between 5 and 14 percent (10, 15).

Table 3 gives the incidence of the different subtypes of depression in our two studies. The importance of the setting in which the study is done can be seen clearly on the table. Depending upon the site of the study, the incidence of the different types of depression varies. The study by Krishnan and colleagues (10) was done primarily on an inpatient pain management program, while the data from France and colleagues (9) was mostly generated at the outpatient level.

The relation between different subtypes of depression and organic pathology is another topic inadequately addressed in the literature on chronic pain. In the study conducted by Krishnan and colleagues, the

Table 3. Subtypes of Depression

Study	Not Depressed (%)	Major Depression (%)	Minor Depression (%)	Intermittent Depression (%)
France et al. (9)	21	21	8	51
Krishnan et al. (10)	21	43	11	25

incidence of major depression was found to be twice as high in patients without organic findings as in those with organic findings (10).

CLINICAL CHARACTERISTICS OF DEPRESSION AND ANXIETY IN CHRONIC PAIN PATIENTS

Krishnan and colleagues (10, 16), in their study of 71 chronic low back pain patients, reported on the item analysis of the modified and expanded Hamilton Depression Rating Scale (Ham-D) (10), the Montgomery-Asberg Depression Rating Scale (MADRS), and the modified and expanded Hamilton Anxiety Scale (Ham-A) (16). A brief summary of the findings from that study will now be presented.

Symptoms of Depression

In general, the degree of guilt was low in chronic low back pain patients with different types of depression. Patients with chronic pain and major depression differed from those without depression on all items of the Ham-D and MADRS (Tables 4 and 5).

Patients with chronic pain and major depression differed significantly from chronic pain patients without depression on the following items of the Ham-D Scale: depressed mood, suicidal ideation, middle insomnia, less involvement with work and interests, somatic anxiety, and general somatic symptoms, all of which were more frequent in the major depression group (Table 4). They differed on almost all of the MADRS (Table 5). Again, chronic pain patients with major depression have an increased frequency of these items than patients without depression.

Chronic pain patients with major depression differed from those with intermittent depressive disorder on almost all items of the Ham-D and MDRS. It is interesting to note that increased appetite was more common in those with intermittent depressive disorders (Tables 4 and 5).

Somatic anxiety and general somatic symptoms were seen more often in patients with minor depression than in those patients with intermittent depressive disorder. Increased appetite and diurnal variation with mood worse in the morning was more common in those patients with intermittent depressive disorder (Table 4).

Depressed mood, guilt, reduced work and interests, psychomotor retardation, gastrointestinal symptoms, and loss of libido are the major Ham-D items that are less frequently seen in chronic pain patients with no depression, as opposed to those with minor depression (Table 4). Apparent sadness, reported sadness, inner tension, reduced appetite, concentration difficulties, lassitude, and reduced interest are the major MADRS items that discriminate between chronic pain patients with

Table 4. HAM-D Items Discriminating Chronic Pain Patients Without Depression and with Different Subtypes of Depression

Item	Major D vs Minor D	Major D vs Inter-mediate D	Major D vs No D	Minor D vs Inter-mediate D	Minor D vs No D	Inter-mediate D vs No D
Depressed mood	x	x	x	ns	x	x
Guilt	ns	x	x	ns	x	x
Suicide	x	x	x	ns	ns	ns
Initial insomnia	ns	ns	x	ns	ns	ns
Middle insomnia	x	ns	x	ns	ns	ns
Delayed insomnia	ns	ns	x	ns	ns	ns
Hypersomnia	ns	ns	ns	ns	ns	ns
Work and interest	x	x	x	ns	x	ns
Retardation	ns	x	x	ns	x	ns
Agitation	ns	ns	ns	ns	ns	ns
Psychic anxiety	ns	x	x	ns	ns	ns
Somatic anxiety	x	x	x	x	ns	ns
GI symptoms	ns	x	x	ns	x	ns
Increased appetite	ns	x	ns	x	ns	ns
General somatic	x	x	x	x	ns	ns
Loss of libido	ns	x	x	ns	x	ns
Increased libido	ns	ns	ns	ns	ns	x
Hypochondriasis	ns	x	x	ns	ns	ns
Loss of insight	x	x	ns	ns	ns	ns
Loss of weight	ns	x	x	ns	ns	ns
Gain of weight	ns	ns	ns	ns	ns	ns
Diurnal variation (PM)	ns	ns	x	x	ns	ns
Diurnal variation (AM)	ns	ns	ns	ns	ns	ns
Depersonalization	ns	ns	ns	ns	ns	ns
Paranoid symptoms	ns	ns	ns	ns	ns	ns
Obsessional symptoms	ns	ns	ns	ns	ns	ns

D = Depression
ns = not significant
x = $p < 0.05$

Table 5. MADRS Items Discriminating Chronic Pain Patients Without Depression and with Different Subtypes of Depression

Item	Major D vs Minor D	Major D vs Inter-mediate D	Major D vs No D	Minor D vs Inter-mediate D	Minor D vs No D	Inter-mediate D vs No D
Apparent sadness	x	x	x	ns	x	x
Reported sadness	x	x	x	ns	x	x
Inner tension	ns	x	x	ns	x	ns
Reduced sleep	ns	x	x	ns	ns	ns
Reduced appetite	ns	x	x	x	x	ns
Reduced concentration	x	x	x	ns	x	x
Lassitude	x	x	x	ns	x	x
Reduced interests	x	x	x	ns	x	x
Pessimistic thoughts	x	x	x	ns	x	ns
Suicidal thoughts	x	x	x	ns	ns	ns

D = Depression
ns = not significant
x = $p < 0.05$

minor depression from those without depression (Table 5), with these items being less frequently seen in patients with no depression.

Depressed mood, guilt, and loss of libido are all items on the Ham-D scale that are more frequently observed in patients with intermittent depressive disorder (IDD) as compared to those without depression. Apparent sadness, reported sadness, concentration difficulties, lassitude, and reduced interests are the items on the MADRS that are likewise more often seen in the chronic pain patient with IDD than those without depression (Tables 4 and 5).

Symptoms of Anxiety

Symptoms of anxiety are frequently seen in chronic pain patients. In general, symptoms of anxiety are more common in chronic pain patients with major depression. Anxious mood, tension, insomnia, cognitive symptoms, general somatic symptoms, gastrointestinal symptoms, genitourinary symptoms, and autonomic symptoms are more common in chronic pain patients with major depression than those without depression (Table 6). Patients with major depression differed from those with minor depression, and reported greater cognitive impairment and a greater number of general somatic and autonomic symptoms (Table 6).

Patients with intermittent depressive disorder reported less anxious mood, tension, fears, general somatic symptoms, autonomic symptoms,

Table 6. HAM-A Items Discriminating Chronic Pain Patients Without Depression and with Different Subtypes of Depression

Item	Major D vs Minor D	Major D vs Intermediate D	Major D vs No D	Minor D vs Intermediate D	Minor D vs No D	Intermediate D vs No D
Anxious mood	ns	x	x	ns	ns	ns
Tension	ns	x	x	ns	ns	ns
Fears	ns	x	ns	ns	ns	ns
Insomnia	ns	ns	x	ns	ns	ns
Cognitive	x	x	x	ns	x	ns
Depressed mood	x	x	x	ns	x	x
General somatic—						
muscular	x	x	x	ns	ns	x
sensory	x	x	x	ns	ns	x
Cardiovascular	ns	ns	ns	ns	ns	ns
Respiratory	ns	ns	ns	ns	ns	ns
Gastrointestinal	ns	x	x	x	x	ns
Genito-urinary	ns	x	x	ns	ns	ns
Autonomic symptoms	x	x	x	ns	ns	ns
Behavior at interview	x	x	x	ns	x	ns

D = Depression
ns = not significant
x = $p < 0.05$

gastrointestinal symptoms, and genitourinary symptoms than those with major depression (Table 6).

Patients with minor depression reported a greater number of gastrointestinal symptoms than those patients with intermittent depressive disorder. Otherwise there is very little difference between the two groups. Chronic pain patients with minor depression differ from those without depression by exhibiting an increase in general somatic, cognitive symptoms and gastrointestinal symptoms, along with more anxious behavior at the time of interview on the Ham-A (Table 6). Patients with intermittent depressive disorder have more general somatic symptoms than those without depression. Other symptoms of anxiety are very similar (Table 6).

Chronic low back pain patients with major depression can be discriminated clearly from those patients without depression and from those patients with other subtypes of depression. Discrimination between minor depression and intermittent depressive disorder is often difficult on symptom analysis alone; a temporal analysis of symptoms tends to be more useful.

Vegetative Symptoms of Depression

The study just referred to points to the importance of assessing neurovegetative symptoms of depression in chronic pain patients. We know little about the neurovegetative changes that accompany chronic pain, and whether these changes have any diagnostic significance in the differential diagnosis of depression and chronic pain. Is chronic pain alone associated with a different neurovegetative profile from that seen in depression? Does depression with pain differ from depression alone? And yet another question arises as to whether the low-grade minor depressions in chronic pain have characteristic neurovegetative symptoms. These questions will be addressed in this section. By vegetative symptoms we mean changes in sleep, weight, appetite, libido, and diurnal variation of mood.

Insomnia has been traditionally accepted as one of the earliest signs of depression, often preceding psychological manifestations of the illness. It is one of the first heralds of recovery (17). Although some authorities consider early awakening to indicate endogenous depression (18), others dispute this (19, 20) and assert that early awakening is a reflection of severity, and not type, of depression (21), or that it is merely a function of age (22). Loss of appetite and loss of weight also are seen characteristically early in depression. Reduced libido is a frequent symptom, as is diurnal variation of mood, with worsening in the morning and improvement in the evening being characteristic of melancholia. There is some evidence that diurnal variation disappears once the illness becomes severe (23, 24), although it is unclear how reliably this can be taken as a measure of severity (25). The importance of neurovegetative symptoms in gauging the severity of depression is reflected by their prominent inclusion in the Ham-D (26).

In 1956, Post (27) described the occurrence of increased appetite as an occasional symptom of depression. Pollitt and Young (28) later dichotomized the vegetative symptoms into typical and atypical types. Typical symptoms comprised early awakening, loss of weight, loss of appetite, loss of libido, and diurnal variation of mood, which was worse in the morning. Atypical symptoms included initial insomnia, increased sleep, increased appetite, increased weight, increased libido, and worsening of mood in the evening. We have presented evidence elsewhere that the symptom of initial insomnia is better regarded as a typical symptom of depression (29), but in this report we will adhere to the traditional view that it is an atypical symptom.

Although traditionally viewed as being characteristic of melancholia, there is little substantial evidence that the typical vegetative symptoms actually have predictive value for this particular diagnosis. Elsewhere (30) we have reviewed and compared five principal sets of diagnostic criteria for melancholia. We noted that no vegetative symptom appeared in more than three of these sets, with anorexia and loss of weight being represented most frequently. We (29, 30) and Nelson and Charney (31) have both concluded that the vegetative symptoms are uncertain diagnostic indicators for melancholia. It may be more appropriate to view them as indicators of major depression, which exist in more severe form in melancholia.

In our survey (29), we found a high incidence of typical vegetative features in both melancholia and nonmelancholia, applicable both to DSM-III and Newcastle diagnostic criteria. Increased appetite had a 100 percent predictive value for the diagnosis of nonmelancholia in the DSM-III diagnosis, and a 99 percent predictive value in the Newcastle scale. Increased weight possessed a predictive value of 83 percent for nonmelancholia by the Newcastle Index, and worsening of mood in the evening carried a 78 percent predictive value for nonmelancholia with the Newcastle scale. When we used selected diagnostic criteria for melancholia derived from our literature review (30), we found that increased appetite had a 78 percent predictive value for nonmelancholia, and worsening of mood in the morning had a 74 percent predictive value for melancholia. Our conclusion is that, by and large, the traditional vegetative symptoms do not usefully predict melancholia as against nonmelancholia, although diurnal variation of mood (worse in the morning) may have some predictive value for melancholia. The atypical symptoms of increased appetite and weight, and worsening of mood in the evening, apparently have some diagnostic utility in nonmelancholia.

Frequency of Vegetative Symptoms

We examined the frequency of each neurovegetative symptom in a population of 92 depressed inpatients and outpatients without chronic pain who entered a series of clinical antidepressant drug trials. Sleep disturbances were the most common symptoms, with initial insomnia appearing in 93 percent and early awakening in 82 percent of cases. Loss of appetite occurred 66 percent of the time, loss of weight 57 percent, and loss of libido 62 percent. Diurnal variation of mood was uncommon, with worsening of mood in the evening being present in 32 percent, while worsening in the morning was present in 24 percent. The four atypical symptoms were uncommon, the 15 percent incidence of increased appetite corresponding to other reports in the literature (32).

This led us to conduct a more detailed study of neurovegetative symptoms in chronic pain patients without depression, with different subtypes of depression, and in control patients with major depression (15). We used the modified and expanded Ham-D and the Vegetative Symptom Scale.

In the chronic pain group, 24 had major depression, 21 had minor or intermittent depression, and 12 had no depression. The frequency of symptoms in each diagnostic group is shown in Table 7. No significant difference was found when patients with minor/intermittent depression were compared with those who were not depressed. Patients with major depression differed significantly from those with minor/intermittent depression in respect to early awakening, weight loss, anorexia, and loss of libido, all of which were more frequent in major depressives. Major depressives also differed from chronic minor/intermittent depressives who had significantly more frequent weight gain. Major depressives differed from the nondepressed group in having more early awakening, more anorexia, loss of libido and initial insomnia.

Other interesting observations include the rarity of diurnal mood variation in chronic pain patients and the unusually high frequency of weight or appetite gain in patients who experience chronic pain and minor/intermittent depression. Weight or appetite gain for these patients was more than twice as frequent as for those with major depression.

One other interesting comparison is that between major depressives without pain and major depressives with pain. As shown in Table 8, the only significant difference cited was that major depressives without pain had more frequent diurnal variation of mood, being worse in the morning ($\chi = 5.71$; df $= 1$; $p < 0.02$).

Table 7. Frequency of Vegetative Symptoms in Chronic Pain

	Type of Depression		
Symptoms	Major $N = 24$	Minor/ Intermittent $N = 21$	None $N = 12$
Sleep: initial insomnia	18**	11	4
early awakening	16*,**	8	3
hypersomnia	0	0	0
Appetite: decreased	12*,**	4	2
increased	3	7	1
Weight: decreased	15*	3	4
increased	3	8***	2
Libido: decreased	16*,**	6	2
increased	0	1	4
Diurnal variation: worse AM	2	2	0
worse PM	4	3	0

  * = $p < 0.05$—Major Depression vs Minor/Intermittent Depression
 ** = $p < 0.05$—Major Depression vs No Depression
*** = $p < 0.05$—Minor/Intermittent Depression vs No Depression

Table 8.   Vegetative Symptoms in Major Depression

	Major Depression	
Symptoms	With Pain $N = 24$	Without Pain $N = 35$
Typical: early awakening	16	30 ns
weight loss	15	20 ns
poor appetite	12	24 ns
decreased libido	16	27 ns
mood worse AM	2	14 p
Atypical: initial insomnia	18	31 ns
weight gain	3	3 ns
increased appetite	4	1 ns
increased libido	0	1 ns
mood worse PM	4	10 ns

ns = not significant
$p = (\chi = 5.71; df = 1; p < 0.02)$

These comparisons suggest that inquiry into neurovegetative changes can be diagnostically useful to the physician confronted with a patient who has chronic pain but denies depressed mood, since these symptoms mirror the neurovegetative symptoms seen in major depression without pain, these symptoms are seen more frequently in chronic pain patients with major depression than in pain patients without depression. However, when a major depression is absent, patients with chronic pain may in many cases admit to atypical vegetative symptoms, and could thus be appropriately considered as having atypical depression. Finally, we have shown that patients who had chronic pain but no depression showed infrequent neurovegetative symptoms. Although weight loss and insomnia occurred in 25 and 33 percent of patients, respectively, loss of appetite, loss of libido, and diurnal variation were rare.

In chronic pain with major depression, the neurovegetative symptoms are very similar to those found in major depression alone. However, the occurrence of diurnal mood variation is rare in chronic pain patients. This interesting observation would merit further study, although it might also be a reflection of the problems associated with rating the symptom. The overall neurovegetative similarities between major depressives with and without pain suggest that inquiry into these items would prove to be diagnostically useful in assessing whether or not a chronic pain patient also has a major depression. Another major finding from this survey is the existence of a significant proportion of females with chronic pain and atypical depression, which is generally of low-grade intensity (minor or intermittent depression). Other evidence supports the view that these patients are frequently seen in pain clinics (33, 34), and that there are important treatment implications since such patients appear to respond well to MAO inhibitors. From two previous studies, it is possible to affirm confidently that phenelzine is therapeutically active in chronic pain syndromes, having been found superior to both placebo (35, 36) and to amitriptyline (36).

NEUROENDOCRINE MARKERS FOR DEPRESSION IN CHRONIC PAIN SYNDROMES

Neuroendocrine strategies are widely used for studying depression. The logic of neuroendocrine strategies is based on the hypothesis that both neuroendocrine function and mood are regulated by the same areas of the brain. These areas are believed to be the limbic system and hypothalamus. Since direct studies of the limbic system are not feasible, the study of neuroendocrine function is used to obtain indirect knowledge about the limbic system. In principle, the study of neuroendocrine function can also be used to test theories about the neurotransmitter bases of the illness, and by extension to study the mode of action of antidepressant medications.

The same strategy is now being used for the assessment of chronic pain syndromes. The strategy was first used to assess whether chronic pain patients were similar to patients with endogenous depression. It was used primarily to try to answer the question of whether the chronic pain was a variant of depression, and whether chronic pain shared common biological characteristics with depression.

Dexamethasone Suppression Test

One of the most widely used neuroendocrine markers for depression is the dexamethasone suppression test (DST). The DST was first introduced by Liddle for the study of Cushing's disease (37). The overnight DST procedure was developed as a screening test for Cushing's disease (38, 39). In this version of the test, a single dose of dexamethasone is given around midnight, and the cortisol level is determined the next morning.

This version of the DST was first applied in patients with depression by Stokes (40, 41) and Carroll and colleagues (42–44). They studied the DST in patients with melancholia because previous studies of the hypothalamo-pituitary-adrenal system in patients with melancholia showed that a number of these patients had high plasma levels of cortisol, increased urine-free cortisol, altered diurnal regulation of cortisol, and increased secretion of cortisol in the evening (45).

Initially it was thought that the abnormal DST results were simply a psychological stress response (46). Carroll showed that the abnormal DST results could not be explained simply as a psychological stress response (47). Carroll and colleagues (48) also showed, using 48-hour venous catheter studies, that the hypothalamo-pituitary-adrenal disturbance seen in patients with melancholia was more subtle. Following dexamethasone, they showed that melancholic patients may suppress cortisol normally in the morning but failed to suppress cortisol in the afternoon or evening. In normal subjects, dexamethasone usually suppresses cortisol from 24 to 36 hours. This result led to the modification of the DST for evaluation of melancholia. Samples of blood following dexamethasone were obtained the next day at 1600 hours and 2300 hours instead of 0800 hours (49, 50).

The specificity of the abnormal DST results in melancholic patients was initially described to be very high by Carroll and colleagues (48–50). Carroll and associates emphasized that a number of factors could cause false positive DST results. Table 9 gives the technical exclusion criteria for the DST.

Shortly after the introduction of the DST as a laboratory test for the diagnosis of melancholia, a number of reports emerged in the literature suggesting that the DST may not be as specific for melancholia as was originally thought. Reports emerged suggesting that the test may be positive in patients with mixed bipolar disorder (51), mania (52), schizophrenia (53), borderline personality disorder (54), dementia (55), and of normal people who are dieting and who have sustained weight loss (56). Blumer and colleagues reported that the DST was abnormal in patients with chronic pain (57). They studied 20 patients with chronic pain and

Table 9. Technical Exclusion Criteria for the DST

Major Physical Illness	Drugs
trauma, fever, nausea, dehydration	estrogens
temporal lobe epilepsy	barbiturates
pregnancy	phenytoin
Cushing's Disease	meprobamate
unstable diabetes	methaqualene
malnutrition	glutethimide
heavy alcohol use	methyprylan
alcohol withdrawal	carbamazepine
hypopituitarism	indomethacin
	cyproheptadine
	steroids
	benzodiazepines (high dose)

stated that the frequency of abnormal DST results in these patients was such that chronic pain could be considered as a variant of depression. However, Blumer and colleagues (57) failed in their study to assess whether the DST results of these patients were related to major depression per se, or were related to chronic pain.

Early studies of cortisol in patients with pain have reported interesting results (58). Shenkin reported that the diurnal variation of plasma cortisol levels was reduced to a greater extent in patients with pain of organic origin (59). On the other end, patients with psychological pain were found to have lower rates of cortisol production than those with pain of organic origin (58, 59). These studies also failed to assess the role of depression in relation to cortisol levels.

To clarify the concept of chronic pain and its relationship to depression, we undertook studies in a uniform group of chronic low back pain patients. Patients were classified into two groups based upon the presence or absence of major depression (using DSM-III criteria) and examined the cortisol response to dexamethasone in each group. Major depression in these patients is best considered as a complication of chronic pain. In a preliminary report of the DST in chronic pain, we found that 40 percent of the patients with depression had an abnormal suppression of cortisol to dexamethasone, but none of the patients without depression had an abnormal test (60). These results were later confirmed in a larger study of 80 patients (61). In addition, patients were assessed as to whether there was any relationship between postdexamethasone cortisol levels and the presence of organic pathology. Organic pathology was defined as including one of the following findings: 1) physical examination positive for a radiculopathy; 2) abnormal radiographic findings (myelogram or CT scans positive for arachnoiditis and bulging of herniated disc); or 3) positive electromyography (EMG).

Of the 80 patients, 35 satisfied criteria for major depression using DSM-III. Forty-five patients did not satisfy criteria for DSM-III major depression. Of these 45 patients, 10 satisfied criteria for dysthymic disorder. Fourteen of the patients with major depression had postdexamethasone cortisol values greater than 5 μg/dl, either at 4 P.M. or at 10 P.M. None of the patients without major depression had postdexamethasone values greater than 5 μg/dl. Of the 24 patients with organic findings and depression, 7 were nonsuppressors; and of the 11 patients with depression without any evidence of organic findings, 7 were not suppressors. The highest postdexamethasone plasma cortisol levels among the diagnostic groups were as follows: major affective disorder with positive DST was 8.24 μg/dl ± 2.9; major affective disorder with a negative DST was 1.44 μg/dl ± 0.53; and no depression was 1.7 μg/dl ± 0.93. In comparison to other groups of patients with major depression, the postdexamethasone plasma cortisol levels were lower.

In an attempt to identify what factor or factors of abnormal DST identifies, we studied postdexamethasone cortisol levels in relation to various items on the Ham-D, the MADRS, and the Ham-A.

Atkinson and colleagues (62) also reported that postdexamethasone cortisol levels were higher in pain patients with major depression. Nonsuppression of cortisol was more frequent (40 percent) in pain patients with associated major depression than in patients without major depression (8 percent). There was no difference between patients with psychogenic and organic pain. Unlike psychiatric controls, pain patients who had nonsuppression of cortisol did not show a nonsuppression of prolactin.

Seventy-one consecutive chronic low back pain patients admitted to the pain service of a major university hospital were studied (63). Twenty-three of the 71 patients were given the DST, which was done with 1 mg of dexamethasone given at 11 P.M. Plasma cortisol was measured by an RIA method at 4 P.M. AND 10 P.M. Eighteen of the patients did not have the DST based on the exclusion factors outlined by Carroll and colleagues. The diagnosis of major depression was made by one of us using the Schedule for Affective Disorders and Schizophrenia (Lifetime) (SADS-L) version, which is modified to include items related to chronic low back pain. Statistical analysis was done by using a stepwise discriminant function analysis. The items that identified nonsuppressors included reported sadness, inner tension, reduced sleep, reduced appetite, concentration difficulty, and some symptoms of anxiety—especially muscular symptoms, autonomic symptoms, and anxious behavior at interview (63). The major symptoms that identified nonsuppressors are listed in Table 10.

Table 10. Major Symptoms Identifying DST Nonsuppressors

Reported sadness
Inner tension
Reduced appetite
Suicidal ideation
Loss of libido
Autonomic symptoms
Anxious behavior at interview
Depressed mood
Hypochondriasis
Paranoid symptoms
Reduced interest
Loss of insight
Weight gain
Concentration difficulties

Thyrotropin-Releasing Hormone Stimulation Test

Thyrotropin-releasing hormone (TRH) is a peptide that is found in the nervous system and in other organs. Thyrotropin-releasing hormone stimulates the release of thyroid-stimulating hormone (TSH). The TRH-stimulation test is the measurement of serum TSH following the administration of a standard amount of TRH. The test also has been used recently as a marker for depression. Unlike the DST, the TRH-stimulation test for depression is reported to be both a trait and a state marker (64). Over 1,000 patients have been studied with various psychiatric conditions. The majority of studies have reported TRH-induced TSH response as blunted in patients with depression. Between 25 and 50 percent of the patients have been reported to be blunted depending upon the assay, the cut-off point used, the psychiatric diagnosis, and the subtyping of depression.

We decided to assess the TRH-induced TSH response in patients with chronic pain in an attempt to further delineate the relationship between depression and chronic pain. We studied 24 patients with chronic pain. Fourteen of the patients had major depression and 10 of the patients did not satisfy DSM-III criteria for major depression. Six of the 24 patients had a blunted TSH response to TRH. Blunted TSH response was defined as Δ TSH (maximum change in TSH levels) less than 5 uIU/ml. Four of 14 with major depression and 2 of the patients without major depression had a blunted TSH response. This was not statistically significant. One of the two patients without depression had a blunted TSH response to TRH and a past history of major depression. Delta TSH response to TRH in the two groups of patients is shown in Figure 2. This study suggests that like the DST, the TRH-stimulation test may be a biological correlate between chronic pain and depression. But it also suggests that chronic pain patients who have this abnormality may be predisposed to developing depression. Further research on this question is warranted.

The study of neuroendocrine markers in chronic pain is in its infancy. Further studies using more sophisticated probes will help to assess the neurochemical and neurobiological bases of both chronic pain and depression in relation to chronic pain. Furthermore, some of these markers may prove to be useful as trait markers for depression in chronic pain patients.

GENETIC FACTORS

At the current time we cannot predict which chronic pain patients will develop major depression. Some preliminary studies indicate that genetic factors may play a role. Schaffer and Donlon (65), in an early study of 20 chronic pain patients, reported that patients with chronic pain had a high familial incidence of depression. Seventy-three percent of chronic pain patients with depression and 40 percent of those without depression had a family history of depressive spectrum disorder (that is, family

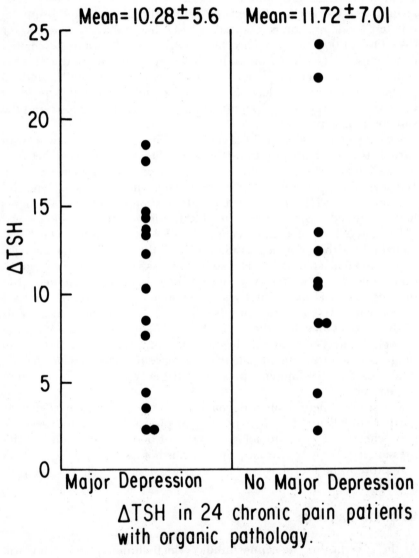

ΔTSH in 24 chronic pain patients with organic pathology.

Figure 2. Thyrotropin-releasing hormone (TRH) stimulation tests: Δ TSH in 24 chronic pain patients with organic etiology

history of depression, alcohol dependency, or sociopathy). Blumer and Heilbronn (66) reported a high incidence of mental disorders such as depression in families of chronic pain patients. They did not use standard criteria for assessing mental disorders in first-degree relatives. They reported that 42 percent of these patients had first degree relatives with a mental disorder.

Recently, we have shown that the incidence of past history of major depression was higher among chronic pain patients with depression than those without depression (10). Using the Family History-RDC method, we studied 50 consecutive chronic low back pain patients admitted to Duke University Inpatient Pain Management Program (67). The inclusion criteria for the study was daily low back pain for more than six months, with pain being the major complaint for which help was sought. Each patient was first interviewed, and a lifetime diagnosis of major depression, using RDC, was first made based on both interview and records. The proband was then interviewed by one of the other authors who used the Family History-RDC method. In addition to psychiatric disorders, a family history of back disorders was also obtained. Morbidity risk was calculated using an abridged Weinberg formula. The age range of risk for alcohol dependence used was 20–40 years and for depression 15–60 years. Of the 50 patients, 34 had major depression, while 16 had no current or past history of major depression. Forty-six percent of chronic pain patients had psychopathology in their families.

The morbidity risk for alcohol dependence was 8.89 percent for parents of probands with major depression, and 6.25 percent for parents of probands without depression. Morbidity risk for alcohol dependence among siblings of probands with major depression was higher (5.31 percent) than for siblings without depression (0). The morbidity risk for recurrent unipolar depression was 6.67 percent for parents and 2.56 percent for siblings of probands with major depression. Twelve percent of the probands with major depression and 13 percent without major depression had first-degree relatives with back problems (67). We confirmed these findings in another 50 patients (68). These studies were limited by the method that was used for obtaining the family history—the RDC method—which has limited sensitivity and high specificity. Increased sensitivity could have been obtained had family members been interviewed. However, the results of these studies suggest that the occurrence of depression in these patients may be related to a genetic vulnerability to depression. As in recent studies of depression, family history of alcohol dependence also might not have a relationship to genetic vulnerability to depression in chronic pain patients. Further study of this question is warranted. Twin studies, adoption studies, and family studies will help further clarify the genetic basis, if any, for depression in these patients.

SOCIOENVIRONMENTAL FACTORS

Systematic studies of socioenvironmental factors in the development of depression in chronic pain patients are not available. France and colleagues, in an early study, compared the demographic characteristics in chronic pain patients with different subtypes of depression. The following characteristics were studied: age, sex, number of years of education, occupational status, litigation status, and medication status. No significant differences between the groups were found (9). Further study of the role of these and other socioenvironmental factors, such as history of prior childhood experiences, is warranted.

THEORIES REGARDING THE DEVELOPMENT OF DEPRESSION IN THESE PATIENTS

Fordyce (69) suggests that the chronic pain patient sustains a major reduction in positive reinforcement as he is forced to curtail previously pleasurable activities. This reduction of positive reinforcement is postulated to lead to the development of depressive symptoms in chronic pain patients.

Seligman's model of learned helplessness also provides a framework within which to understand the development of depression in these patients. Chronic pain can be viewed as a state leading to learned helplessness and depression.

Beck's cognitive theory of depression (70) has been studied in relation to pain. Lefebvre has shown that chronic pain patients with depression show a greater number of cognitive distortions than do depressed patients with pain (71). However, the relationship between pain and cognitive distortions and depression is yet to be understood. It is possible that the development of depression in these patients may be secondary to disturbances of serotonin and opioid regulation that are postulated to occur in pain, since the same neurotransmitters are implicated in the pathophysiology of depression. For the present, any theory on the development of depression in chronic pain patients must remain speculative.

SUMMARY

Depression is frequently seen as a complication of chronic pain. Depressed mood may be part of the normal illness behavior or may be part of a psychopathological disorder. The incidence of depression as a psychopathological disorder varies considerably across different studies. This may be secondary to the clinical setting and the different criteria used. Different subtypes of depression, such as major depression, minor depression, and intermittent depressive disorder (dysthymia), may be clearly identified in chronic pain patients. Symptoms of depression, especially neurovegetative symptoms and symptoms of anxiety, serve as useful discriminators of these subtypes. Abnormal DST results are frequently seen in chronic pain patients with major depression, but not in those patients without major depression. The abnormal DST results are not related to pain alone or to the presence or absence of organic pathology.

Depression is more often seen among relatives of chronic pain patients with major depression than among those without major depression. This suggests that genetic factors may play a role in the development of depression in these patients. Further study is needed to establish the role of both genetic and socioenvironmental factors in the etiopathogenesis of depression in chronic pain patients.

Assessing depression among chronic pain patients is important because the therapeutic management and response, especially to antidepressants, may be different. For further discussion of the role of antidepressants in chronic pain, see Chapter 19.

REFERENCES

1. Hendler N: The four stages of pain, in Diagnosis and Treatment of Chronic Pain. Edited by Hendler N, Long D, Wise TN. Littleton, MA, John Wright PSG, 1983
2. Hendler N: Depression caused by chronic pain. J Clin Psychiatry 45:30–34, 1984
3. Blumer D, Heilbronn M: The pain prone disorder: a clinical and psychological profile. Psychosomatics 22:395–402, 1981
4. Hill OW, Blendis L: Physical and psychological evaluation of non-organic abdominal pain. Gut 8:221–229, 1967
5. Large R: The psychiatrist and the chronic pain patient. Pain 9:253–263, 1980
6. Lascelles RG: Atypical facial pain and depression. Br J Psychiatry 122: 651–659, 1966
7. Lindsey P, Wyckoff M: The depression pain syndrome and response to antidepressants. Psychosomatics 22:511–517, 1981
8. Maruta T, Swanson DW, Swenson WM: Pain as a psychiatric symptom: comparison between low back pain and depression. Psychosomatics 17:123–127, 1976
9. France RD, Houpt JL, Scott A, et al: The phenomenology of depression in chronic pain. Paper presented at the 137th Annual Meeting of the American Psychiatric Association. Los Angeles, CA, May 1984
10. Krishnan KRR, France RD, Pelton S, et al: Chronic pain and depression, I: classification of depression in chronic pain patients. Pain 22:279–287, 1985
11. Kramlinger KG, Swanson DW, Maruta T: Are patients with chronic pain depressed? Am J Psychiatry 140:747–749, 1982

12. Pilowsky I, Chapman CR, Bonica JJ: Pain, depression and illness behavior in a pain clinic population. Pain 4:183–192, 1977
13. Turkington RW: Depression masquerading as a diabetic neuropathy. JAMA 243:1147–1150, 1980
14. Wilson WD, Blazer DG, Nashold BS: Observations on pain and suffering. Psychosomatics 17:73–76, 1976
15. Davidson JRT, Krishnan KRR, France RD, et al: Neurovegetative symptoms in chronic pain and depression. J Affective Disord 9:213–218, 1985
16. Krishnan KRR, France RD, Pelton S, et al: Chronic pain and depression, II: symptoms of anxiety in chronic pain patients. Pain 22:289–294, 1985
17. Slater E, Roth M: Clinical Psychiatry. London, Bailliere, Tindall and Cassell, 1970
18. Costello CG, Selby MM: The relation between sleep patterns and reactive and endogenous depressions. Br J Psychiatry 111:497–507, 1965
19. Hinton JM: Patterns of insomnia in depressive states. J Neurol Neurosurg Psychiatry 24:184–188, 1963
20. Carney MWP, Roth M, Garside RF: The diagnosis of depressive syndromes and the prediction of ECT response. Br J Psychiatry 111:659–672, 1965
21. Hamilton M: Rating depressed patients. J Clin Psychiatry 41:21–24, 1980
22. Foulds GA: The design of experiments in psychiatry, in Methods of Psychiatric Research. Edited by Sainsbury P, Kreitman N. New York, Oxford University Press, 1975
23. Waldman H: Die Tagesschwankung in der Depression als rhythmisches Phanomena. Fortschritte der Neurologie-Psychiatrie 40:83–104, 1972
24. Ede A, Gravitz A, Templer D: Diurnal variation and endogenous components of depression. Br J Psychiatry 128:509–510, 1976
25. Stallone F, Huba G, Lawlor WG, et al: Longitudinal studies of diurnal variation in depression: a sample of 643 patient days. Br J Psychiatry 123:311–318, 1973
26. Hamilton M: A rating scale for depression. J Neurol Neurosurg Psychiatry 23:56–62, 1960
27. Post F: Body weight changes in psychiatric illness: a critical review of the literature. J Psychosom Res 1:219–230, 1956
28. Pollitt JD, Young J: Anxiety state or masked depression? a study based on the action of monoamine oxidase inhibitors. Br J Psychiatry 119:143–150, 1971
29. Davidson JRT, Turnbull CD: The diagnostic significance of vegetative symptoms in depression. Br J Psychiatry 148:442–446, 1986
30. Davidson JRT, Turnbull CD, Strickland R, et al: Comparative diagnostic criteria for melancholia and endogenous depression. Arch Gen Psychiatry 41:506–511, 1984
31. Nelson JC, Charney DS: The symptoms of major depressive illness. Am J Psychiatry 138:1–13, 1981
32. Paykel ES: Depression and appetite. J Psychosom Res 21:401–409, 1977
33. Davidson JRT, Raft D: Atypical symptoms, chronic pain and response to MAO inhibitors. Arch Gen Psychiatry 42:635, 1985
34. Feinmann C, Harris C, Cawley R: Psychogenic facial pain: presentation and treatment. Br Med J 288:463–468, 1984

35. Lascelles RG: Atypical facial pain and depression. Br J Psychiatry 112:651–659, 1966
36. Raft D, Davidson JRT, Maddox A, et al: Double-blind evaluation of phenelzine, amitriptyline and placebo in depression associated with pain, in Monoamine Oxidase: Structure, Function and Altered Functions. Edited by von Korff R, Singer E, Murphy D. New York, Academic Press, 1979
37. Liddle GW: Tests of pituitary-adrenal suppressibility in the diagnosis of Cushing's syndrome. J Clin Endocrinol Metab 20:1539–1560, 1960
38. McHardy-Young S, Harris PWR, Lersoff MH, et al: Single dose dexamethasone suppression test for Cushing's syndrome. Br Med J 1:740–744, 1967
39. Nugent CA, Nichols T, Tyler H: Diagnosis of Cushing's syndrome: single dose dexamethasone suppression tests. Arch Intern Med 116:172–176, 1965
40. Stokes PE: Alterations in hypothalamic pituitary adrenocortical function in man during depression. Endocrine Society, 52nd Meeting (Abstract), 337, 1970
41. Stokes PE: Studies on cortisol of adrenocortical function in depression, in Recent Advances in the Psychobiology of Depressive Illness. Edited by Williams TA, Katz MM, Shield JA. Washington, DC, U.S. Government Printing Office, 1972
42. Carroll BJ: The hypothalamic pituitary adrenal axis in depression, in Depressive Illness: Some Research Studies. Edited by Davies B, Carroll BJ, Mowbray RM. Springfield, Ill, Charles C Thomas, 1972
43. Carroll BJ, Davies BM: Clinical association of 11-hydroxy-corticosteroid suppression and nonsuppression in severe depressive illness. Br Med J 1:789–791, 1970
44. Carroll BJ, Martin FIR, Davies BM: Resistance to suppression by dexamethasone of plasma 11-OHCS levels in severe depressive illness. Br Med J 3:285–287, 1968
45. Sachar EJ, Hellman L, Fukushima DK, et al: Cortisol production in depressive illness: a clinical and biochemical classification. Arch Gen Psychiatry 23:289–298, 1970
46. Mason JW: A review of psychoendocrine research on the pituitary-adrenal cortical system. Psychosom Med 30:586–607, 1968
47. Carroll BJ: Limbic system pituitary adrenal cortex regulation in depression and schizophrenia. Psychosom Med 38:106–121, 1976
48. Carroll BJ, Curtis GC, Mendels J: Neuroendocrine regulation in depression, I: limbic system adrenocortical dysfunction. Arch Gen Psychiatry 33:1039–1044, 1976
49. Carroll BJ, Curtis GC, Mendels J: Neuroendocrine regulation in depression, II: discrimination of depressed from nondepressed patients. Arch Gen Psychiatry 33:1051–1057, 1976
50. Carroll BJ, Feinberg M, Greden JF, et al: A specific laboratory test for the diagnosis of melancholia. Arch Gen Psychiatry 38:15–22, 1981
51. Krishnan KRR, Maltbie AA, Davidson JRT: Abnormal cortisol suppression in patients with simultaneous manic and depressive symptoms. Am J Psychiatry 140:203–205, 1983

52. Graham PM, Booth J, Baranga G: Dexamethasone suppression test in mania. J Affective Disord 4:201–211, 1982
53. Dewan MJ, Pandurangi AK, Boucher ML: Abnormal dexamethasone suppression test results in chronic schizophrenic patients. Am J Psychiatry 139:1501–1503, 1982
54. Krishnan KRR, Davidson JRT, Rayasam K, et al: The dexamethasone suppression test in borderline personality disorder. Biol Psychiatry 19:1149–1153, 1984
55. Spar JE, Gerner R: Does the dexamethasone suppression test distinguish dementia from depression? Am J Psychiatry 139:238–240, 1982
56. Edelstein CK, Roy Byrne P, Fawzy FI, et al: Effects of weight loss on the DST. Am J Psychiatry 140:338–341, 1983
57. Blumer D, Zorick F, Heilbronn M: Biological markers for depression in chronic pain. J Nerv Ment Dis 170:425–428, 1981
58. Lascelles PT, Evans PR, Merskey H, et al: Plasma cortisol in psychiatric and neurological patients with pain. Pain 97:533–538, 1974
59. Shenkin H: The effect of pain in the diurnal pattern of plasma cortisol levels. Neurology 14:1111–1117, 1964
60. France RD, Krishnan KRR, Houpt JL, et al: Differentiation of depression from chronic pain with the dexamethasone suppression test and DSM-III. Am J Psychiatry 141:1577–1580, 1984
61. France RD, Krishnan KRR: The dexamethasone suppression test as a biological marker of depression in chronic pain. Pain 21:49–55, 1985
62. Atkinson J, Kremer E, Risch S, et al: Neuroendocrine markers of affective disorders in chronic pain. Abstract 310 Pain Supplement 2:1–474, 1984
63. Krishnan KRR, France RD, Pelton S, et al: What does the DST identify? Biol Psychiatry 20:957–964, 1985
64. Loosen PT, Prange AJ: Serum thyrotropin response to thyrotropin releasing hormone in psychiatric patients: a review. Am J Psychiatry 139:405–416, 1982
65. Schaffer CB, Donlan PT, Bittle RM: Chronic pain and depression: a clinical and family history survey. Am J Psychiatry 137:118–120, 1980
66. Blumer D, Heilbronn M: Chronic pain as a variant of depressive disease: the pain prone disorder. J Nerv Ment Dis 170:381–406, 1981
67. Krishnan KRR, France RD, Houpt J: Chronic pain and depression. Psychosomatics 26:299–304, 1985
68. France RD, Krishnan KRR, Trainor M: Chronic pain and depression, III: family history study of depression and alcoholism in chronic low back pain patients. Pain 24:185–190, 1986
69. Fordyce WE: Behavioral methods for control of chronic pain and illness. St. Louis, CV Mosby, 1976
70. Beck AT: Cognitive therapy and emotional disorders. New York, International Universities Press, 1976
71. Lefebvre M: Cognitive distortion and cognitive errors in depressed psychiatric and low back pain patients. J Consult Clin Psychol 49:517–525, 1981

Chapter 12

Substance Abuse in Chronic Pain Patients

K. Ranga Rama Krishnan, M.D.
Una D. McCann, M.D.
Randal D. France, M.D.

It is a common notion among physicians that substance abuse is frequently seen in chronic pain patients. This arises from confusing the use of analgesics with their abuse and addiction. This often leads to underestimation of pain and underutilization of analgesics. Conversely, there is the overuse of analgesics with subsequent abuse and addiction; although rare, it is an important problem. In this chapter we will discuss the various definitions pertaining to drug abuse with special reference to chronic pain. We will also briefly describe the various kinds of drug abuse seen in chronic pain patients.

DEFINITIONS

The term abuse has many connotations, although in simple terms the definitions given in Table 1 usually suffice. DSM-III defines substance abuse in a more rigorous fashion (Table 2)—that is, as a pattern of pathological use causing impaired social or occupational functioning lasting one month or more. It is important to realize that drug abuse *does not* necessarily mean the same thing as drug dependence. A simple definition of drug dependence is given in Table 1, as is a definition for addiction (which, while still employed, is a term not used to the same extent as in the past). Abuse liability refers primarily to that quality of the drug that leads to drug-seeking behavior. Most drugs of this type are now scheduled as controlled substances. Table 2 also gives the DSM-III definition of drug dependence. The distinction between drug abuse and drug dependence is especially important as it relates to chronic pain patients.

Table 1. Definitions

Misuse	Inappropriate drug use; often unintentional
Abuse	Using a drug for effects other than the one the drug is indicated for; and Taking drugs at dose levels in circumstances and settings that significantly augment their potential for harm
Dependence	A syndrome manifested by a behavioral pattern in which the use of a given psychoactive drug, or class of drugs, is given a much higher priority than other behaviors that once had a higher value
Abuse Liability	Quality of a drug that can lead to its abuse by an individual
Addiction	Compulsive and repetitive use of an abusable drug, usually accompanied by physiological dependence and the occurrence of adverse consequences in the individual

Table 2. DSM-III Definitions

Substance Abuse	Substance Dependence (requires evidence of either 1 or 2)
1. A pattern of pathological use 2. Impairment in social and occupational functioning caused by the pattern of pathological use 3. Duration of pathological use should be at least one month	1. *Evidence of Tolerance:* Markedly increased amounts of the substance are required to achieve the desired effects, or there is a marked effect with regular use of the same dose 2. *Withdrawal:* In withdrawal, a substance-specific syndrome follows cessation of a reduction in intake of a substance that was previously regularly used by the individual to induce a physiological state of intoxication

Drug abuse and drug dependence can occur independently of each other. For example, chronic pain patients may abuse drugs such as nonopioid analgesics without becoming dependent on them. Maruta and colleagues have defined drug abuse and drug dependency in a manner they consider suitable for the chronic pain population (1). They define drug abuse as the use of a drug when there is no medical indication for its sustained use, and when one of the following conditions is present: a) daily opioid use for more than one month; b) nonopioid analgesic use at near-maximum or greater-than-maximum recommended use for more than a month; or, c) simultaneous use of four or more pain medications on a daily basis for more than one month. Drug dependency, on the other hand, is defined as the sustained use of a drug when there is no medical indication for its use and at least one of the following is present: a) an increasing daily dose of opioids for more than one month; b) use of more than one opioid daily for more than one month, along with a past history of opioid dependency; or c) increasing daily use of nonopioid drugs for more than one month with evidence of physical dependence (1).

Both definitions revolve around the medical indication for analgesics in chronic pain. Although many authorities believe that chronic use of opioids and other analgesics is not warranted in pain of idiopathic origin, we have found that in some patients low-dose opioids can be very useful in both relieving pain and in returning the patient to society without any development of tolerance to the drug (2, 3). Thus, an important criterion we use in assessing drug abuse in chronic pain patients is whether the drug relieves the pain *and* helps the patient return to a reasonable level of functioning. If the drug relieves the pain but impairs functioning to an extent greater than did the pain, then the drug should not be taken, and doing so may be construed as abuse.

OPIOID ABUSE AMONG CHRONIC PAIN PATIENTS

In trying to determine the extent of opioid abuse among patients with chronic pain syndromes, it is important to keep in mind that opioid *use* should not be misconstrued as opioid *abuse,* since many chronic pain patients do benefit from the use of opioids. In certain pain syndromes, such as phantom-limb pain, opioids, in combination with tricyclics and other psychotropic medications, alleviate pain (3). Furthermore, tolerance is rarely seen in these patients. When observed, tolerance tends more toward a euphoric effect than to an analgesic effect. Another chronic pain syndrome for which opioids are used with considerable benefit is cancer pain (4).

When opioids are used in pain syndromes of psychological origin, they are of limited benefit; that is, in such syndromes as psychogenic pain or conversion disorder. A pattern of abuse can soon develop, which in turn can lead to both psychological and physiological dependence. Opioid abuse is more common in pain syndromes of psychiatric or idiopathic origin than in pain syndromes that are primarily organic in origin. Table 3 lists some of the characteristics exhibited by chronic pain patients who abuse opioids or other drugs.

When a psychiatrist is called in to evaluate a chronic pain patient because of alleged drug abuse, it is often because the patient is in conflict with the staff or physician who is treating the condition. The staff or physician often views the patient's request for opioid drugs as undue and in excess of what is really required for the pain, and a negative countertransference may occur (5). In evaluating chronic pain patients for opioid abuse, these factors must be kept in mind.

Chronic pain patients who abuse opioid drugs fall primarily into three classes:

Table 3. Common Characteristics Which Lead to Drug Abuse in Chronic Pain Patients

Past history of drug/alcohol abuse/dependence
Idiopathic pain or pain of psychiatric origin
Premorbid personality—antisocial, dependent
Family history of alcohol/drug abuse
Associated depression and anxiety patient self-treats

1. patients with a history of drug dependence who use pain as a complaint to obtain opioids (6)

2. patients with ongoing depression and anxiety who use opioids to alleviate their depressive symptoms

3. patients with idiopathic pain, who may have been initially treated with opioids for the pain but who have developed a drug abuse/dependence pattern. This response is secondary to the interaction between the inherent high abuse liability of the drug and the personality of the individual. Patients with a past history of drug/alcohol abuse are perhaps more predisposed towards this pattern

Few studies are available that clearly identify opioid abuse among chronic pain patients. Ziesat and colleagues (7), in a study of 440 patients, assessed the relationship between various types of drug use and two different classes of pain patients—those with operant pain and those with nonoperant pain. Operant pain was defined as: a) pain in which cause is not identified by the physician; b) pain for which the physician can provide no relief; and c) secondary gain that reinforces pain and pain behavior. It was noted in the Ziesat study that chronic pain patients with operant pain used opioids more often than did patients with nonoperant pain. However, this study did not address the issue of use versus misuse and dependence in these patients (7).

Maruta and colleagues have reported on substance abuse in chronic pain patients in a series of publications (1, 8–10). They have discovered that codeine and oxycodone are the drugs most frequently abused by these patients and that outcome was poor among patients who abused opioid drugs. Oxycodone was found to be associated with both cognitive impairment and poor outcome (9, 10). Approximately 25 percent of the 144 chronic pain patients were dependent on drugs, 41 percent were drug abusers, and 35 percent were nonabusers as per the criteria mentioned above.

Evans (4) reported an incidence of opioid abuse of 97 percent, but only 7 percent of those were considered to be dependent (that is, addicted) to opioids. Opioid *addiction* (dependence) was not seen in cancer patients. This may be secondary to the short length of time they were on opioids. Furthermore, indices of psychological dependence—for example, euphoria and elation—are usually considered to be beneficial; therefore, psychological dependence is often underestimated in these patients. Among headache patients on codeine, the incidence of abuse was low, less than 10 percent (6). Abuse was defined in these patients as the use of codeine more than 50 percent above the maximal recommended dose.

Specific Drugs Abused by Chronic Pain Patients

Ergotamines

Patients using ergot alkaloids can fall into the pattern of using the drug for headache relief, developing what are called ergotamine headaches from the drug itself (11–13), and then increasing the use of the ergot alkaloid. Soon a vicious circle is in place. These patients develop withdrawal symptoms when taken off ergotamine (11). Such a pattern of ergotamine use can be construed as abuse of the drug. Treatment of this abuse includes withdrawal using chlordiazepoxide (11) followed by treatment with tolfenamic acid.

Benzodiazepines

In Chapter 18, we briefly review the lack of utility of benzodiazepines in *chronic* pain syndromes. However, we commonly see chronic pain patients who are on these drugs. Since the benzodiazepines do not help the patient and often may contribute to depression and a reduction of cognitive capacity, their use in chronic pain may be construed as abuse. A problem with benzodiazepine abuse is the effect these drugs have on memory. Further, many pain patients may become dependent on benzodiazepines, both physically and psychologically. Although the abuse liability of the drug is relatively low, dependence has been shown to occur with relatively low doses (14, 15). Withdrawal symptoms are more common following high-dose benzodiazepine treatment (16) and include anxiety, both psychic and somatic insomnia, dizziness, nausea, vomiting, postural hypotension, muscle twitches, and hallucinations. Propranolol may be effective in alleviating the mild withdrawal symptoms (14). The best method of treating benzodiazepine abuse is by gradual withdrawal of the drug. It must be noted that seizures have been reported as a side effect of these drugs.

Nonsteroidal Analgesics

Chronic pain patients are often on salicylates, acetaminophen, and other nonsteroidal nonopioid analgesics. Whether this is a legitimate use of these drugs or whether it constitutes abuse is difficult to determine. In general, use of these drugs when there is no obvious benefit in terms of reduction in analgesia, and when the well-being of the individual is affected, can be construed as abuse. The incidence of abuse of these drugs has not been well documented.

CONCLUSIONS

From the brief discussion above, it can be seen that several questions remain poorly described or answered concerning drug abuse in chronic pain patients. While it is generally accepted that drug abuse is common among these patients, studies of the incidence of drug abuse in chronic pain syndromes is hampered because of two major problems. First, there is lack of agreement on the definition of drug abuse in chronic pain patients. In addition, definitions of the different chronic pain syndromes are also lacking. Well-defined criteria need to be developed, and careful epidemiological studies using these criteria are needed, in order to resolve the controversy regarding the nature and incidence of drug abuse in chronic pain patients.

For effective patient management, it is important to keep in perspective the distinction between use and abuse. Chapter 20 examines the pharmacology and clinical use of analgesics; Chapter 21 explores the management of opioid dependence in chronic pain patients.

REFERENCES

1. Maruta T, Swanson DW, Finlavson RE: Drug abuse and dependency in patients with chronic pain. Mayo Clin Proc 54:241–244, 1979
2. France RD, Urban BJ, Keefe FJ: Long-term use of narcotic analgesics in chronic pain. Soc Sci Med 19:1379–1382, 1984
3. Portenoy RK, Foley KM: Chronic use of opioid analgesics in non-malignant pain: report of 38 cases. Pain 25:171–186, 1986
4. Evans PJD: Narcotic addiction in patients with chronic pain. Anesthesia 36:597–602, 1981
5. Schoof KG, Buck R, West P: Psychiatric consultation for the chronic pain patient who abuses drugs. Psychiatric Annals 14:801–807, 1984
6. Medina JL, Diamond S: Drug dependency in patients with chronic headaches. Headache 16:12–14, 1977
7. Ziesat HA, Angel HV, Gentry WD, et al: Drug use and misuse in operant pain patients. Addict Behav 4:263–266, 1979
8. Maruta T: Substance abuse by patients with chronic pain. Curr Psychiatr Ther 21:15–168, 1982
9. Maruta T: Prescription drug induced organic brain syndrome. Am J Psychiatry 135:376–377, 1978
10. Maruta T, Swanson DW: Problems with the use of oxycodone compound in patients with chronic pain. Pain 11:389–396, 1981
11. Ala-Hurula V, Myllyla VV, Hokkanen E, et al: Tolfenamic acid and ergotamine abuse. Headache 21:240–242, 1981
12. Hokkanen E, Waltimo O, Kallanranta T: Toxic effects of ergotamine used for migraine. Headache 18:95–98, 1978
13. Lippman CW: Characteristic headache resulting from prolonged use of ergot derivatives. J Nerv Ment Dis 121:270–273, 1955

14. Tyrer P, Rutherford D, Huggett T: Benzodiazepine withdrawal symptoms and propranolol. Lancet 1:520–522, 1981
15. Abernethy DR, Greenblatt DJ, Shader RI: Treatment of diazepam withdrawal with propranolol. Ann Intern Med 94:354–355, 1981
16. Pevnick SJ, Jasinski DR, Haertzer CA: Abrupt withdrawal from therapeutically administered diazepam. Arch Gen Psychiatry 39:995–998, 1978

Learned Responses to Chronic Pain: Behavioral, Cognitive, and Psychophysiological

Suzanne L. Ross, M.A.

Karen M. Gil, Ph.D.

Francis J. Keefe, Ph.D.

Preparation of this manuscript was supported by NIMH grant number 1 RO3 MH38407–01 (Behavioral Assessment of Chronic Low Back Pain), NIADDK grant number 1 RO1 AM35270–01 (Coping with Osteoarthritic Knee Pain), and a grant from the John D. and Catherine T. MacArthur Foundation.

In Chapter 8, we introduced concepts of learning important in understanding chronic pain. We emphasized that responses to pain are learned in the same manner that all behavior is learned. The individual's past history, his or her current environment, and the reactions of family members and physicians all play an important role in the learning process. As with any learned behavior, responses to pain are shaped or changed gradually over time as the person has more experience with pain. Changes are observed in the way the individual acts, feels, and thinks. Someone who is socially active may become withdrawn. Someone who is optimistic and easy-going may become depressed and irritable. A relaxed, physically fit person may become tense and out of shape. These changes occur slowly. Patients, family members, and health-care providers are frequently unaware that they have occurred.

In this chapter, we consider the development of learned maladaptive behaviors in people having chronic pain. We consider learning influences affecting three major response systems—overt behavioral, cognitive-affective, and psychophysiological. To understand the changes that occur, we feel it is useful to consider stages in the learning process. Thus, for each response system, we will discuss three stages patients go through in dealing with chronic pain: the acute, prechronic, and chronic. The acute stage refers to behavior patterns usually seen with the first 6 months of persistent pain, the prechronic state with 6 to 12 months of pain, and the chronic stage with 12 months or longer of pain. It should be noted that the learning process is a highly individualized phenomenon, and the precise amount of time a patient takes to progress through the stages is likely to vary.

CHANGES IN OVERT BEHAVIOR

The behavior patterns of chronic pain patients are well known by most primary-care physicians. These individuals often adopt a sedentary and restricted lifestyle that makes them extremely dependent on those around them. Some rely excessively on narcotic medications and are difficult for physicians to manage because of their increasing demands for medication and other treatments. These characteristic behavior patterns are usually entrenched and difficult to modify. It often seems to the clinician that the patient has always displayed these behavior patterns. A careful behavioral analysis, however, usually reveals that these habitual behaviors are learned over a long period of time.

Acute Stage

In response to the acute onset of pain most individuals show a marked change in their behavior. These changes include alterations in activity level, restrictions of movement, changes in facial expression, and modified patterns of social interactions. Changes in facial expression in response to pain occur in many primate species, and common facial expressions of pain have been recorded in diverse cultural groups (1). Much of the individual's behavioral response to acute pain, however, is linked to social and cultural factors (2)

Patients presenting with pain complaints have had numerous experiences with pain throughout their lifetime. As children, they observed how their parents responded to pain and how other children reacted. These models provided vicarious learning experiences that teach them about appropriate behavioral responses to painful stimuli (3). The individual's own prior experiences with pain and the responses of others to these experiences are equally important parts of each patient's learning history (4).

In Western societies, such as the United States, a typical reaction to acute pain is to take palliative steps to deal with the cause of the pain and, if this fails, to seek medical attention. Palliative interventions could include taking minor analgesics, resting in bed, or using moist heat. When pain persists or is related to an injury or disease, patients will seek out the advice of physicians. The patient typically is asked by the physician to describe as accurately as possible the intensity, frequency, and quality of the pain. Frank and open descriptions of pain are encouraged, since they can aid in arriving at a proper diagnosis. Treatment suggestions given often require significant changes in behavior on a temporary basis in an effort to relieve pain. Patients may be encouraged, for example, to spend more time reclining, and to decrease their involvement in social, vocational, and recreational pursuits. They are also often asked to make time in their day for treatment regimens such as taking medications, using moist heat, or exercising.

It should be noted that the changes in behavior described above are viewed by both the patient, the family, and the medical community as quite adaptive. In most cases, these behavioral responses are associated with successful treatment and relief of pain. The behavior pattern is thus a strongly reinforced one that is socially sanctioned and supported. One of the major reasons for this is that the behavior pattern is considered to be a temporary change which will be abandoned once pain is relieved. The problem becomes more complicated, however, when pain persists and the individual enters a prechronic stage in dealing with pain.

Prechronic Stage

When pain continues past the acute stage, more permanent changes in behavior need to be made to adjust and cope. Coping with pain that persists for a matter of months requires the ability to set limits, to develop new interests, to learn new ways of approaching home and work responsibilities, and to communicate feelings and concerns to others directly. When these behavioral coping skills are adequate, patients are able to adapt successfully to pain and continue to lead functionally effective and rewarding lives.

A poor behavioral adaptation to chronic pain is evident in extreme variability in behavior (5). For example, on one day the individual may appear to be quite functional, whereas on the next, the same person is confined to bed and taking increasing doses of narcotics. Other signs of dysfunctional adaptation are a progressive decrease in pleasurable activities and increased social isolation. Social interactions that do occur become strained and are marked by extremely unassertive or aggressive behavior.

The pain cycle is a key concept to the understanding of how maladaptive reactions to chronic pain develop at the prechronic stage. The basic elements of this cycle are depicted in Figure 1. As can be seen, the cycle starts with overactivity such as prolonged sitting, standing, or walking. This activity is continued until pain becomes intolerable, at which time the person rests and/or takes pain medication. Each time the pain cycle is repeated it is a learning trial. Because activity is repeatedly paired with extreme pain, patients come to fear simple activities and begin to avoid them. If they do engage in activity, they may do so in an overly anxious, tense, and cautious fashion that only increases pain. This anxiety is apparent to observers (such as a spouse or family members) as increased body posturing or painful facial expressions. The pain cycle also teaches patients to associate extreme pain with an opportunity to get relief from that pain. Rest and pain medication serve as positive reinforcers that come to reward pain and pain behavior because they invariably are withheld until pain becomes extreme.

To spouse and family members the behavior patterns seen in the pain cycle are quite confusing (5). On one day the patient seems to feel fine in that he or she is out and active. The next day the pain becomes extreme

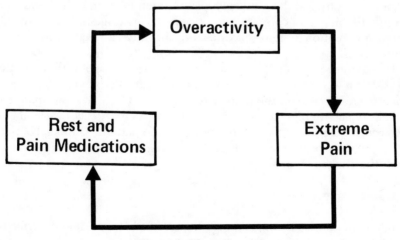

Figure 1. The pain cycle

and the patient reverts to a sedentary and more dependent lifestyle. One factor that contributes to confusion on the part of the spouse and family is that the chronic pain sufferer finds it hard to admit to others that the pain is persistent and to accept behaviorally the chronic nature of his or her pain. Being overactive may actually be a behavioral form of denial through which the individual is trying to deny to others the reality of the persistent pain. Denial is not a very effective coping strategy in the long-run, and when pain becomes severe, patients swing to the opposite extreme, becoming overly preoccupied with pain. At these times, social interactions may be characterized by hypochondriacal complaints, aggressiveness, and irritability.

As is true with behavioral reactions to acute pain, the patient's response to the more persistent pain in the prechronic stage is also influenced by sociocultural factors. Some persons have had clear models for chronic pain and chronic sick-role behaviors (4). A parent, for example, may have suffered from a long-standing illness or pain problem. When faced with persistent pain, many of the behaviors previously learned through observing others may be exhibited.

At this prechronic stage there often is less social support and sanction for continued pain and sick-role behavior. Family members and physicians may become frustrated by the lack of improvement and less tolerant of pain complaints and pain behavior. Demands to return to vocational or social pursuits are made that may motivate the patient to resume these activities too abruptly.

Individuals who fail to gradually build up their activity and who are unable to return to their jobs become involved in the disability and workmen's compensation settlement process. In many cases financial status is contingent on continuing to report pain and disability. Chronic pain patients quickly learn that if they improve, they are expected to return to work and forfeit disability payments. If they are unable to handle the physical demands of work, it often takes months or years to secure disability and compensation payments once again. Unfortunately, the compensation system serves as a disincentive for return to work in many cases.

In summary, patients who are attempting to cope with pain that persists for several months need to make more permanent changes in their behavior to keep the pain under control. Those who are unable to develop effective pain-coping responses show a great deal of variability in behavior and frequently fall into a pain cycle pattern. Ultimately, many go on to develop the very entrenched, maladaptive patterns associated with the chronic pain stage.

Chronic Stage

When pain persists for years and patients have failed to develop effective ways of coping with it, they enter what might be called a chronic pain stage. Behavior patterns at this stage are characterized by an overly sedentary and restricted lifestyle maintained mainly because it seems to minimize pain and is thus rewarding in the short term. The long-term consequences of this behavior pattern, however, are quite negative.

Extreme inactivity often develops with patients only spending two to four hours a day up and out of bed. Many patients fail to dress, eat regularly, or engage even in passive recreational activities such as watching television. They become extremely dependent on family and spouse and spend virtually all of their time in the house. Communication, even with close family members, is often minimal or absent. Long periods of silence may be broken by angry outbursts which the patient later regrets.

At this chronic stage, the individual typically has great difficulty interacting with physicians and other medical personnel. He or she is perceived as being quite demanding and manipulative, particularly in regard to the need for narcotic medications. Doctor shopping is common. Many pursue nonconventional means of medical treatment in hopes that it will provide a complete cure or at least some relief.

Family members often reinforce maladaptive forms of coping without being aware that they are doing so. Positive reinforcement may take the form of increased sympathy or attention whenever the patient seems to be having more pain and showing more pain behavior. At the same time, the family members may be paying less attention to the patient when the patient seems to be doing well. This *differential reinforcement* for pain behavior and lack of reinforcement for well behavior is believed to be a major factor promoting the maintenance of maladaptive pain behaviors (4).

CHANGES IN COGNITION AND AFFECT

Cognitive and affective responses comprise the subjective component of the chronic pain experience. Maladaptive cognitions and negative affects such as depression, anxiety, and fear can readily be identified in a substantial portion of the chronic pain population (6). These responses are believed to be due both to having to deal with the discomfort of pain, and difficulties patients have in coping with widespread disruptions in social, recreational, and vocational patterns. A recognition and consideration of these psychological changes is integral to the understanding of the chronic pain patient.

Acute Stage

The onset of acute pain triggers a wide variety of cognitions. Initially, pain is conceptualized as a warning signal of impending danger or harm (7). When pain is viewed as a warning signal it arouses feelings of anxiety and fear, which in turn motivate the individual to take action. Frequently the action involves seeking out medical assistance for diagnosis and treatment. Since these cognitions initiate appropriate actions they may be considered to be adaptive or functional. Moreover, contact with health-care professionals usually serves to decrease anxiety and fear, as patients are frequently told that through their own efforts, such as bedrest and complying with medical regimes, they can successfully relieve the pain. Anxiety regarding the future course of the pain often enhances compliance with treatment interventions (for example, taking mild analgesics). Generally, there is a decrease in anxiety as the pain abates.

In some cases, the patient may experience continued anxiety and fear that is perpetuated when there is unremitting pain despite attempts to ameliorate the problem. For example, a patient with intractable headaches may question the validity of the diagnosis if he or she harbors the belief that there is a brain tumor or other type of malignancy. Therefore, the cognitions associated with more intractable pain should be examined carefully.

In summary, acute pain patients usually interpret pain as a warning signal and often experience anxiety. Feelings of anxiety serve to motivate the individual to engage in health-seeking behaviors, which decrease the probability that the pain will continue. Finally, these cognitive-affective responses are initially quite adaptive since they increase the likelihood that the acute pain patient will initiate the appropriate steps to return to a state of health.

Prechronic Stage

Further changes in cognition and affect become evident when pain persists for months. Irrational cognitive responses often occur (8). For example, an anxious low back pain patient may be convinced that by positioning himself in a rigid posture the back will be protected, and thereby the back pain will be decreased. This posturing, however, only exacerbates the pain. Moreover, it is frequently the case that cognitions and affects that were functional in the acute stage become dysfunctional as the pain persists. For example, a patient with intractable pain may continue to believe that the pain is an acute problem that will quickly resolve when the "right" physician or cure is found. Such an individual may refuse to comply with treatment recommendations designed to help him manage a chronic pain problem (for example, lose weight, engage in a regular exercise program, or use medications on the time-contingent schedule) (7).

The recognition that the pain might be a chronic problem often triggers substantial anxiety. For example, the thought, "I will not be able to live with this pain," is common and leads to high levels of tension and anxiety. Often there is also an increasing focus on bodily symptoms, such as numbness and tingling (7). Selective attention to these symptoms can trigger cognitions, such as "I need to avoid sitting, it always makes my pain worse," as well as a passive orientation. Inactivity itself results in increased fatigue that further alarms an individual with a predisposition toward a hypochondriacal orientation. As patients become increasingly focused on their symptoms, they are perceived by others as excessively worried, tense, and anxious (5).

Guilt often occurs in the prechronic stage as patients begin to have cognitions such as, "I am a burden on my family." It is not uncommon for the patient who has been the "breadwinner" to fear that he or she can no longer financially support dependent family members. This situation can become worse if there is an absence of the requisite skills needed to pursue alternative vocational choices. Likewise, a housewife may maintain the belief that she will never be able to handle domestic chores, and this is likely to produce negative affects such as guilt and depression.

Patients are likely to have fault-finding and blaming cognition as they become increasingly ineffectual. Hostility is often directed toward the physician, the insurance company, the person responsible for the accident, or at family members. The family may respond to this hostility by withdrawing further from the patient (9). This social isolation in turn generates new fears of being abandoned by the spouse at a time when the pain patient experiences pervasive underlying feelings of dependency. Additionally, patients may perceive their need to utilize pain medications and rest as evidence that they are inherently weak or worthless, which, in turn, leads to depression. Depression frequently is exacerbated by the recognition that there has been a significant reduction in participation in important social and recreational activities.

Chronic Stage

By the time the patient moves into the chronic pain stage, he or she often develops a cognitive response pattern that is deeply embedded and resistant to change. Over time, thoughts focus almost exclusively on pain and pain-related issues. This restriction of cognition is believed to be responsible, in part, for the development of depression that is often seen in chronic pain patients (8).

Beck (10) examined the role of cognition in the development and maintenance of depressive states. He proposed that the depression-prone person is vulnerable to the extent that the self, the world, and the future are viewed in a negative manner. These depressive cognitions are automatic and involuntary, and, as a result, they are uncritically accepted even when the thoughts do not objectively correspond to reality. Ellis (11) asserts that "irrational" ideas are central to the initiation and perpetuation of emotional distress. It is now recognized that dysfunctional cognitions are instrumental in the development and maintenance of depression in chronic pain patients (8).

Chronic pain patients may endorse a wide variety of pain-related cognitions that result in depression. Examples of such maladaptive cognitions include, "The pain will always be this bad," "I cannot control the pain," and "It doesn't matter what I do because nothing works to alleviate the pain." All of these cognitions are maladaptive to the extent that they create the illusion of helplessness and hopelessness. Likewise, hypochondriacal and hysterical cognitions tend to become stronger with the continuation of the pain, and this increases anxiety. Many patients harbor the cognition that "The pain will get worse," and this leads to generalized anxiety which often accompanies low mood.

Chronic pain patients who have not functioned within the home and work environment for an extended period of time perceive themselves as "disabled." This perspective lowers self-esteem and elicits questions about self-worth. Likewise, decreased involvement in recreational or leisure time activities removes the feeling of pleasure from experience, and patients may begin to feel useless.

Finally, if the cause of continued pain cannot be identified, the patient is confronted by frustrated physicians and confused family members who seem to suggest that the pain may be psychological, imaginary, or "all in the head." The validity of the pain and pain complaints may then be questioned even though the pain subjectively persists. The inability to identify an underlying cause for a long-standing pain problem increases fear, anxiety, and frustration. This can create and lead to counterproductive behaviors such as excessive reliance on bedrest or narcotics. These passive ways of coping with pain may be further encouraged by frustrated and anxious family members (9).

In summary, in the chronic pain stage, major reductions in social, recreational, and vocational activities, along with the tendency to respond to this with faulty information processing (for example, "Only bedrest and a large dose of narcotics will relieve the pain") and cognitive errors (for example, "I am unable to function") contribute greatly to depression and other negative affective states such as anxiety, frustration, guilt, anger, and fear. Cognitive-behavioral treatment interventions (12) are designed to help control these maladaptive cognitions. This intervention involves training patients to recognize distorted cognitions and to replace them with more rational coping statements. These interventions reverse the tendency toward passivity and inactivity, and encourage a more rational appraisal and response to the chronic pain experience.

CHANGES IN PSYCHOPHYSIOLOGICAL RESPONSES

Physiologically, chronic pain patients present with a number of problems. Often, they have undergone multiple surgeries. Some of these may have been directed at repairing the tissue damage itself, whereas in some cases, neurosurgical procedures may have attempted to interrupt or modify the pain pathways (that is, neuroaugmentation and neurodestruction techniques). Iatrogenic effects of these interventions may be present and may partially explain the pain problems. Neurological tests (for example, EMG, CT, myelogram) and physical examinations may reveal that scar tissue or other pathophysiologic factors are present. However, physical findings are often insufficient to explain the severity of the individual's condition (4). Psychophysiological responses to pain play an important role in increasing pain in many patients.

Chronic pain patients are often obese. They usually have significant disturbances in sleep patterns, and they complain of chronic fatigue. Abnormal muscle activity is a factor in chronic pain syndromes (13). Muscle spasms (14) and generalized muscle tension (15) are common. Physical therapy evaluation often reveals extreme deficits in muscle strength, flexibility, and endurance. People with chronic pain are often hyperresponsive to certain situations, and they experience heightened physiological arousal when engaged in or anticipating certain activities (16). For example, Glynn and colleagues (17) found that hyperventilation was a problem for chronic pain patients. During physical exam, these patients may flinch when touched, or become tense and physically aroused when instructed to walk or move in a particular fashion. These psychophysiological responses develop over time and are closely related to changes in overt behavior.

Acute Stage

Whenever injury or disease occurs, there is the possibility that tissue pathology will lead to acute pain sensations at or near the site of damage or irritation. For example, a herniated disc injury may result in acute pain due to impingement on a nerve. In other cases, physiological changes may occur even without an injury or disease per se. For example, vasoconstriction and vasodilation of cranial blood vessels may lead to acute migraine headache pain.

In addition to local changes, individuals may display two psychophysiological reactions that are dependent upon higher nervous system activity. First, skeletal muscle changes such as muscle spasms, generalized muscle tension, and inappropriate use of muscles may often occur during an acute pain episode. These bodily responses to the onset of acute pain have some initial adaptive value. Through them, the individual may be protected from further injury. Second, autonomic arousal occurs in response to acute pain. Arousal is characterized by increases in pulse rate, blood pressure, stroke volume, respiratory changes, inhibition of gastrointestinal responses, and changes in skin resistance (16). These responses are part of a "fight-flight" reaction that prepares the individual physically to deal with emergency situations. Thus, this autonomic arousal is also initially adaptive.

Researchers have attempted to determine whether there are separate and unique patterns of autonomic arousal for experiences such as anxiety, fear, and pain across individuals, or whether there is a more generalized response to stress (18). Overall, the data suggest that there is no separate and unique pattern for these experiences. There is some indication that a given individual may respond consistently across different stressors with an idiosyncratic pattern of autonomic activity (19). However, some individuals display different autonomic reactions across stressors. Regardless, there is considerable overlap in physiological responses to anxiety and pain (20). Therefore, in the acute pain episode, it is impossible to determine which psychophysiological responses are due to acute pain and which are a result of anxiety or fear.

As with behavioral responses to acute pain, sociocultural and cognitive factors may influence a person's physiological response to acute pain. For example, in one early study, Sternbach and Tursky (21) found that ethnic background was related to palmar skin potential response to experimental pain. In this study, white, Anglo-Saxon Protestants were found to have significantly lower skin responses as compared to Italian, Irish, and Jewish individuals. Also, these four groups differed with regard to their thresholds for experimental pain.

During the acute stage of pain, surgical and medical interventions provide remedies for many patients in pain by directly correcting the underlying tissue pathology. However, in some cases, pain persists despite these efforts, and some patients enter a prechronic phase.

Prechronic Stage

As pain persists beyond the acute stage, patients begin to show variability in psychophysiological response. Occasionally, attempts to engage in certain movements and activities may lead to exacerbation of underlying tissue pathology and flare-ups of pain. During flare-ups, patients experience heightened autonomic arousal and increased muscle tension. The person's response to flare-ups is critical. Some will adapt by pacing themselves and finding alternative ways to manage their work and family lives. These patients will likely experience a decrease in autonomic arousal and muscle tension over time. Others will have problems managing these flares in pain. There are a number of possible reasons why they are unable to adapt. They may have personality problems (for example, hypochondriacal tendencies), be under extreme situational stress (for example, recent loss of loved one or job), have poor models of coping with pain (for example, another family member with a chronic pain problem), or may lack pain coping skills (for example, inability to pace appropriately). This latter group becomes vulnerable to certain learning experiences which characterize the prechronic stage.

Considerable learning occurs each time a person attempts an activity, such as walking or bending, and feels increased pain. An association between that activity and pain occurs. This association can be thought of as a learning trial. Following repeated exposure to such trials, an almost automatic physiological reaction occurs whenever the individual attempting the activity experiences pain, in a manner similar to that in which an individual develops a phobic reaction (22). In addition, through a process of classical conditioning, the environmental stimuli associated with that particular activity begin to elicit this autonomic reaction. For example, a man with a back injury may begin to feel better and go for a long car ride. After sitting for a prolonged period, he develops severe pain, autonomic arousal, and muscle tension. An association between pain, sitting, and environmental stimuli such as the car itself occurs. The association becomes stronger and physiological arousal becomes more intense after repeated exposure to pain following prolonged sitting in the car. Although he may take some car rides without increased pain, intermittent episodes of extreme pain following car rides will result in a very strong learned association between pain and the environmental stimuli. Over time, the car and even thoughts of taking a drive elicit strong anticipatory reactions characterized by anxiety and arousal. The pain that results from exacerbation of underlying tissue pathology is a key factor in the development of this learned response. However, the learned response to stimuli associated with increased pain will often continue long after tissue pathology resolves. In our example, the man may continue to experience physiological arousal to the car even after the back injury heals.

According to reinforcement theory (23), intermittent associations between events are very powerful learning experiences, and learning that occurs under an intermittent reinforcement schedule is highly resistant to change. Even greater resistance to change occurs once intense anticipatory fear leads to avoidance of the situation. Avoidance learning has two steps (24). First, an association is made between a stimulus and a response such as fear or pain. Second, the individual escapes or avoids the stimulus to reduce the fear or pain. Avoidance learning is particularly resistant to change when the emotional response is intense (25).

In our example, the patient anticipates pain and physiological arousal occurs. He or she increasingly avoids sitting or getting in the car. When "forced" to engage in these feared activities (for example, the patient must go to the doctor's office), the patient typically experiences extreme anticipatory arousal and high levels of muscle tension that, in fact, does increase his pain. The patient may continue to wear braces (for example, a back brace or cervical collar), use a cane, and take muscle relaxants to avoid pain long after he or she needs to do so. All of these habits are learned and highly resistant to change. Over time they may lead to progressive decreases in muscle strength, flexibility, and endurance.

Patients whose pain fits the psychophysiological model described in Chapter 8 also undergo important learning experiences in the prechronic stage as described above. In these patients, stress directly elicits a physiological response responsible for pain. For example, a woman under extreme job stress may develop a migraine headache and experience pain associated with cerebral vascular changes and increased autonomic arousal. Exposure to repeated job stress and subsequent migraines results in a learned association. Job-related stimuli as well as other stressful situations may elicit physiological symptoms. Thus, she may become hypersensitive physiologically to stress and overrespond to minimally stressful situations. She develops anticipatory avoidance patterns similar to those previously described, and she may begin to avoid stressful situations such as work.

Although anxiety and fear are key contributory features to the physiological arousal experienced by both of these groups of patients, individuals in the prechronic stage typically do not report feeling anxious, but rather seem more preoccupied with pain and a variety of physical symptoms. They do not perceive their physiological arousal as anxiety or fear, but rather as increased pain. This is probably due to the fact that all of these experiences result in a nonspecific increase in arousal, and the individual labels the experience (for example, fear, pain, anxiety) according to the environmental context (26).

In addition to progressive muscle weakness, muscle spasms, and decreases in muscle strength and flexibility, prechronic patients develop generalized muscle tension. Episodes of muscle contraction headaches, bruxism, or pain in a second site other than the original one may occur. For example, someone with low back pain may develop neck and shoulder pain due to awkward posture. Decreases in activity and exercise may further contribute to general levels of fatigue. Disturbance in sleep patterns and eating habits are common problems. Others reduce food intake drastically because of depression. Some become progressively more dependent upon analgesics and narcotics, placing them at risk for long-term narcotic addiction.

Chronic Stage

In the chronic pain stage, evidence of underlying tissue damage may be minimal or out of proportion to the severity of the pain complaint. Experiences with pain that occurred during the prechronic stage result in highly learned psychophysiologic responses. These learned patterns are quite resistant to change. Patients avoid activities and movements that they have learned to associate with pain. Decreases in activity and exercise results in a deteriorating physical condition. Significant deficits occur in muscle strength, flexibility, and endurance. Muscle tone is often reduced. In addition, chronic pain patients may become habitual overresponders to stress, and they may experience intense physiological arousal whenever confronted with or anticipating a stressful event. Chronic fatigue is a frequent complaint. Significant disturbances in sleep such as nighttime insomnia and daytime naps are common. Patients often experience drastic changes in their weight, either substantial weight gain or loss.

Research has suggested that there is a link between exercise and activity and the body's natural pain regulatory substances; that is, the endorphins. Exercise appears to increase endorphin activity (27). In the chronic pain stage when patients are very sedentary, the body may actually fail to produce much needed endorphins. The individual may therefore rely heavily on analgesics and narcotics, and physical and psychological addictions become serious risks in this stage.

The learning process is also a critical factor in the development of addictive behavior. Patients learn to associate narcotics as well as the stimuli associated with them (for example, syringe, pills, capsules) with reductions in their pain level and physiological arousal. Reductions in pain level and arousal are powerful consequences of taking medications, and thus patients readily acquire strong learned patterns (almost rituals) around taking medications. These learning factors are quite important during withdrawal from medications. Over time, the stimuli associated with taking medication become powerful and there are physiological withdrawal symptoms from these stimuli in addition to withdrawal symptoms from the drugs themselves (28). These considerations provide the rationale for using a pain cocktail (7) as a means to taper medications.

Some people who have persistent pain problems show somewhat different patterns from the group described previously. Rather than continuous pain, these individuals experience repeated acute flares in pain. These flare-ups may be the result of exacerbation of underlying tissue pathology (as explained in the muscle reeducation model), increases in emotional stress (psychophysiological model), or increased autonomic arousal and muscle tension following an attempt to engage in a particular anxiety-provoking task (conditioned-fear model). These patients may continue for years alternating between relatively normal pain-free periods, and distinct periods of increased pain, reduced activity, and physical function. It is these individuals who usually show the most pronounced pain responses to stressful life events.

CONCLUSION

In summary, in this chapter we have reviewed the changes that occur over time in overt behavior, cognitive-affective responses, and psychophysiological responses to persistent pain. While it is helpful to conceptualize the learning process in three stages (acute, prechronic, and chronic), it is important to realize that people do not progress through these stages in a set manner. Some reach the chronic stage quite rapidly, for example, in a matter of weeks or months. Others demonstrate a prechronic pattern even after years of continuous pain. The first major task of the assessment procedure is to determine where each individual falls in the learning process. In other words, is the development of the pain syndrome in an early stage or a more advanced stage?

Although this chapter has separated the changes that occur in the three response systems (overt behavioral, cognitive, psychophysiological), it is important to realize that these three areas interact and influence each other. For example, a man with thoughts that he is useless and worthless may become inactive. Likewise, his inactivity may result in physiological changes such as muscle weakness and atrophy. Thus, most people will experience changes in all three response areas. The second major task of the assessment is to determine which response system is affected most.

Assessment has important implications for treatment planning. For example, if the assessment determines that the patient is dependent upon family members and narcotics, and these are the most significant factors contributing to the pain problem, then treatment must be geared specifically to these problems. In other cases, cognitive-affective responses will be determined as the most significant. For example, a person with significant depression will require behavioral treatment aimed at altering irrational cognitions and increasing pleasant activities.

In conclusion, it is important to recognize that chronic pain patients are a heterogeneous group. Patients are at different points in the development of pain behavior patterns, and some behavioral problems are more entrenched than others. For each individual, the problems occurring in the three response systems (overt behavioral, cognitive-affective, psychophysiological) are somewhat different. Problems often occur in more than one response system. The assessment process is aimed at determining which response system(s) need to be targeted for treatment and what treatment techniques are most likely to help. Patients whose problems are at the acute or prechronic stage often respond well to training in self-control methods. Those at the chronic stage usually require more structured, operant conditioning programs in which staff and family take a primary role in behavior change efforts. Chapter 17 explores the specifics of behavioral assessment in greater detail, and Chapter 19 describes the four behavioral treatment protocols used in our pain management program.

REFERENCES

1. LeResche L, Dworkin SF: Facial expression accompanying pain. Soc Sci Med 19:1325–1330, 1984
2. Tursky B, Sternbach R: Further physiological correlates of ethnic differences in response to shock. Psychophysiology 4:67–74, 1967
3. Craig KD: Social modeling influences on pain, in The Psychology of Pain. Edited by Sternbach RA. New York, Raven Press, 1978
4. Fordyce WE: Behavioral Methods for Chronic Pain and Illness. St. Louis, C.V. Mosby, 1973
5. Keefe FJ, Brown C: Behavioral treatment of chronic pain, in Behavioral Medicine in General Medicine Practice. Edited by Boudewyns P, Keefe FJ. Menlo Park, CA, Addison-Wesley, 1982
6. Keefe FJ: Behavioral assessment and treatment of chronic pain. J Consult Clin Psychol 50:896–911, 1982
7. Sternbach RA: Pain patients: Traits and Treatment. New York, Academic Press, 1974

8. Lefebvre MF: Cognitive distortion and cognitive errors in depressed psychiatric and low back pain patients. J Consult Clin Psychol 49:517–525, 1981

9. Block AR, Boyer SL: The spouse's adjustment to chronic pain: cognitive and emotional factors. Soc Sci Med 19:1313–1318, 1984

10. Beck AT, Rugh AJ, Shaw BF, et al: Cognitive Therapy of Depression. New York, Guilford Press, 1979

11. Ellis A: Humanistic Psychotherapy: The Rational-Emotive Approach. New York, McGraw-Hill, 1973

12. Turk D, Meichenbaum D, Genest M: Pain and Behavioral Medicine: A Cognitive Behavioral Perspective. New York, Guilford, 1983

13. Kraus H, Raab W: Hypokinetic Disease. Springfield, IL, Charles C Thomas, 1961

14. Travell J, Rinzler S, Herman M: Pain and disability of the shoulder and arm. Treatment by intramuscular infiltration with procaine hydrocholoride. JAMA 120:417–422, 1943

15. Holmes TH, Wolff HG: Life situations, emotions and backache. Psychosom Med 14:18–33, 1952

16. Bonica JJ: Neurophysiologic and pathological aspects of acute and chronic pain. Arch Surg 112:750–761, 1977

17. Glynn CJ, Lloyd JW, Folkhard S: Ventilatory responses to chronic pain. Pain 11:201–212, 1981

18. Selye H: The general adaptation syndrome and diseases of adaptation. Journal of Clinical Endocrinology 6:217–230, 1946

19. Lacey J, Lacey J: Verification and extension of the principle of autonomic response stereotype. Am J Psychiatry 71:50–73, 1958

20. Gross RT, Collins FC: On the relationship between anxiety and pain: a methodological confounding. Clinical Psychological Reviews 1:375–386, 1981

21. Sternbach RA, Tursky B: Ethnic differences among housewives in psychophysical and skin potential responses to electric shock. Psychophysiology 1:241–246, 1965

22. Marks IM: Fears and Phobias. London, Heinemann Medical Books, 1969

23. Ferster CB, Skinner BF: Schedules of Reinforcement, New York, Appleton Century Crofts, 1957

24. Mowrer OH: On the dual nature of learning—A reinterpretation of "conditioning" and "problem-solving." Harvard Educational Review 17:102–148, 1947

25. Solomon RL, Wynne LL: Traumatic avoidance learning: the principle of anxiety conservation and partial irreversibility. Psychol Rev 61:353–385, 1954

26. Schacter S, Singer JE: Cognitive and social and physiologic determinants of emotional state. Psychol Rev 69:379–399, 1962

27. Olausson B, Rydenhag B, Ericksson E, et al: Naloxone effect on dental pain thresholds after muscle exercise and low frequency TNS: a comparative study in humans. Paper presented at the IVth World Congress on Pain of the International Association for the Study of Pain, Seattle, WA, August 31–September 5, 1984

28. Siegel S: The role of conditioning in drug tolerance and addiction, in Psychopathology in Animals: Research and Clinical Applications. Edited by Keehn JD. New York, Academic Press, 1979

Chapter 14

Musculoskeletal Changes in Chronic Pain Patients

Linda M. Lawrence, L.P.T.

Physical therapy should be an important part of the comprehensive treatment program provided for patients with chronic pain. Patients, as well as physicians and therapists, need to recognize that complete alleviation of the pain may not always be possible. In many cases, pathology is present and no amount of exercise, medication, or other modalities can change abnormal structures back to preinjury states. Goals of treatment may be to help reduce the stresses on the structures involved, prevent secondary losses, educate patients about methods of pain reduction, and/or maximize their functional capabilities. In many cases, the patient's functional outcome is far from what society terms normal, but compared to his or her pretreatment level, the patient has improved, as evidenced by improved sleep, less pain medication, decreased hours in bed, more pleasurable activities, improved work capacity, or just more independence in activities of daily living. In order to be successful with chronic pain patients, traditional treatment plans and goals need to be adjusted. Success cannot always be judged in terms of returning to work, being able to play ball, or lifting 50 pounds.

The body consists of an intricate system of balances that control the stresses on body parts. Abnormal postures can place additional stresses on the anatomical structures. Just as abnormal muscle strength can cause extra stresses by failing to maintain the balance, so too can muscle tightness or loss of range of motion prevent muscles from maintaining the body in normal alignment. Pain can be caused by normal stress on unprepared or abnormal tissues, or by irregular stress on normal or abnormal tissues (1). For example, in bending the index finger backwards, there is a range of motion in which no pain is elicited. Continuing to bend the finger backwards until there is tension on the anterior structures will not immediately produce pain. If this position were to be held for an undue length of time, however, pain would eventually develop. If the finger should be bent past its normal range, pain is felt sooner, since the nociceptive receptors in the joint will be stimulated to limit further injury. Abnormal muscle and tendon shortening will reduce the normal range of motion, and the stress from motion will cause pain readily during normal activity. Excessive lengthening of the muscles produces an unstable support structure against mechanical stress, making pain noticeable with normal activity. The stretch reflexes of the muscles are ineffectual in stabilizing the joint from excessive motion.

Abnormal stress can cause muscle weakness, shortening of muscle fibers, or habitual postural malalignments. For example, the accentuated forward head position seen in depressed or chronic pain patients causes malalignment of the vertebrae. Excessive muscle tone results when the intricate balance of the spine is lost. The forward leaning of the head must be restrained by muscle action or be balanced against abnormally stretched ligaments. This creates a situation in which tissue is stretched on one side of the joint and compressed on the opposite side. Furthermore, additional muscle contraction is needed to raise the head or maintain normal posture. The overstretched ligaments and muscles then lead to a stretch weakness (1). Hence, both normal and abnormal stress increases muscle tension and activity. The increased metabolic needs of the muscle groups involved increase the build-up of toxic waste products in the muscle. The resulting fatigue and muscle ache generate and promote the pain cycle. Thus, as we have just seen, pain of musculoskeletal origin is multidetermined.

It is the physical therapist's job to determine how pain, posture, tissue condition, and pathophysiology affect the strength, range of motion, flexibility, and posture of the chronic pain patient. Only after obtaining an understanding of which abnormal structures and stresses are common to these patients can treatment interventions be designed. It must be emphasized that individual variations occur in response to injury, abnormal stress, and pain. Since no clinical diagnosis can accurately predict how a particular patient's body will respond to a pathophysiological disorder, each patient must be assessed in terms of the stresses and balances just mentioned. This chapter provides an overview of some common musculoskeletal and other pain syndromes seen in chronic pain patients and the clinical problems they encounter frequently. For a brief description of major pain syndromes, see Chapter 10.

MUSCULOSKELETAL DISORDERS OF THE SPINE

Postural Pain

In the patient with a purely postural problem, pain is caused by static postures (1) and decreases with activity and exercise. These patients experience less pain in the mornings or on days when their normal routine is altered. As poor postures are assumed, however, the pain begins. Patients frequently have days without pain, especially when they are more active. Normally, however, they lead sedentary lifestyles and rarely exercise. At first these patients have no deformities, but as their normal postures become habitual, dysfunction (adaptive shortening) and weakness develop. Patients then experience pain at the end range of motion or with static postures. Usually patients feel better when they rest in a position with good support and alignment (for example, lying flat on their back with pillows under the knees). These patients may need to change positions frequently.

The treatment goal for patients with postural pain is to correct faulty posture and body mechanics. If dysfunction has occurred, the structures that have adaptively shortened and the resulting weak muscles will need to be addressed. Patients must be taught the range of motion their muscles are able to tolerate, and to avoid positions that would maximally stretch them. Such patients can benefit from activity rest cycles, exercise, and back school.

In patients with dysfunction (adaptive shortening), pain is brought on by stretching a tight structure (1). Repeated flexion or extension does not increase the peripheral symptoms except at the endpoint during the range of motion. When the stretch is released, pain diminishes unless the structure is stressed to such a degree that there is micro-tearing of the muscle fibers or a chemical irritation. These patients may have a form of postural pain, or they may be in the healing phase of a derangement of the disc. Frequently loss of joint motion will eventually lead to tightness of ligaments and muscles on the concave, with weakness on the convex side of the joint. These patients lose strength as their range of motion is lost; treatment is thus directed at the adaptive shortening. In evaluating the patient with dysfunction, we must first identify what structures are involved, such as facet joint capsule, ligaments, and/or muscles. Once normal length is obtained with treatment, then the weakness must be addressed. Exercise programs for stretching should be frequent throughout the day. Poor posture can be rectified after correction of length and strength. Improvement usually will take weeks or months of participation in a specific exercise program. Mobilization procedures are very helpful in gaining specific joint mobility. Frequently, motion beyond the dysfunction will become hypermobile to compensate for the loss of motion in other parts. This area can also become painful because of the excessive motion, especially during normal activities of daily living.

Derangement

Derangement of the disc needs to be differentiated from the dysfunction syndrome. This is done by identifying the pathological structure (using a myelogram or CT scan) and/or the movements and positions that intensify or diminish the peripheral pain. This analysis helps the therapist design an appropriate exercise program. Any activity that increases peripheral pain needs to be adjusted or discontinued for a period of time. Frequently, with posterior lateral disc protrusions (annulus intact), prolonged or repeated flexion increases the anterior pressure on the nucleus, which forces the protrusion further posterior or at least increases the pressure in that direction (1). These patients will stand with a flat back, prefer walking short distances over sitting, and feel increased leg pain with flexion and decreased pain with extension. They need to increase their passive extension range and frequently go into extension throughout the day to help move the nucleus forward. The patient should avoid all flexion and flexion with rotation activities/exercises until the peripheral pain is under control.

After the leg pain has been resolved, a balance of flexion, strength, range of motion, and extension should be achieved. All exercise and flexion activities are followed by passive extension. A lumbar roll should be utilized while sitting. Patients should maintain a normal lordosis with all activities, especially lifting. If the patient has a lateral shift of the pelvis, this needs to be corrected prior to any extension. If extension increases the peripheral symptoms as well as flexion, then the patient may be a candidate for mechanical traction (approximately one-half the patient's body weight) and/or bedrest until a slow, gradual extension range can be restored. Abdominal strengthening exercises can eventually be done if they are followed with spine extension. Full curl-ups are not encouraged. Patients should attend back school to learn proper body mechanics. It is extremely important that these patients lie in a completely flat position since sitting or reclining positions increases disc pressure, which was pointed out in Nachemson's study (2). If new or progressive neurological signs are found, the patient should be referred to the physician for further evaluation and diagnosis.

Degenerative Joint Disease

Patients with degenerative joint disease will frequently show a loss of spinal motion in all directions. The history of these patients often includes greater pain with extension of the spine, such as occurs during standing, lying on the stomach, walking, or extension exercise. Patients may feel better while sitting, doing knee-to-chest exercise, curling up on their sides, or lying on their backs with the hip and knees flexed. Each patient's posture needs to be evaluated for excessive lordosis or other postural problems that might decrease the size of the intervertebral foramen or cause compression of the facets, either of which would increase the pain (3).

Frequent problems seen with these patients are: 1) muscle weakness of abdominals and hip extensors; 2) tightness of the lumbar extensors, hip flexors, or hamstrings; and 3) decreased joint mobility. Exercises should be based on the findings elicited from the evaluation. Postural exercises should be stressed, especially in the standing positions. Lifting and activities of daily living should be done with a posterior pelvic tilt to decrease compression of the posterior structures of the spine. These patients should not sleep on their stomachs or do excessive extension exercises if these cause pain. Patients should be discouraged from wearing high-heeled shoes. Shock-absorbing soles help to decrease the impact of heel strike. Back school may be valuable in helping patients understand the rationale behind exercise and in learning body mechanics. Weight reduction is emphasized to help reduce the movement of the center of gravity forward.

Facet Pathology

The facet joints can cause spine pain, with or without radiating pain (4). This pain syndrome is not associated with neurological compression signs. When doing standing active truck movements, the trunk will frequently deviate to one side, or a juttering of movement can be seen in a specific area. Lateral flexion and rotation of the lumbar spine is frequently limited in the opposite directions. This could be caused by a nipping of the meniscoid structure in the facet, joint stiffness (dysfunction) due to immobilization caused by guarding, and/or scarring from a sprain of the facet joint following a vigorous or violent activity. Evaluation of passive joint mobility is essential to assess for hypo- or hypermobility of each spinal segment. Exercises are then prescribed to either increase or decrease mobility, whichever is necessary. Mobilization techniques can be beneficial to the hypomobile joint in conjunction with exercise treatments. Manual or mechanical traction can frequently help increase motion, decrease pain, and decrease compression on the joint structures (5). Corsets, strengthening exercises, and posture are the major physical therapy treatments for the hypermobile joints (6).

Compression Fractures

Compression fractures of the spine usually involve a wedging of the anterior vertebral body. Patients usually show a forward flexion in the trunk and increase in the dorsal kyphosis, forward head, and rounded shoulders. These patients must reduce the forward flexed position, as this puts even more compression on the anterior bodies. They need to be encouraged to use as few pillows as possible when lying supine. If the patient has a hospital bed, the head should be flat. The patient should sit in a firm chair, with buttocks slid to the back, and maintain a normal lordosis. The spine should be straight, with the head over the spine; this should be the case whether sitting on the side of the bed, on the toilet, or in the car—the spine must remain straight. The therapist should review with the patients methods of getting in and out of a chair and up and down from the supine position. Patients need to know how they can maintain extension of the spine.

These patients also need to learn to stoop or squat with a straight spine, making their legs do the work. Reachers (an adaptive piece of equipment) should be considered for persons who are unable to squat. Patients should not do any heavy lifting or lifting of objects that are large and bulky. Exercises are designed to increase thoracic extension range and strength. It is valuable to increase the strength of the scapulae, shoulders, and the legs in order to increase their efficiency during functional activities. It has been shown in osteoporosis that weight-bearing exercises help maintain calcium in the bone, so such exercises should be incorporated into the patient's program. Exercises to help correct postural problems might include stretching the pectoralis, stretching the hip flexors or the hamstrings, isometric abdominal strengthening, hip extensor strengthening, and against-the-wall posture exercises (7). Because of the forward head position, cervical and shoulder range of motion are frequently limited and can be incorporated into the program. Body mechanics and back care principles must be learned.

Spinal Fusion

Spinal fusions that are at least one year postoperative can be handled without precaution regarding spinal motion. A patient's program is directly related to the outcome of the musculoskeletal evaluation. Frequently, abdominal weakness is seen because of the immobility during the postoperative phase, postural habits, and use of corsets during this period of time. Often, hip flexor tightness may be seen since these muscles arise from the anterior body of the lumbar vertebrae and are associated with increased lumbar lordosis, tightness in the back, and anterior pelvic tilting. Hamstring tightness and adhesions of the nerve root and scar tissue also can be seen. These respond to very slow, gradual stretching over a period of months.

Increasing hip strength to help give the lumbar area stability and to make the lower extremities do the work frequently helps reduce stress on the lumbar complex. Increasing flexibility of the lumbar muscles, stretching of the scar tissue, and increasing joint mobility above the fusion is considered on an individual basis. Without doing any treatment at all in this area, you can still often obtain relief of pain through the strengthening of the lower extremities, increasing the stability of the trunk, and stretching of the muscles that span the trunk and the extremity. Quadricep muscles need to be strong enough to allow the patient to stoop and squat during normal daily activities that require bending and lifting. Posture and gait exercises can further help reduce the stresses on the lumbar complex. Back school is essential. Patients are encouraged to reduce their weight, and cardiovascular exercise programs can help by encouraging activity. High-heeled shoes are discouraged and shock absorbing soles can sometimes help reduce some of the stresses of walking on concrete surfaces.

Patients with broken or unstable fusions often exhibit pain with spinal motion. Since physicians will usually prescribe that patients restrict their spinal motion, physical therapy programs must be geared toward that goal. In addition to what is done for the stable fusion, more time is spent increasing the stability of the trunk while working on the strength and mobility of the lower extremities. The goal is to reduce the stresses on the lumbar complex and allow the extremities to do the work. Programs usually consist of increasing abdominal strength, slowly stretching hip flexors or hamstrings, and strengthening hip flexors, quadriceps, hamstrings, hip extensors, and hip abductors. Pelvic tilting while doing exercises of the lower extremities helps improve stability of the trunk during mobility of these extremities. Strengthening of the upper back is started using theraband to resist upper extremity motion. Standing and posture exercises help to reinforce these changes. Working on gait patterns to decrease trunk and pelvic motions also helps reinforce the goals. Positioning, transferring, and activities of daily living should be reviewed to insure mastery of the skills.

Strengthening of the upper and lower extremities can be done as long as the back is well supported and the weights that are used are light enough so as not to cause excessive trunk motion during the exercise. An exercycle can help with endurance and burning of calories for weight reduction. The patient should position the seat high enough to prevent excessive hip flexion and the handle bars high enough to allow the spine to stay straight. A corset may be needed during difficult stress and work situations, where the patient may not remember good body mechanics. Continual corset use is not encouraged since it produces loss of abdominal strength, a false sense of security, and does not actually prevent patients from bending their backs, especially when sitting slumped.

Arachnoiditis

Patients with excessive arachnoiditis are often treated as if they had unstable fusions. Most of the exercises are geared toward the extremities and do not include spinal motion. These patients frequently need to be started on a very slow and gradual program, starting with an active range of motion of legs and arms. Slowly, over a period of a few months, weights and more vigorous exercises can be added. These patients must be shown that they can succeed with an exercise program. If they are overwhelmed at the beginning they will give up, since exercise seems impossible given their amount of pain. These patients must be convinced of the benefit of exercising, even though it does not take away the pain. They must realize that they had pain without exercising and that they were only growing weaker and reducing their activity. With an activity–rest program and a few simple exercises, these patients can hope to gain strength and increase their level of activity within that same level of pain.

Postoperative Scarring

Excessive scarring may develop postoperatively in patients. If these people could be seen immediately following their operations and started on some gentle stretching over a period of time, long-term problems might be reduced. Once scarring has bound the nerve root, however, benefits from stretching will only occur with a very slow and gradual stretch. Patients must keep the stretch below a level that causes pain. The stretch must be slow and held long enough and done frequently enough so as to achieve flexibility. It is important to find a method of stretching that is comfortable to the patient and which he or she is able to do at home, and the patient must understand the needs, reason for, and effect of the exercise program.

Other problem areas identified during the musculoskeletal evaluation are addressed in the appropriate sequence.

Spondylolithesis

Patients with spondylolithesis should not be given extension exercises. For them, a program should be designed that increases abdominal tone, corrects posture, stretches tight muscles, and increases lower extremity strength (6). Back school is important. A corset or surgery is needed in severe cases. Corsets should not take the place, however, of good abdominal strength.

Pyriformis Syndrome

Pyriformis syndrome is sometimes encountered in patients with low back and buttock pain. The sciatic nerve travels under the pyriformis muscle. In a certain percentage of patients the nerve travels through the pyriformis muscle. If the muscle is tight or goes into spasm, pressure on the nerve results and this produces leg pain. Treatment involves stretching the muscle in hip flexion, adduction, and internal rotation. Hip joint capsule tightness may be a secondary problem as a result of the lower extremity being held in external rotation. Pain patients frequently ambulate with excessive external rotation and circumduction, which leads to tightness of the pyriformis, and which then could be a secondary problem to the back pain.

Cervical Spine Pain

Cervical spine pain frequently begins in one specific area, but over time becomes more diffuse as muscle tension increases. Gradually, this tension increases the cervical lordosis and causes greater compression on the cervical spine and postural malalignments. The increased lordosis produces compression of posterior elements, narrowing of intervertebral foramen, and shortening of posterior ligaments and muscles. Frequently these problems lead to irritation of upper cervical nerve roots and hence cause headaches. Thoracic kyphosis causes constant stretching of the thoracic muscles, which leads to weakness and decreased range of motion in the shoulder. Full shoulder range of motion is not possible because the acromion is lowered and the humerus internally rotates, causing subacromial impingement. This increases bursitis and thinning of the rotator cuff as the acromion is lowered and impingement occurs. These can all lead to increased shoulder pain mimicking cervical radicular symptoms.

Constant neck pain can also cause increased clenching of the teeth and bruxism. Associated symptoms from neck pain can include giddiness, swallowing difficulties, fullness or ringing in the ears, and blurred vision. Evaluation of the patient must include the cervical spine, a shoulder screen, jaw function, muscle evaluation of the thorax and scapula, and a posture evaluation to include the low back and lower extremities. Occasionally, even distant structures such as tight hamstrings or weak hip extensors will affect the cervical spine. Treatment must be designed in response to the evaluation results. All secondary problems must be corrected before an effect can be achieved on the cervical spine problems. Patients must understand the rationale behind the need to change their postural habits and exercise distance structures. As with low back pain patients, proper body mechanics during all activities of daily living must be enforced. For this reason, we include these patients in the back school program and again review on an individual basis.

OTHER PAIN SYNDROMES

Reflex Sympathetic Dystrophy

Patients with reflex sympathetic dystrophy frequently cannot tolerate movement of the affected limb. Successful therapy is based on a thorough evaluation of the patient's range of motion, strength, activity level, skin condition, and passive joint mobility. Once the evaluation is complete, the patient is then started on a series of sympathetic blocks and medication, after which vigorous activity is encouraged that emphasizes weight bearing, function activities, and an active range of motion. Muscle activity of the affected part is usually minimal, bone density is decreased, and there is no functional use of the part. Joint mobilization is tried gently (without pain) to stimulate the joint nociceptors, and desensitizing techniques are started. Modalities are used with great caution and education on skin protection is reviewed. General activities for noninvolved extremities are encouraged to help with general conditioning, to decrease depression, control body weight, and increase activity. Contrast baths, massage and electrical stimulation, and neuroprobe may be tried to help increase circulation, decrease pain, and desensitize the involved area.

Postherpetic Neuralgia

Chronic pain from postherpetic neuralgia is another very difficult condition for the physical therapist to treat. A few patients will respond favorably to transcutaneous nerve stimulators, neuroprobe, ice, or heat. With some patients the pain is increased or no effect occurs from these cutaneous stimulators. Postherpetic pain patients exhibit decreased activity secondary to the pain. Loss in range of motion and strength of muscle shortening, postural adaptations, and decreased activity are seen. An example would be lesions in the T4 dermatome, causing pain with shoulder elevation. The patient begins to protect the arm by holding it across the abdomen, which soon leads to tightness in the pectoral muscles and roundness in the shoulders. As a result, the head comes forward and soon the patient develops secondary neck pain. Treatment involves educating the patient in ways to maintain normal range of motion and strength, as well as keeping the patient as active as possible. Exercises to the painful part should be limited to a few repetitions at one time but should be done frequently during the day. The other extremities are exercised to help cardiovascular endurance and maintain activity.

Amputation

The chronic pain suffered by amputees has multiple sources and the physical therapy treatment with these pains varies accordingly. Phantom limb pain may be reduced with compression dressings or the wearing of a prosthesis. General conditioning or range of motion exercises do little to decrease the pain. Immediate postoperative compression with casting or fitting with a temporary prosthesis has been said to help control this type of pain. Once started, however, the pain does not respond to physical treatment. Pain caused by an extremely sensitive limb and which increases with cutaneous stimulation may improve upon initiation of a desensitizing program that includes tapping, rubbing of different textures over the stump, and using different stimuli to change sensitivity.

Another type of pain experienced by amputees comes from pressure of the prosthesis on a bony protuberance or irregular scar formation. The amputee begins to develop gait deviations to avoid pressures, which leads to muscle weakness and tightness. Patients may require a device that will assist in taking some of the weight off the stump. This may lead to the patient no longer wearing the prosthesis. Functions and activities of daily living are then decreased secondary to the pain. Treatment is aimed at changing the pressure areas in the prosthesis, checking the prosthesis for proper fit, or possibly trying a new type of socket or suspension system. Muscle and joint contractures need to be stretched and muscles strengthened to a normal grade before the gait deviations can be corrected. An assistive device may need to be prescribed to change the weight-bearing pattern so that the patient can stay more active and experience less pain. Sometimes a wheelchair or motorized cart may be recommended for long-distance outings. At times we must accept these devices as a way for the patient to be more functional and independent. Generalized conditioning, and maintaining range of motion and strength, are extremely important for these patients.

Chronic Abdominal Pain

Chronic abdominal pain can start after abdominal surgery (hysterectomy, exploratory laparotomy, cholecystectomy) for unknown reasons and is often attributed to scar tissue or adhesions. These patients walk with trunk flexion for six to eight weeks following surgery because of incisional pain and they do not use their abdominal muscles during this time. As a consequence, they develop abdominal weakness, postural malalignments, shortness of the hip flexors, and tightness of the back extensors. Along with the abdominal weakness, the contents of the cavity have a weakened retaining wall, and normal spacial relationships are changed. Due to the forward tilt of the pelvis, the hip extensors are stretched for a prolonged time, which creates a stretch weakness. Frequently patients experience a gradual increase in back pain as well as abdominal pain, and their normal activity is reduced secondary to the surgery and pain. Often the patient gains weight and gradually loses muscle strength and cardiovascular endurance. Treatment is based on a full musculoskeletal evaluation.

SUMMARY

Many pain syndromes are caused by or produced from dysfunction of the musculoskeletal systems. Various psychiatric disorders associated with chronic pain syndromes invariably lead to inactivity. An understanding of the altered pathophysiology, physical endurance, and structural adaptations is essential to formulate a physical therapy program that will reverse these changes. The physical therapy evaluation is incorporated into the overall assessment of the chronic pain patient to facilitate its integration into the multidisciplinary treatment of the chronic pain patient.

REFERENCES

1. McKenzie R: The Lumbar Spine. Waikonae, New Zealand, Spinal Publications, 1981
2. Nachemson A: The lumbar spine: an orthopaedic challenge. Spine 1:50–71, 1976
3. Kirkaldy-Willis WH, Wedge JH, Yong-Hing K, et al: Pathology and pathogenesis of lumbar spondylosis and stenosis. Spine 3:319, 1978
4. Paris S: Anatomy as Related to Function and Pain: The Orthopedic Clinics of North America. Philadelphia, W.R. Saunders, 1983
5. Gould J, Davies G: Orthopaedic and Sports Medicine, Saint Louis, C. V. Mosby, 1985
6. Saunders HD: Evaluation, Treatment and Prevention of Musculoskeletal Disorders. Minneapolis, Viking Press, 1985
7. Kendall F, McCreary E: Muscles Testing and Function. Baltimore, Williams & Wilkins, 1983

Chapter 15

Sexual Dysfunction
and Chronic Pain

John S. Jordan, Ph.D.
Francis J. Keefe, Ph.D.

Recent estimates of sexual dysfunction among chronic pain patients place the prevalence as high as 75 percent (1). Moreover, because sexual functioning is often central to psychological and marital adjustment, it is typically an area of major concern to chronic pain patients and their spouses. Despite its high prevalence and importance, however, the sexual functioning of this population has been largely ignored. Indeed, to date there are no reported controlled studies of sexual rehabilitation with chronic pain patients.

We begin this chapter with a summary of the limited research on sexual functioning in chronic pain patients. Next we examine some of the complex interrelationships between sexuality and chronic pain. Finally, we offer practical suggestions for preventing and/or treating the sexual dysfunction of chronic pain patients.

CURRENT STATUS OF RESEARCH ON SEXUAL FUNCTIONING AND CHRONIC PAIN

Little has been written about the prevalence of sexual dysfunction among chronic pain patients. There are also no reported studies of sexual rehabilitation with this population, either through direct intervention or as an indirect result of other intervention strategies.

Among the possible reasons for the paucity of data are: a general underestimation of the degree of importance of sexual functioning to chronic pain patients and their spouses; frequent reluctance to enter into discussions of such "sensitive" material by both the patient and health care provider; a lack of understanding about what can be done to alter the course of sexual dysfunction once identified in this population; and the difficulties one faces with research on a problem with multiple etiologies and complex interactions with other factors. Nevertheless, the little research conducted on this problem does suggest that sexual dysfunction is of great magnitude and importance to chronic pain patients and their spouses.

LaBan and colleagues (2) studied 43 men who had sustained back injuries from industrial accidents. Using a narrow view of sexual functioning—ability to satisfactorily perform intercourse—they found that 63 percent were impotent. In a study of 66 married patients referred to a pain management center, Maruta and Osborne (3) found that almost two-thirds reported deterioration in sexual adjustment, and more than one-third reported deterioration of the marriage itself. Although 20 percent of the females and none of the males reported sexual dysfunction prior to the onset of pain, approximately one-half of each group reported sexual dysfunction after the onset of the pain problem. A similar prevalence of sexual dysfunction was found in a subsequent study by Maruta and colleagues (1). In independent interviews of 50 patients and their spouses, these researchers found that 78 percent of patients and 84 percent of spouses reported either reduction or elimination of sexual activity.

Although these studies provide important and interesting first facts about the extent of sexual and marital dysfunction and dissatisfaction among chronic pain patients, they have significant shortcomings. The measures of sexual dysfunction and marital satisfaction employed are quite cursory (often single questions) and do not permit comparison with studies of normal couples (4). The whole definition of sexuality in these studies is severely restricted; no regard is given to the multiple possible modes of sexual expression other than intercourse. Absent are clear measures of the degree to which chronic low back pain patients view their sexual functioning as an important area for rehabilitation. Nor has the contribution of depression or the patient's beliefs about the relation of his or her sexual functioning to the pain syndrome been explored.

RELATION BETWEEN CHRONIC PAIN AND SEXUALITY

The relation between chronic pain and sexuality is complex. In chronic pain patients, sexual activity may increase or decrease pain. The underlying pathophysiology, psychological sequelae, or even the treatment of chronic pain can cause sexual dysfunction. To grasp the sometimes complex relation between chronic pain and sexuality it is first necessary to understand the relevant organic, conditioning/learning, dyadic, and intrapsychic components.

Organic Factors

In chronic low back pain, both the underlying pathophysiology and certain treatment methods can adversely affect sexual functioning. A primary reason is that the portions of the lumbar and sacral spine most often involved in chronic low back pain are those in close proximity to the nerve roots responsible for transmission of sexual stimulation (5). For example, because the hypogastric plexus is located in front of the L5 disk, the risk of iatrogenic effects on sexuality from surgical interventions for low back pain is significantly increased, particularly with anterior fusions.

Many of the medications employed with chronic pain patients can affect sexual functioning. For example, antidepressant medications occasionally cause male erectile dysfunction and a decrease in the clitoral erectile response. Narcotic analgesics may decrease libido. Neuroleptics also have been related to erection and ejaculatory problems.

Because the most commonly used positions for sexual intercourse involve hyperextension of the spine, such positions can exacerbate pain.

Conditioning and Learning Factors

Individuals learn quickly which behaviors worsen their pain and which make them feel better. Those that increase pain tend to be avoided in the future, whereas those that reduce pain are likely to be repeated. Sexual activity in chronic pain patients can have either effect.

Physiologic tension may be the primary determinant of whether sex will increase or reduce pain—the greater the tension, the greater the pain. Some sexually related activities (for example, massage, caressing) may specifically reduce tension; others, particularly performance-directed activities, may typically increase tension. Whether a particular sexual activity will actually increase or reduce tension, however, depends on many factors. These include one's cultural and religious values, attitudes about one's partner, and expectations regarding pain. The latter may be particularly important. If prior sexual activity has resulted in pain increases, the patient is likely to be especially avoidant, guarded, and tense regarding future sexual activity. Such anticipatory tension results in a self-fulfilling prophecy of increased pain. Often, as a result of this kind of tension-pain cycle, sexual activity comes to be avoided altogether.

Other aspects of chronic pain patients' prior sexual learning histories also may influence their sexual functioning. Basically, the more restricted an individual's repertoire of sexual behavior and goals, the more difficulty he or she is likely to experience with sexuality. Those chronic patients most prone to sexual dysfunction may be those who do not know how to (or choose not to) engage in foreplay, alternative positions for sexual intercourse, nonorgasm-oriented mutual pleasuring, and nonintercourse stimulation to orgasm (for example, oral or manual). Individuals who either lack the skills or flexibility for alternative sexual satisfaction will have difficulty when the sole or primary sexual behavior pattern results in pain.

Anxiety related to faulty beliefs or "myths" about sexuality sometimes has adverse consequences for chronic pain patients. For example, the onset of a pain disorder may heighten awareness of altered sexual functioning that actually stems from the normal aging process. In the female, age-related changes may include a reduction in the distensibility of the vaginal barrel, marked thinning of the vaginal mucosa, and delay in the production of vaginal lubrication. These changes may result from declining postmenopausal estrogen secretion and cause significant discomfort (6). In the aging male, normal changes include significant delays in attaining and maintaining a full penile erection, decreased ejaculatory force and volume, and longer refractory periods (7). These changes may be misperceived by the chronic pain patient as signs of impending impotence. While these age-related changes frequently require minor alteration of sexual patterns for both the male and female (for example, increased foreplay time), they certainly need not result in sexual dysfunction. Note, however, that the anxiety and discomfort surrounding these changes may be sufficient to lead to avoidance of sexual activity or sexual dysfunction.

Dyadic Factors

Chronic pain occurs within the context of a network of social relationships. These relationships are almost invariably stressed. For the chronic pain patient, few areas of daily functioning remain unaffected. Family role changes are common. The "breadwinner" is often no longer able to fulfill his or her role as family provider and the nonafflicted spouse is then typically forced to assume both household and money-earning responsibilities. Patients may be angry with what they perceive to be the family's lack of understanding or support. Spouses and family members of chronic pain patients (as well as the patients themselves) may become frustrated with their inability to effect any change in the pain syndrome. To avoid making the situation any worse, the frustration and anger with this situation is often hidden under a superficial harmony.

Relationship conflicts, especially when inhibited from direct expression, have adverse effects on sexual relations. Both patients and spouses may withhold sexual contact as an indirect expression of their anger and frustration. Sometimes spouses' concerns about hurting the chronic patient are indirect expressions of their anger. Minimally, the presence of such concerns suggests some inadequacy in the couples' communication.

Any preexisting relationship problems are also likely to be potentiated under the stress of chronic pain. Some writers (8) have actually suggested that chronic pain patients are characterized by a high prevalence of preexisting marital distress. For some couples, chronic pain may provide a "legitimized" excuse for avoidance of a previously unsatisfactory sexual relationship.

Intrapsychic Factors

The severe depression observed in some chronic pain patients is often responsible for sexual dysfunction. Depression may sufficiently reduce sexual interest to preclude sexual functioning even in the absence of organic, dyadic, or learning deficits. Similarly, decreased self-esteem (represented in concerns about body image and attractiveness, meeting role expectations) may be a factor in reduced sexual interest.

Individuals' basic attitudes about sexuality sometimes inhibit their capacity for satisfactory sexual relations. In the extreme, individuals may acquire the belief that sexual behavior is morally wrong, a disgusting and/or unpleasant but necessary evil, or intended exclusively for procreation. Traumatic or unpleasant prior sexual experiences may be similarly brought forward into new and otherwise potentially rewarding sexual opportunities (9).

PREVENTION AND TREATMENT OF SEXUAL DYSFUNCTION IN CHRONIC PAIN PATIENTS

Detailed sex therapy techniques are clearly beyond the scope of this chapter and the competence of most practitioners involved in the treatment of chronic pain. There are, however, a number of intervention strategies that may usefully be applied in many treatment settings. On a continuum of effort and expertise required, these include educational, behavioral, and marital interventions. Patients and spouses are often quite concerned about their sexual functioning. However, until someone is comfortable and straightforward in their willingness to discuss these issues, they will often go unaddressed (9).

Educational Interventions

At the most basic level is permission-giving, letting the patient and partner know that it is O.K. to engage in sexual relations. When combined with an openness to patients' and partners' specific concerns, permission-giving is often sufficient to counter negative beliefs and unnecessary fears (for example, about "sick people" having sex, or fears about permanent physical harm being done). Sometimes a health "authority" figure can be instrumental in helping the patient/partner expand their sexual repertoire and goals merely by indicating that this is appropriate. Specific information on positions for intercourse is often welcomed. Generally, the likelihood of pain seems to be reduced with the pain patient in a nondominant (nonthrusting) position. Because of hyperextension of the spine, face-to-face positions are not recommended. However, many clinicians highly recommend the "spoon" position for intercourse. In this position, both partners lie on their sides (often with the knees slightly tucked in a fetal position). The male lies behind the female and enters the vagina from the rear.

Behavioral Interventions

Behavioral interventions are geared toward reducing the anxiety and tension often associated with sex. Often patients' concerns about exacerbating pain with sexual behavior are so great that their avoidance of sex is near phobic proportions. Some patients indicate that they will rarely even allow partners to touch them. One useful intervention is to have the couple contract not to engage in intercourse or attempts to achieve orgasm. Instead, they are encouraged to engage in a graded series of exercises beginning with massage and light (that is, nongenital) caressing. With the performance pressure thus removed, both partners often become extremely sexually aroused, so aroused in some cases that they violate the rule against intromission and thereby (paradoxically) effect a cure. More typically, however, recovery is not spontaneous. Couples are guided through a series of "sensate focus" exercises intended to heighten awareness of pleasure from a wide variety of body sensations—both as giver and receiver. Kaplan (7) provides a comprehensive description of these procedures.

Marital Interventions

When anger and frustration are intense and marital communication is quite poor, educational and behavioral sex therapy interventions by themselves may have little effect. Such couples can be helped to work on agreed-upon pain management goals, communicate needs more directly, engage in problem-solving, and focus on positive aspects of the relationship. As a way of enhancing communication, mutual understanding, and pleasant activity, couples sometimes benefit from encouragement to reinstate "dating." Jacobson and Margolin (10) describe a brief and apparently effective form of behavioral marital therapy that may be particularly appropriate for this patient population.

REFERENCES

1. Maruta T, Osborne D, Swanson, DW, et al: Chronic pain patients and spouses: marital and sexual adjustment. Mayo Clin 56:307–310, 1981
2. LaBan MM, Burk RD, Johnson EW: Sexual impotence in men having low–back syndrome. Arch Phys Med 47:715–723, 1966
3. Maruta T, Osborne D: Sexual activity in chronic pain patients. Psychosomatics 19:531–537, 1978
4. Frank E, Anderson C, Rubinstein D: Frequency of sexual dysfunction in "normal" couples. N Engl J Med 299:111–115, 1978
5. Infante MC: Sexual dysfunction in the patient with chronic back pain. Sexuality and Disability 4:173–179, 1981
6. Kay B, Neelley, JN: Sexuality and the aging: a review of current literature. Sexuality and Disability 5:38–46, 1982
7. Kaplan HS: The New Sex Therapy. New York, Brunner/Mazel, 1974
8. Waring EM: The role of the family in symptom selection and perpetuation of psychosomatic illness. Psychother Psychosom 28:253–259, 1977
9. Thorn-Gray BE, Kern LH: Sexual dysfunction associated with physical disability: a treatment guide for the rehabilitation practitioner. Rehabilitation Literature 44:138–144, 1983
10. Jacobson NS, Margolin G: Marital Therapy. New York, Brunner/Mazel, 1979

Assessment

Chapter 16

Assessment of Chronic Pain

Randal D. France, M.D.
K. Ranga Rama Krishnan, M.D.

An accurate evaluation of the chronic pain patient is important since multiple factors can produce or modify the pain complaints. The evaluation usually includes an assessment of the precipitating illness that has led to the chronic pain state, and the patient's present state of health and functioning. In the preceding chapters, different aspects of the chronic pain state were described and formulated according to four different but related approaches—phenomenological, psychological, behavioral, and biological. If the assessment is based on a multidimensional perspective that takes into account all four approaches, a more comprehensive and effective treatment plan can then be implemented. Furthermore, the label chronic pain syndrome does not imply or state the etiological cause of the persistent pain. This diagnosis is merely descriptive of the duration of the pain complaint. It is, therefore, essential in evaluating these patients that the physician obtain a thorough description of the pain, present and past medical history, as well as a determination of past and present psychological functioning.

Since pain is the presenting and major complaint, the initial assessment of this symptom should be done. An organized approach to the assessment of the pain is recommended to glean an understanding of the clinical state and to formulate a diagnosis. While an open-ended style of interviewing elicits associations among psychologically related data, there is the danger that the interviewer will be left with a large amount of seemingly unrelated clinical data. Often the task with a chronic pain patient is to understand the associations or relationships that exist between the various physical and psychological symptoms. As noted earlier, most chronic pain patients have both a psychological and physiological cause of the persistent pain. If only the psychological complaints are addressed, an erroneous assessment of the pain will likely result. When the pain complaints are assessed from a purely psychological perspective with a failure to assess the presence or absence of physical causes, the interviewer will formulate a psychological diagnosis on the assumption that there are no physical problems.

An organized assessment of the chronic pain patient begins with a description of the presenting complaint and pain, and proceeds to the psychiatric assessment of the patient. Such an approach highlights the pain complaint both to the patient and to the examiner. In this method, questions concerning psychological functioning are reserved until late in the interview. The initial questions concern the pain complaint itself and thus help establish rapport between the patient and physician, as these questions mark the pain complaint as important. After a rapport has been established, the more sensitive questions concerning psychological functioning can be addressed.

SITES

Analysis of the pain complaint is initiated by locating the site of the pain (Table 1), which may be either single or multiple. If a patient complains of multiple pain sites, a determination is made as to whether the sites are constant in location or are migratory. In addition, in patients with multiple pain complaints, individual discrepancies among the various pain sites are rated to determine to what extent the pain sites are part of the same pathophysiological process.

Patients whose pain is psychological in origin usually complain of multiple sites, the description of which varies greatly. When analyzing migratory pain, the circumstances causing the appearance of pain in a new location are examined. Frequently these patients complain of one pain site at a given time, but the location of the pain may vary over time. Events precipitating any associated symptoms are considered for possible causative factors. To determine whether the pain follows a radicular pattern or is diffused, the distribution of the pain site needs to be elicited. Psychological pain rarely follows a radicular distribution. The site of the pain is examined for any evidence of swelling, tenderness, skin color changes, temperature differences, texture of the skin, or presence of trigger points. Swelling, skin changes, temperature differences, and changes in the texture of the skin are commonly seen in causalgia, reflex sympathetic dystrophy, and vascular insufficiency. Pain complaints in these patients may or may not follow a dermatomal pattern. In patients with longstanding reflex sympathetic dystrophy, the skin becomes thin and paper-like. The physical changes may occur over time or can be absent for various intervals. Precipitating events causing the physical

Table 1. Analysis of Pain Complaints: Site

Number	Associated physical changes
single	swelling
multiple	tenderness
constant	skin color changes
migratory	temperature changes
	texture of skin
Constancy of site	trigger points
	irritation of peripheral nerves
Physiological/autonomical correlation	
present	Sensory changes
absent	decrease hypoalgesia
	increase hyperalgesia
	exaggerated (hyperpathic)
	abnormal (paresthesia)
	unpleasant (dysesthesia)

changes should be assessed. Trigger points within the muscles are present in patients with myofascial pain syndrome. Inflamed or irritated peripheral nerves elicit pain on palpation (Tinel's sign). Sensory changes (increased, decreased, exaggerated, or abnormal) near or on the pain site are assessed.

ONSET

The onset of the pain should be determined (Table 2). Did the pain begin rapidly, over time (gradually), or over an unknown period of time? Precipitating factors, both physical and psychological, are assessed. Physical events can include such things as trauma, infection, malignancy, medication intake, and medical or surgical treatment. Assessment is made of the patient's social setting and psychological distress level at the time the physical factors initiated the pain syndrome. A determination of what psychological factors preceded or were present at the onset of the pain is made. Death of a close relative, anniversary reaction, loss of employment, divorce or marriage, or birth of a child are all life events that may be contributing factors.

CHARACTER

The character of the pain includes the sensory, emotional (affective), and intensity descriptions of the pain (Table 3). Sensory words include such adjectives as burning, hot, aching, shooting, cramping, sore, and sharp. Emotional or affective descriptors frequently cited are tiring, fearful, cruel, binding, tortuous, and annoying. Intensity descriptors often heard include weak, mild, moderate, intense, severe, or excruciating. An important question to be asked is whether the pain radiates to specific or

Table 2. Analysis of Pain: Onset

Time of onset	Psychological events preceding pain
	death of a close relative
Speed of onset	anniversary reaction
rapid	loss of job
gradual	divorce/marriage
insidious	birth of a child
Precipitating factors	
trauma	
infection	
malignancy	
medication	
operation	

Table 3. Analysis of Pain Complaints: Character

Pain Descriptors

Sensory:	aching	pinching	sore
	burning	pulling	tingling
	cramping	scalding	stabbing
	crushing	sharp	stinging
	hot	shooting	throbbing
Emotional:	agonizing	exhausting	sickening
	binding	fearful	suffocating
	cruel	killing	tiring
	dreadful	punishing	torturing
Intensity:	weak	mild	moderate
	strong	intense	severe
	excruciating		

0–10 pain scale:

0 = no pain
10 = pain they could not tolerate

Radiation: specify vague, clear, generalized

---

vaguely described areas. To quantify measures of these descriptors, Melzack (1) developed the McGill Pain Questionnaire (Table 4). The word descriptors for pain are divided into three major groups of words—sensory, affective, and evaluative. Numerical values are assigned to each word descriptor. A score can be computed for each major group of words and a total score can be determined. The number of words chosen can also be used. These data provide quantitative information of a patient's pain complaint that can be treated statistically. Dubuisson and Melzack found that specific groups of words could correctly identify certain acute pain states (toothache, labor pain) (2). However, in a study of chronic pain patients (cancer, arthritis, benign chronic pain), Atkinson and colleagues (3) found that patients suffering from chronic pain caused by different illnesses do not use pain words in a systemic fashion. It has also been shown that the level of psychological distress affects the way in which patients describe their pain (3, 4). The intensity of the pain can be assessed on a 0–10 pain scale. For example, the patient can be asked to rate the intensity of his or her pain on a 0–10 scale, with 0 representing no pain and 10 being the worst it can be. The patient should rate the level of pain at the present time as well as at its highest and lowest levels. The words the patient uses to describe the intensity of the pain does not help us differentiate whether the pain is of psychologi-

Table 4.   McGill Pain Questionnaire

What does your pain feel like?
Tell which words best describe your present pain.
Use only a single word in each appropriate group—the one that applies best.
Indicate answer with (✔)

1		2		3		4	
1. flickering	☐	1. jumping	☐	1. pricking	☐	1. sharp	☐
2. quivering		2. flashing		2. boring		2. cutting	
3. pulsing		3. shooting	☐	3. drilling		3. lacerating	☐
4. throbbing				4. stabbing			
5. beating				5. lancinating			
6. pounding	☐						

5		6		7		8	
1. pinching	☐	1. tugging	☐	1. hot	☐	1. tingling	☐
2. pressing		2. pulling		2. burning		2. itchy	
3. gnawing		3. wrenching	☐	3. scalding		3. smarting	
4. cramping				4. searing	☐	4. stinging	☐
5. crushing	☐						

9		10		11		12	
1. dull	☐	1. tender	☐	1. tiring	☐	1. sickening	☐
2. sore		2. taut		2. exhausting	☐	2. suffocating	☐
3. hurting		3. rasping					
4. aching		4. splitting	☐				
5. heavy	☐						

13		14		15		16	
1. fearful	☐	1. punishing	☐	1. wretched	☐	1. annoying	☐
2. frightful		2. grueling		2. blinding	☐	2. troublesome	
3. terrifying	☐	3. cruel				3. miserable	
		4. vicious				4. intense	
		5. killing	☐			5. unbearable	☐

17		18		19		20	
1. spreading	☐	1. tight	☐	1. cool	☐	1. nagging	☐
2. radiating		2. numb		2. cold		2. nauseating	
3. penetrating		3. drawing		3. freezing	☐	3. agonizing	
4. piercing	☐	4. squeezing				4. dreadful	
		5. tearing	☐			5. torturing	☐

cal or physical origin. Another measure of pain intensity is the Visual Analog Scale (VAS). This consists of a 100 mm line with end-points described as "no pain" and "pain as bad as it can be." The patient is asked to mark the point which represents his intensity of pain (5).

COURSE

Patients can describe the time course of their pain as continuous or intermittent (Table 5). The intensity of continuous pain can either fluctuate or be constant. Factors associated with fluctuations in the intensity of the persistent pain should be solicited. Sensory and emotional descriptors themselves can be either continuous or changing. Again, it is important to determine what factors change the descriptors of the pain. Intermittent chronic pain can be periodic (changing at regular intervals) or varying irregularly. Cyclic types of pain complaints are often seen with chronic pelvic pain in women. Diurnal and seasonal fluctuations in pain complaints can occur. With mechanical types of pain, the intensity usually increases as the pain continues throughout the day as a result of physical activity. Pain complaints in patients with recurrent major depression or manic-depressive illness may show a seasonal variation. Pain that is initiated on a specific date or time not associated with illness or trauma may indicate an underlying anniversary reaction when chronic pain is of psychological origin.

Factors Modifying Pain

Any factors that modify the pain complaint need to be noted. As is shown in Table 6, these factors can be clustered into four major groups:

Physical factors include movement, posture, coughing, sneezing, weather and temperature, eating, defecation, micturition, sex, and fatigue. Certain movements in posture can either intensify or attenuate

Table 5. Analysis of Pain Complaints: Course

Continuous	constant
Intensity:	fluctuate
Description:	constant
	change
Intermittent	(regular intervals)
	irregular
Diurnal	seasonal fluctuation

Table 6. Analysis of Pain Complaints: Factors Modifying Pain

	Aggravating	Relieving
Physical:		
movement	+	+
posture	+	+
coughing	+	
sneezing	+	
weather	+	+
eating	+	+
temperature	+	+
defecating	+	
micturiting	+	
sex	+	
fatigue	+	
Emotional:		
stress	+	
anxiety	+	
depression	+	
relaxation		+
Treatment:		
Medication		
narcotic analgesic		+
nonnarcotic analgesic		+
minor tranquilizer	+	+
neuroleptic		+
antidepressant		+
steroids		+
Physical treatment		
local treatment	+	+
nerve stimulators	+	+
traction	+	+
management	+	+
exercise program	+	+
brace	+	+
operation	+	+
nerve block		+
Socioenvironmental:		
compensation	+	
litigation	+	
disability	+	
social support system	+	+

pain complaints. Patients are usually quite aware of these factors. Coughing and sneezing both increase pain, especially when there is nerve root irritation. Damp, cold weather or drop in barometric pressure are associated with increase in pain. Temperature or eating can either increase or decrease the level of pain. Eating is increased in chronic pain patients when the intensity of the pain is elevated. The act of defecation and micturition increases pain. Sexual intercourse usually increases pain complaints, especially in patients with low back pain and females with pelvic pain. Fatigue is reported to increase pain for most all chronic pain patients.

Emotional reactions, such as depression or anxiety, exaggerate the pain. Emotional stress of any kind will also increase the pain complaints. Relaxation or mental distraction will decrease pain complaints.

Treatment with opioid analgesics, nonopioid analgesics, neuroleptics, antidepressants, and steroids are often associated with lessening of pain. Minor tranquilizers, however, exaggerate the complaints of chronic pain patients. Physical treatment (exercise or localized physical therapies) can either increase or decrease pain, as do operations or bracing. Nerve blocks attenuate chronic pain complaints in patients with nerve root irritation.

Socioeconomic factors such as compensation, litigation, and disability, often exaggerate the level of pain and disability from the pain complaint. Social support systems can either intensify or help attenuate the pain.

Effects of Pain

The effects of pain on the patient's level of activity at home, work, or social setting should be assessed (Table 7). Examples of questions that

Table 7. Analysis of Pain Complaints: Effect of Pain

Activity	Neurovegetative signs
home	sleep
work	appetite
social	weight
	sex
Psychological	
depression	Mentation
anxiety	concentration
maladaptive behavior	memory
Substance abuse	
alcohol	
drugs (minor tranquilizers,	
narcotics, nonnarcotics)	

should be asked include: What type of activity does your pain keep you from doing? Does the pain keep you from working? How much time do you spend resting (lying in bed) to control the pain level? Estimations of sitting and walking tolerance are made. How far the patient can walk and how long he or she can sit before the pain level is increased should be determined. To what extent the pain isolates the patient from family and friends is also important to learn.

An assessment of the psychological and behavioral reaction caused by the chronic pain comes next. Determining the severity of the depression and anxiety symptoms helps us decide whether the patient is experiencing an emotional reaction or has a psychophysiological disorder resulting from the persistent pain. The patient's misuse or abuse of alcohol or drugs to control the effects of the chronic pain must be examined. Type and severity of neurovegetative signs (sleep, appetite, sex) should be assessed, as should be any alterations in concentration, mentation, and memory. Psychoactive drugs and pain medications used in chronic pain states will alter a patient's ability to mentate.

Prior History

Questions relating to any current and past treatments for chronic pain are an integral part of the assessment (Table 8). The patient's response to each treatment should be noted, as well as how long each treatment has continued. A history of previous painful and/or major illnesses is taken, with examination of the cause, duration, treatment, and outcome of each illness. Any prior history of psychiatric illness or substance abuse is also recorded. Since medications and behavioral treatments used to treat

Table 8. Analysis of Pain Complaints: Prior History

Current and past treatment	History of previous painful,
traction	major illnesses
braces	course
physical therapy	duration
ice pack/heat	treatment
massage	outcome
electrical stimulation	
pain medications	History of previous psychiatric
hypnosis	illnesses or substance abuse
acupuncture	
nerve blocks	
psychotherapy	
operations	
physical manipulation	
biofeedback	
psychotropic drugs	

chronic pain may be similar to the ones used to treat psychiatric disorders, a patient's reaction to previous psychiatric treatment should be carefully assessed.

Premorbid Personality and Interpersonal Behavior

Specific premorbid personality traits are associated with chronic pain that originates from psychological causes (Table 9). These patients have personality traits that involve excessive dependency needs, masochistic character, self-punitive behavior, excessive somatic concerns, poor impulse control, and limited ability to regulate self-esteem. In addition, these patients usually lack psychological-mindedness. Traditional insight-oriented psychotherapy fails even if the pain generates out of psychological causes. However, these patients often do respond to a structured and supportive pain management program. The goal for these patients is management and control of the pain symptoms and avoidance of unnecessary medications and elective operations.

The sociopathic patient who complains of chronic pain has a limited response to treatment. Patients with paranoid ideation and psychotic thought processes should be assessed carefully, especially when invasive treatments have been recommended by their physicians, since such invasive procedures or operations are, in general, to be avoided in these patients. This group of patients also has a limited response to pain management treatment approaches. For some people with poor impulse control, pain serves as a defense against their aggressiveness. Treatment specifically aimed at their pain complaints can precipitate aggressive types of acting-out behavior.

Emotional reactivity and hysterical traits are frequently associated with psychological causes of pain, but alone are not pathognomonic of psychological pain. In fact, in patients with hysterical personality traits/disorders, pain is distressing since it and the resulting disability limits their attractiveness and exhibitionism. While patients with such personality traits/disorders may develop psychologically based chronic pain, there are other aspects of their personalities (immaturity, excessive dependency, somatization, and masochistic character) that can also account for the development of pain symptoms.

In patients whose chronic pain is organic-based, an assessment of their premorbid personality is important for predicting their response to treatment. Once again, elective operations or procedures should be avoided in chronic pain patients with psychotic thought processes, paranoid ideation, sociopathic traits, self-punitive behavior, poor impulse control, excessive somatic concerns, or masochistic character. These patients, too, will show poor response to pain management programs. As pain management occurs, these patients often display defenses in the form of regression or acting out behavior.

Table 9. Analysis of Pain Complaints: Premorbid Personality and Interpersonal Behavior

Premorbid personality traits	Interpersonal behavior
dependency	stability of relationships
masochistic character	type of relationship
self-punitive behavior	interpersonal themes:
self-esteem regulation	excessively dependent
narcissistic traits	masochistic
excessive somatic concerns	overly independent
histrionic traits	hostile–demanding
degree of emotionality	suspicious
intro/extroversion	explosive
impulse control	self-reliant
ability to sublime	good-directed
psycho/sociopathic traits	adaptive
paranoid ideation	
psychotic thought	

For chronic pain patients who have had a history of stable and mature interpersonal relationships, the pain is less likely to be psychological in origin. On the other hand, when patients describe relationships that are characterized by excessive or overt dependency, masochism, hostile demanding, or exploitation, the possibility is likely that the chronic pain is psychological or has significant psychological components. Patients who tend to be self-reliant, goal-directed, and adaptive tend not to have pain as a psychological defense; and if these patients do develop a chronic pain state based on organic causes, then they respond well to pain management approaches.

Family History

The family's medical history should be examined for occurrence of major illness, chronic illness, disability resulting from chronic illness or trauma, and age and cause of death of first-degree relatives (Table 10). These data cannot, obviously, tell us whether the patient's current pain problem is genetically or environmentally determined, but the impact of such chronic or major illnesses can be assessed. A family history assessment for psychiatric disorders should be done, especially for depression and alcoholism, as these disorders are commonly seen in chronic pain patients.

Chronic pain patients generally come from large family units. The relationship the patient has had and presently has with his or her parents and siblings needs to be explored. The reaction of the family members to the chronic pain patient should be examined. Behaviors and attitudes on the part of family members that promote or generate the patient's pain

Table 10. Analysis of Pain Complaints: Family History

Medical family history
   major illnesses
   chronic illnesses
   disabilities
   age and death of first degree relatives

Psychiatric family history
   psychiatric disorder
   alcohol or substance abuse/
     addiction

History of family structure and function
   size of family
   relationship with parents and siblings
   family's reaction to chronic pain and illness
   age and reason for leaving home

behaviors need to be assessed. Such behaviors would include over-solicitous concern, denial of the problem, need for a cure to the problem, emotional or physical exclusion of the pain patient from the family, and failure of the family to support pain control or management approaches. The patient should be asked to describe the circumstances and reasons for leaving home and at what age he or she first did so. These issues are especially pertinent in women whose chronic pelvic pain is without obvious organic pathology.

Marital History

The marital status of the chronic pain patient should be determined (Table 11). Most chronic pain patients are married. It is important to question the medical and psychiatric history of the spouse to discover whether he or she has a chronic pain or disability problem. The employment status and source of income of the spouse should be established. A description of the marital relationship and the spouse's reaction to the chronic pain patient is vital, since the spouse's attitude and behavior toward the patient is often significant in the rehabilitation process. If a spouse does not support pain therapy, it will be difficult for the patient to comply with treatment.

Social History

The patient's employment status and occupation should be elicited (Table 12), along with current work status and source of income, either from employment or disability payment (and which type). Many patients

Table 11. Analysis of Pain Complaints: Marital History

Marital status	Medical history of spouse
single	Psychiatric history of spouse
married	
widowed	Employment status of spouse
separated	Spouse's source of income
divorced	Type of marital relationship
	Spouse's reaction to chronic pain

whose pain has persisted for longer than one year are either on a medical leave of absence or are unemployed. These patients are often on disability payments and have experienced a loss of income since the onset of their illness. In some cases, the spouse has begun work to support the family, and the family now depends on this income. Inquiries into whether the patient is involved in the process of litigation for Workmen's Compensation claims, Social Security disability, or a liability suit for personal injury are appropriate. Patients who are in the process of litigation for personal injury have a poor prognosis for pain management. Even though questions concerning pending litigation are not part

Table 12. Analysis of Pain Complaints: Social History

Occupation	Pending litigation
	compensation
Employment	Social Security disability
full time	liability suit for personal injury
part time	
medical leave of absence	Social support system
retired	family
retired on disability	friends
student	church
unemployed seeking work	community
unemployed not seeking work	medical support groups
Source of income	Patient's reactions to social
employment	environment
Social Security	
Social Security disability	
Workmen's Compensation insurance	
long-term disability	
none	
spouse's income	

of the usual medical or psychiatric evaluation, the process of litigation for personal injury has a strong negative correlation to treatment outcome. Litigation for Social Security and Workmen's Compensation claims are not as significant in predicting a poor outcome for pain management as for personal injury litigation. If the chronic pain is a result of a job-related injury, documentation of the injury and/or its relationship to the present pain problems is important from both a legal (Workmen's Compensation) and clinical standpoint.

A brief history of the patient's social support system should be examined. Medical support groups for chronic pain patients are rarely found in communities. However, with the growing number of pain centers around the country, medical support groups have been established in communities near such centers. Many chronic pain patients withdraw from family, friends, and fellow members of church and community groups. This isolation heightens their depression and despair. Patients who poorly manage their pain often describe emotionally stressful interactions with family members or friends. As the chronic pain patient manages the condition more effectively, he or she is increasingly able to use the support of surrounding persons.

A complete review of systems should be included in the evaluation. The chronic pain patient may have an ongoing and/or undetected illness that may not be part of the original problem connected with chronic pain. Over a four-year period, two percent of the chronic pain patients admitted to Duke University's Pain Management Program were discovered to have an undiagnosed malignancy at the time they began the program. This is noteworthy since all patients were physician-referred and had extensive evaluations prior to their referral to the pain management program. The incidence of newly diagnosed thyroid dysfunction in the same program is approximately four percent. It is important to determine whether medical illnesses promote or exaggerate the chronic pain problem (that is, hypothyroid dysfunction). Due to the consuming nature of the chronic pain problem itself, other illnesses are often not thought of by the treating team. In addition, since the primary problem of these patients is chronic pain over extended periods of time, other illnesses certainly may have had time to present themselves.

The examiner should review the previous medical or surgical evaluation in chronic pain patients who have been referred by other physicians (Table 13). This review may include the results of metabolic laboratory studies (erythrocyte, sedimentation rate, thyroid panel, complete blood count, liver panel, calcium, phosphorus, blood chemistries, plasma creatinine, fluorescent antinuclear antibodies), electromyogram, myelogram, plain x-ray films, computerized tomograms, and somatosensory evoked potentials. If it appears that the work-up is incomplete, further evaluation and special consultation is warranted.

Table 13. Analysis of Pain Complaints: Laboratory Evaluations

Blood analysis	Electromyelogram
complete blood count	
chemistries	Somatosensory evoked potentials
creatinine	
liver panel	Radiography
thyroid panel	plain film x-rays
calcium, phosphorus	myelography
erthyrocyte sedimentation rate	computerized tomography
fluorescent antinuclear antibodies	

Mental Status

A thorough mental status examination should be performed. Deficiencies in mentation are often seen in chronic pain patients, and mainly occur in two groups: those patients overmedicated for their pain complaints, and demented patients whose mentation defects are masked by their pain complaints. It may be helpful to use a standardized mental status examination that can be scored, such as the Folstein and Folstein Minimental state exam (6). Since the incidence of psychotic disorders is uncommon, mental status testing for psychotic thought, delusions, hallucinations, and abstract thinking yields limited useful data. It is important to ask questions relating to the presence or absence of suicidal ideation, intent, or plan since depression is commonly seen in chronic pain patients, many of whom are experiencing a debilitating illness with significant degrees of social isolation and suffering.

Psychiatric Assessment

The psychiatric evaluation should determine whether or not the patient has a psychopathological disorder, a reactive psychiatric illness, or emotional factors that would affect a physical illness. Occasionally, clinicians state that it is difficult to assess for the presence of a psychopathological disorder in chronic pain patients since the symptoms of the chronic pain illness may be similar to ones observed in psychiatric disorders. This confusion certainly has been applied to chronic pain and affective disorders because both types of patients complain of neurovegetative symptoms (alterations in sleep, energy, appetite, and sex). However, if one of the standard diagnostic schemes for depression is used, it is relatively easy to differentiate the presence or absence of depression in chronic pain patients. The depressed patient not only exhibits neurovegetative symptoms but, in addition, displays the cognitive and mood disturbances associated with affective disorders. If poorly defined criteria for depression are used or if depression is diagnosed on a severity continuum (no depression to severe depression), then the confusion is increased between what is depression and what is chronic pain.

Assessment of Current Psychiatric Disorders

In Chapter 9, we discussed the occurrence of pain complaints in various psychiatric disorders. In that chapter, we focused on the diagnosis and differential diagnosis of these conditions. In Chapters 11 and 12, we noted the occurrence of depression and substance abuse as complications of chronic pain syndromes. The focus of the psychiatric interview with chronic pain patients should be directed toward an assessment of symptoms so as to aid in the diagnosis of those disorders discussed in Chapter 9. Sometimes it may be important to obtain a history from a patient's relative and from a careful chart review. Differentiation of somatoform disorder and affective disorder in patients presenting with pain as a major complaint can be based on the symptoms as discussed in Chapter 9, but clinical characteristics of pain can also be used to differentiate between the disorders (Table 14).

Symptoms of depression can occur in all disorders but are most prevalent in patients with major depression. When depressive symptoms are seen in patients with somatoform disorder, they are secondary. Chapter 11 delineates and discusses the clinical characteristics of depression in the various forms of affective disorders seen in chronic pain patients. The major types of depressive illnesses are dysthymic disorder, major affective disorder, and minor depression. They can occur secondary to the pain or may be primary. Depressed mood is likely to be less often reported in patients with major affective disorder secondary to pain than when major depression is primary. Terminal insomnia is also more likely to be seen in patients with major depression secondary to chronic pain than in primary major depression. Weight loss, decreased appetite, decreased concentration, decreased libido, guilt, irritability, social withdrawal, and suicidal thoughts are less often seen in patients with major depression secondary to chronic pain than in primary major depression. Increased appetite is more common in patients with dysthymic disorder secondary to pain than in other subtypes of depression. Patients with minor depression have more intense but less persistent symptoms of depression than patients with dysthymic disorder.

Symptoms of anxiety also serve to differentiate subtypes of depressive syndromes and anxiety disorders. It is interesting to note that anxious mood and tension is often as severe in patients with major depression as in patients with generalized anxiety disorder. Autonomic symptoms of anxiety are generally higher in patients with generalized anxiety disorder as compared to depressed patients.

The presence of delusions, hallucinations, decreased memory or forgetfulness should be carefully assessed during the evaluation. Pain complaints may be a presenting symptom of psychosis and occasional dementia. In addition, it is important to assess the present and past history of substance abuse, especially in relation to prior records of psychological distress and physical illness. This not only includes the assessment of opioid dependence, but also alcohol, barbiturates, benzodiazepines, and

Table 14. Differentiation of Somatoform Disorders and Major Depression in Relation to Chronic Pain

Clinical Characteristics of Pain	Somatization Disorder	Conversion Disorder	Psychological Pain Disorder	Hypochondriasis	Major Depression
Onset:					
acute	−	+	+	−	+
insidious	+	−	−	+	+
Site:					
single	−	+	+	+	−
multiple	+	+	−	+	+
variable	+	−	−	+	+
Duration:					
transient	−	+	+	−	+
intermittent	+	+	+	+	+
chronic	+	+	+	+	+
Presence of organic finding:	+ −	−	−	+ −	−
Factors decreasing pain:	−	−	−	−	−
Temporal psychological correlation:	−	+	+	−	−
Presence of other medical symptoms:	+	+	−	+	+
Symptoms of primary depression:	−	−	−	−	+

Key: − = absence
   + = presence

other sedative hypnotics. For a further discussion, see Chapters 12, 21, and 22.

Rating instruments to measure the patient's level of psychological distress can aid in the assessment of chronic pain patients. The Symptom Checklist-90-R, a self-rating instrument measuring the level of psychological distress, can be easily administered in a clinical setting and is tolerated well by pain patients (7). The Beck Depression Inventory (8), a self-rating instrument for depressive symptomatology, can be readily and reliably used with chronic pain patients (9). Observer-rating instruments for depressive symptomatology used in the chronic pain population include the Hamilton Depressive Rating Scale (10) and Montgomery-Asberg Depression Rating Scale (11, 12). It has been shown that both self-rating and observer-rating instruments for depressive symptomatology accurately measure the intensity of depressive symptomatology among the various subtypes of depression (9) and are not falsely elevated by the chronic pain syndrome.

The Minnesota Multiphasic Personality Inventory (MMPI) has traditionally been used to evaluate the level of psychological distress and personality profile for chronic pain patients (13). It should be noted that patients with a pathophysiological-based pain disorder (for example, postherpetic neuralgia, reflex sympathetic dystrophy) will have a positive response to many questions on this test. These responses will inappropriately elevate the MMPI scales leading to an overstatement of the psychological distress or psychopathology in the pain patient.

Psychiatric Interview of the Chronic Pain Patient

Generally, the chronic pain patient does not personally initiate the psychiatric assessment. These patients are usually referred to the psychiatrist for evaluation by a referring physician. In some instances, the referral is at the request of an insurance carrier and/or social or governmental agency. Psychiatric assessment occurs after the chronic pain patient has been in contact with various other physicians and health care agencies. Due to these circumstances, the interview with the chronic pain patient must be modified to ensure a worthwhile assessment. It is helpful for the psychiatrist to be aware of the circumstances surrounding the referral of the patient for evaluation. If these matters are not addressed, the interview can be taxing for both the patient and the psychiatrist. A brief description follows of the various ways in which a chronic pain patient presents to a psychiatrist, the accompanying reactions, and techniques that may be used to deal with such patients.

I don't need a psychiatrist, my pain is real. The patient who comes in with this statement often feels at the end of his or her rope. He or she is angry and frustrated at the inability of doctors to find a cause for the pain and to prescribe adequate treatment. The patient is resentful because a psychiatrist is being consulted. He or she is thinking that the doctors do not believe the pain is real. It will be necessary to emphasize to such a patient that the psychiatrist believes that the pain is indeed real. Often it is useful to tell the patient that the psychiatrist is there to help. The methods sometimes used by psychiatrists, including those drugs commonly prescribed, may be helpful for the chronic pain. It is useful to make such a comment if the psychiatrist is reasonably sure that the chronic pain syndrome is more multifactorial than psychiatric in origin.

They have given up on me. This type of patient, unlike the first patient, is likely to be experiencing covert rather than overt anger. He or she is also likely to be depressed and may project this hopelessness onto physicians. He or she feels as if no one can help with the pain. As in the patient above, being asked to see a psychiatrist is almost like a final blow to the patient. Our approach to this type of patient is similar to the one above. It is also useful to address the patient's sense of defeat. Statements concerning a message of interest and realistic hope will be supportive to the patient. To address the rejection felt by the patient, we can point out that the referring physician is interested in identifying treatments that may be helpful to the patient.

Why am I seeing a psychiatrist when my doctor has been a surgeon? The patient under these circumstances is often quite confused by having been evaluated by a surgeon or treated surgically for his or her pain problem and now, suddenly, talking to a psychiatrist. A direct response to the patient's query is effective in lessening some of this confusion. The explanation offered is that, at present, the patient's doctor (surgeon) could not detect any surgically correctable lesion or problem, and so the psychiatrist wants to see if a conservative, noninvasive treatment approach using medications, exercise techniques, and activity programs could control the pain level. Since most of these interventions offer only symptomatic treatment, the psychiatrist should state that these treatments are generally not curative but that they can afford symptomatic relief. This statement applies to patients with a combination of organic and psychological causes of their pain syndrome.

My doctor says the test (x-rays) do not show anything, so I guess he thinks it's in my head. Self-doubt and rejection are common themes in this statement by chronic pain patients. They are faced with the fact that tests or a group of tests could not explain their pain complaints, and that their physician is unable to give a clear explanation for the persistence of the pain. The patient often believes that since the tests are negative and that the physician has referred the patient to a psychiatrist, the physician thinks the patient is "making up" the pain. This perception further confuses the patient as to the cause of the pain and increases self-doubt. The psychiatrist can respond by stating that even though the tests are negative, that does not preclude the patient from being helped, and that x-ray tests usually mean there is no *surgical* treatment for the pain. The patient should be reminded that medications and other treatments are available and may be of help. Some patients defend against this situation by directing their anger toward the referring physician, family, or evaluating psychiatrist. These patients will often state that they are not interested in seeing a psychiatrist and that their physicians did not "do enough" or perform the "right tests" to determine the cause of their pain. If these patients are willing to continue with the interview, an empathetic statement from the psychiatrist may alleviate some of the tension. For instance, the psychiatrist might say, "I can understand your confusion over what is causing your pain since the tests don't show any cause. But this doesn't exclude other causes or problems which may be increasing your pain." The words should be followed with some statement like, "From the assessment, maybe I can determine some other cause or problem that is intensifying your pain and offer suggestions which may be of help to you and your doctor."

In summary, the psychiatric interview must be modified and modeled after a structured interview approach as opposed to an open-ended psychological interview. Initially, the psychiatrist should address the presenting problem, which is chronic pain. The assessment should focus on the location, character, modifying factors, and precipitating causes of the chronic pain. The influences of the chronic pain state on the marriage, family, social support system, work, and employment of the patient should be made. This is followed by a careful psychiatric assessment of the clinical state and past psychiatric history. The psychiatrist should determine whether a psychopathological disorder, psychiatric reactive illness, or any psychological factors affecting a patient's physical illness are present. The psychiatric assessment should focus on signs and symptoms of depression, generalized anxiety disorder, somatoform disorders, and substance and alcohol abuse, since these are the major psychiatric illnesses found in chronic pain patients. The psychiatrist should also be alert to the presence of other medical illnesses because it is not uncommon to discover undetected medical illnesses in chronic pain patients.

After the collection of the clinical data and obtaining other ancillary data (laboratory, EMG, x-rays, and so on), it is necessary to integrate this information with that obtained by behavioral assessment and physiotherapy assessment in order to formulate a treatment program for the patient. To accomplish this, we need to have a clinical data base. A segment of such a data base dealing with the pain complaint, past pain therapies, and demographic information is shown in the Appendix.

REFERENCES

1. Melzack R: The McGill pain questionnaire: major properties and scoring methods. Pain 1:277–299, 1975
2. Dubuisson D, Melzack R: Classification of clinical pain description by multiple group discriminant analysis. Exp Neurol 51:480–487, 1976
3. Atkinson JH, Kremer EF, Ignelzi RJ: Diffusion of pain language with affesturbance confounds differential diagnosis. Pain 12:375–384, 1982
4. Kremer EF, Atkinson JH: Pain language: affect. J Psychosom Res 28:125–132, 1984
5. Huskisson EC: Measurement of pain. Lancet 2:1127–1131, 1974
6. Folstein M, Folstein S, McHugh PR: Minimental state: a practical method for grading the cognitive state of patients for the clinician. J Psychiatr Res 12:289–298, 1972
7. Derogatis LR: Symptom Checklist-90-R (Revised). Baltimore, MD, Johns Hopkins University School of Medicine, 1977
8. Beck AT, Beamsderfer A: Assessment of depression: the depression inventory, in Psychological Measurements in Psychopharmacology, Modern Problems in Pharmacopsychiatry, vol. 7. Edited by Pichot P. Basel, Karger, 1974
9. France RD, Houpt JL, Skott A, et al: Depression as a psychopathological disorder in chronic low back pain patients. J Psychosom Res 30:127–133, 1986
10. Hamilton M: A rating scale for depression. J Neurol Neurosurg Psychiatry 23:53–62, 1960
11. Montgomery SA, Asberg M: A new depression scale designed to be sensitive to change. Br J Psychiatry 135:382–389, 1979
12. Krishnan KRR, France RD, Pelton S, et al: Chronic Pain and Depression, I: classification of depression in chronic low back pain patients. Pain 22:279–287, 1985
13. Sternbach RA: Pain Patients: Traits and Treatment. New York, Academic Press, 1974

APPENDIX 1
CHRONIC PAIN
CLINICAL DATA BASE

NAME _____   PATIENT HISTORY NO. _____

ADDRESS _____   SOCIAL SECURITY NO. _____

_____   TELEPHONE NO. (Home) _____

_____   TELEPHONE NO. (Work) _____

SEX: Male _____ Female _____ AGE _____ BIRTHDAY _____

MARITAL STATUS: Single____ Married ____ Widowed ____ Divorced ____ Separated ____

RACE: White __ Black __ Oriental __ Spanish American __ American Indian __ Other __

EDUCATION: None _____ 0-8 _____ High school incomplete _____ High school complete _____
        Business/trade school _____ College _____ Postgraduate college _____

RELIGION: Type _____ Active _____ Inactive _____ None _____

OCCUPATION _____ EMPLOYER _____

EMPLOYMENT: Full-time _____ Part-time _____ Medical leave of absence _____
        Retired _____ Retired on disability _____ Student _____
        Unemployed seeking work _____ Unemployed not seeking work _____
        Self-employed without income _____

SOURCE OF INCOME: Employment __ Social Security __ Social Security disability __
        VA disability ____ Disability (Workmen's Compensation Insurance) __
        Long-term disability _____ Spouse's income _____

SPOUSE'S OCCUPATION _____ SPOUSE'S EMPLOYER _____

SPOUSE'S EMPLOYMENT: Full-time __ Part-time __ Medical leave of absence __
        Retired _____ Retired on disability _____ Student _____
        Unemployed seeking work _____ Unemployed not seeking work _____
        Self-employed without income _____

SPOUSE'S SOURCE OF INCOME:
        Employment _____ Social Security _____ Social Security disability _____
        VA disability _____ Disability (Workmen's Compensation Insurance) _____
        Long-term disability _____ Spouse's income _____

PROCESS OF LITIGATION for Compensation, Social Security disability, liability suit
        for an injury: YES _____ NO _____

REFERRING PHYSICIAN _____

LOCATION OF PAIN

PAIN IS:
Deep _____
Superficial _____
Constant _____
Intermittent _____

TYPE OF PAIN:
Aching _____
Burning _____
Shooting _____
Other _____

DURATION OF PAIN SINCE INITIAL ONSET:

Hours _____ Days _____ Weeks _____ Months _____

PRECIPITATING FACTORS:

Metabolic _____   Infection _____   Malignancy _____
Degenerative _____   Iatrogenic _____   Unknown _____
Trauma (home) _____   Trauma (work) _____   Other _____

DURATION OF CONTINUOUS PAIN _____

PAIN LEVEL (0 TO 10 SCALE: 0 = No Pain, 10 = pain as bad as it can be):

Present _____ Lowest _____ Highest _____ Average _____

FACTORS MODIFYING PAIN (circle increasing ↑, decreasing ↓, no change θ):

Activity	↑ ↓ θ	Eating	↑ ↓ θ	Coughing/sneezing	↑ ↓ θ
Sitting	↑ ↓ θ	Defecation	↑ ↓ θ	Sexual intercourse	↑ ↓ θ
Lying	↑ ↓ θ	Micturition	↑ ↓ θ	Weather	↑ ↓ θ
Standing	↑ ↓ θ	Anxiety	↑ ↓ θ	Change in temperature	↑ ↓ θ
Walking	↑ ↓ θ	Depression	↑ ↓ θ	Menstrual period	↑ ↓ θ
Fatigue	↑ ↓ θ	Stress	↑ ↓ θ	Other	↑ ↓ θ

LIFE EVENTS AT TIME OF ONSET:

Death of relative _____   Marriage _____   Divorce _____
Loss of employment _____   Birth of a child _____
Anniversary reaction _____   Other _____

COURSE: Intermittent _____ Continuous _____

TIME PATTERN OF PAIN:

Number of Hours in Pain Per Day _____
Diurnal Variation: Worse AM _____ Worse PM _____ Specific Time _____
                Better AM _____ Better PM _____ Specific Time _____

EFFECTS OF PAIN (Increase ↑, Decrease ↓, No Change θ):

Satisfaction with work	↑	↓	θ	Sleep	↑	↓	θ
Efficiency at work	↑	↓	θ	Appetite	↑	↓	θ
Change in work	↑	↓	θ	Weight	↑	↓	θ
Interest in leisure activities	↑	↓	θ	Mood	↑	↓	θ
Restriction in leisure activities	↑	↓	θ	Tension	↑	↓	θ
Interest in family activities	↑	↓	θ	Libido	↑	↓	θ
Restriction in family activities	↑	↓	θ	Energy	↑	↓	θ
Interest in social activities	↑	↓	θ	Mentation	↑	↓	θ
Restriction in social activities	↑	↓	θ	Memory	↑	↓	θ
Change in income	↑	↓	θ	Fatigue	↑	↓	θ

LIMITATIONS ON ACTIVITY:

Activity tolerance (duration of activity without increase in pain)

Lying _____ Sitting _____ Standing _____ Walking _____

Activity endurance (duration of activity limited by pain)

Lying _____ Sitting _____ Standing _____ Walking _____

TREATMENT FOR PAIN:

Treatment	Tried (yes/no)	When (year)	Helped (yes/no)
Chiropractor	————	————	————
Traction	————	————	————
Braces	————	————	————
Nerve block	————	————	————
Physical therapy	————	————	————
Hypnosis	————	————	————
Acupuncture	————	————	————
Biofeedback	————	————	————
Ice packing/heating	————	————	————
Opioid analgesics	————	————	————
Massage	————	————	————
Religious counseling	————	————	————
Psychological counseling	————	————	————
Electrical stimulation	————	————	————
Surgery	————	————	————
Antidepressants	————	————	————
Neuroleptics	————	————	————
Minor tranquilizers	————	————	————
Nonopioid analgesics	————	————	————

OPERATIONS FOR PAIN _____

_____

OTHER OPERATIONS _____

_____

MOST EFFECTIVE TREATMENT _____

_____

PRESENT MEDICATIONS (drug name, amount, frequency)

_____

_____

OTHER CURRENT MEDICAL ILLNESSES _____

_____

_____

PAST MEDICAL HISTORY _____

_____

_____

_____

_____

PAST SURGICAL HISTORY _____

_____

_____

_____

_____

PAST PSYCHIATRIC HISTORY _____

_____

_____

SUBSTANCE ABUSE/ADDICTION HISTORY

	USE	ABUSE	ADDICTION
Alcohol	_____	_____	_____
Tobacco	_____	_____	_____
Opioids	_____	_____	_____
Sedative-hypnotics	_____	_____	_____
Stimulants	_____	_____	_____
Hallucinogens	_____	_____	_____

DRUG SENSITIVITIES (Drug and reaction) _____

_____

_____

_____

DRUG ALLERGIES (Drug and reaction) _____

_____

_____

_____

HISTORY OF BLOOD TRANSFUSIONS _____

_____

FAMILY HISTORY:

Medical illnesses _____

_____

_____

Physical disabilities _____

_____

_____

Pain disorders _____

_____

_____

Psychiatric disorders _____

_____

Alcohol/drug abuse _____

_____

_____

Parents:
    Father—Living ( )   Deceased ( ), Age _____
    Mother—Living ( )   Deceased ( ), Age _____

Number of Siblings _____ Ages _____

Marriages _____

Children _____

MEDICAL REVIEW OF SYSTEMS

OPHTHALMOLOGY AND OTORHINOLARYNGOLOGY

EYES:
    Visual acuity _____
    Diplopia _____
    Scotoma _____
    Ocular pain _____
    Glasses _____
    Other _____

EARS:
    Hearing loss _____
    Otalgia _____
    Tinnitus _____
    Discharge _____
    Hearing aid _____
    Other _____

NOSE:

Nasal obstruction _____

Discharge _____

Epistaxis _____

Pain _____

Sinus pain _____

Anosmia _____

Deformity _____

Other _____

MOUTH AND THROAT:

Dental _____

Sore throat _____

Dysphagia _____

Hoarseness _____

Soreness of tongue _____

Taste _____

Dentures _____

Other _____

CARDIOPULMONARY:

Dyspnea _____

Cough _____

Orthopnea _____

Shortness of breath _____

Chest pain _____

Cyanosis _____

Asthma _____

Palpitation _____

Irregular heart rate _____

Hemoptysis _____

Edema _____

Night sweats _____

Sputum _____

Other _____

GASTROINTESTINAL:

Appetite _____

Nausea _____

Vomiting _____

Hematemesis _____

Weight change _____

Abdominal pain _____

Dysphagia _____

Regurgitation _____

Jaundice _____

Constipation _____

Diarrhea _____

Eructation _____

Obstipation _____

Melena _____

Stools _____

Other _____

GENITOURINARY

URINARY:

Frequency _____

Nocturia _____

Urgency _____

Dysuria _____

Incontinence _____

Flank Pain _____

Hematuria _____

Pyuria _____

Hesitation _____

Stones _____

Polyuria _____

Other _____

MENSTRUAL:

Menarche _____

Last menstrual period _____

Regularity _____

Menstrual cycle _____

Menorrhagia _____

Premenstrual dysphoria _____

Menopause _____

Birth control _____

Vaginal discharge _____

Mittelschmerz _____

Dysmenorrhea _____

Other _____

SEXUAL:
FEMALE:
Anorgasmia _____

Dyspareunia _____

Frigidity _____

Vaginismus _____

Libido _____

Other _____

MALE:
Impotence _____

Premature ejaculation _____

Retrograde ejaculation _____

Priapism _____

Libido _____

Other _____

NERVOUS SYSTEM:
Memory _____

Seizures _____

Vertigo _____

Paresthesias _____

Paralysis _____

Tremor _____

Numbness _____

Myoclonus _____

Dyskinesias _____

Headaches _____

Syncope _____

Dysarthria _____

Anhidrosis _____

Other _____

MUSCULOSKELETAL:
Myalgia _____

Arthralgia _____

Joint swelling _____

Joint stiffness _____

Muscle atrophy _____

Deformity _____

Limitation of movement _____

Muscle hypertrophy _____

Other _____

Disease _____

ENDOCRINE:
Habitus change _____

Pigmentation _____

Weakness _____

Temperature sensitivity _____

Polydypsia _____

Polyuria _____

Polyphagia _____

Myxedema _____

Striae _____

Exophthalmos _____

Goiter _____

Skin Change _____

Other _____

Disease _____

PHYSICAL EXAMINATION

VITAL SIGNS:

	Lying (3 min.)	Standing (3 min.)
Temperature _____		
Height _____	Pulse (R) _____	_____
Weight _____	(L) _____	_____
Respiratory rate _____	B/P (R) _____	_____
	(L) _____	_____

GENERAL APPEARANCE:

Habitus—size _____

deformity _____

Hygiene _____

Gait _____

Stigmata _____

Posture _____

Facial expression _____

Physical aids _____

SKIN:

Pigmentation _____

Texture _____

Temperature _____

Lesions _____

Hair _____

Nails _____

HEAD:

Lesions _____

Scalp _____

Hair pattern _____

Other _____

EARS:

Pinna _____

External canal _____

Tympanic membrane _____

Mastoid _____

Hearing _____

Rinne _____

Weber _____

Other _____

EYES:

Eyelids _____

Conjunctiva _____

Sclera _____

Iris _____

Anterior chamber _____

Pupil _____

Lens _____

Nystagmus _____

Fundus _____

EOM _____

Visual fields _____

Visual acuity _____

Consenual reaction _____

Corneal reflex _____

Lacrimal gland _____

Other _____

NOSE:

Muscous membrane _____

Nasal septum _____

Discharge _____

Turbinates _____

Sinuses _____

Other _____

MOUTH:

Lips _____

Mucous membrane _____

Teeth _____

Gums _____

Tongue _____

Breath _____

Pharynx _____

Other _____

NECK:

Nuchal rigidity _____

Movement _____

Thyroid _____

Carotid arteries _____

Masses _____

Lymph nodes _____

Trachea _____

Other _____

THORAX AND LUNGS:
    Inspection _____
    Palpation _____
    Percussion _____
    Auscultation _____

BREASTS:
    Inspection _____
    Palpation _____
    Nipples _____

HEART:
    PMI _____
    Parasternal pulsations _____
    Heart sounds _____
    Murmurs _____ Gallops _____

ABDOMEN:
    Scars _____
    Hernias _____
    Pulsations _____
    Veins _____
    Masses _____
    Liver _____ Spleen _____
    Bowel sounds _____ Bruits _____
    Flank pain _____ Tenderness _____

MUSCULOSKELETAL:
  TRUNK:
    Spine curvature _____
    Tenderness _____ Spasm _____
    Spine ROM _____
    Trigger points _____
    Deformities _____
    Scars _____
  CERVICAL SPINE: Flexion _____ Extension _____ Lateral Bending _____
  LUMBAR SPINE: Flexion _____ Extension _____ Lateral Bending _____
  EXTREMITIES:
    ROM _____
    Tenderness _____ Spasm _____
    Joint redness _____
    Crepitation _____
    Pulses _____
    Lymph nodes _____
    Clubbing _____

Cyanosis _____

Deformity _____

SLR: right _____ Left _____

Figure of Four: right _____ Left _____

Other _____

NEUROLOGICAL:

Cranial Nerves (I–XII) _____

_____

Motor:

Strength (Right upper) _____

(Left upper) _____

(Right lower) _____

(Left lower) _____

Size _____ Tone _____

Involuntary Movements _____

Gait and Station:

Gait _____ Walking on toes _____ Walking on heels _____

Static ataxia _____ Tandem walking _____

Coordination _____

_____

Sensory (note change in pinprick, light touch, position, vibration, temperature) ___

_____

_____

Deep Tendon reflexes:

	Triceps	Biceps	Brachoradialis	Patella	Ankle
(R)	_____	_____	_____	_____	_____
(L)	_____	_____	_____	_____	_____

Pathological Reflexes _____

Aphasia _____

Tinel's Sign _____

popliteal compression test _____ sciatic stretch test _____

Stereognosis _____ Two-point discrimination _____

GENITAL (MALE):

Penis _____ Masses _____

Discharge _____ Prostate _____

Scrotum _____ Testis _____

PELVIC (FEMALE):

Perineum _____ Cervix _____

Vulva _____ Uterus _____

Vagina _____ Ovaries _____

Adnexa _____ Other _____

RECTAL _____ sphincter tone _____

MENTAL STATUS:

Orientation: Time _____ Place _____ Person _____

Level of consciousness: Alert _____ Drowsy _____ Stupor _____ Coma _____

Abnormal movements _____

_____

Mannerisms _____ Posturing _____

Psychomotor activity: Agitated _____ Retarded _____ Normal _____

Speech and thought:

Rate _____ Rhythm _____ Articulation _____

Flight of ideas _____ Looseness of association _____

Thought content _____

Suicidal ideation:

Thoughts of dying _____

Ideation _____

Plan _____

Delusions _____

Hallucinations _____

Illusions _____

Affect: Flat _____ Blunted _____ Full Range _____

Mood: Low _____ Euthymic _____ Elevated _____

Irritable _____ Other _____

Concentration _____

Memory: Recent _____ Remote _____

Recall _____

Confabulation _____ Perservation _____

Judgment _____ Insight _____

Chapter 17

Behavioral Assessment Methods for Chronic Pain

Francis J. Keefe, Ph.D.

One of the major tasks confronting any clinician working with a chronic pain patient is analyzing the patient's behavior. To understand this behavior, the clinician must consider overt behaviors, cognitive and affective responses, as well as physiologic response patterns. In the past 10 to 15 years, important advances have been made in behavioral assessment methods for evaluating chronic pain syndromes. These advances include systematic methods for observing and recording nonverbal expressions of pain (1), methods for evaluating how patients cope with pain (2), psychophysiological approaches to studying the impact of stress on pain phenomenon (3), and more sophisticated methods for measuring pain perception (4). These methods make possible a more objective and comprehensive analysis of the pain experience. They appeal not only to behavioral psychologists but also to the medical community for several reasons. First, they allow one to identify the behavioral problems of chronic pain patients in a much more precise and objective fashion. Second, they can provide a data base which allows the physician and patient to make a more educated decision about medical, surgical, or behavioral treatment alternatives. Third, these assessment methods often help clarify the role that social, environmental, and intrapersonal factors play in controlling pain behavior. Finally, behavioral assessment methods allow one to identify specific behavioral problems likely to respond to intensive behavioral pain management. Early identification and treatment of these problems can prevent them from becoming entrenched and speed up the patient's return to vocational and social pursuits.

This chapter provides an overview of behavioral assessment methods used in our pain management program. The chapter is divided into two sections. In the first section, behavioral assessment methods are described; in the second section, the ways in which assessment information gathered is used to match treatment to the patient's needs are examined (Figure 1).

BEHAVIORAL ASSESSMENT METHODS

Chronic pain patients are a heterogeneous group having a wide range of behavioral problems (5). A comprehensive behavioral assessment is needed to identify behavioral problems in particular patients and to understand the behavioral and psychological variables that may affect those problem behaviors. Figure 2 depicts the basic elements of our behavioral assessment approach. The assessment process begins with a structured interview designed to identify the patient's presenting behavioral problems. Following this, more detailed information on problem behaviors is gathered using five assessment methods. These are: self-monitoring, standardized pain behavior observations, psychophysiologic

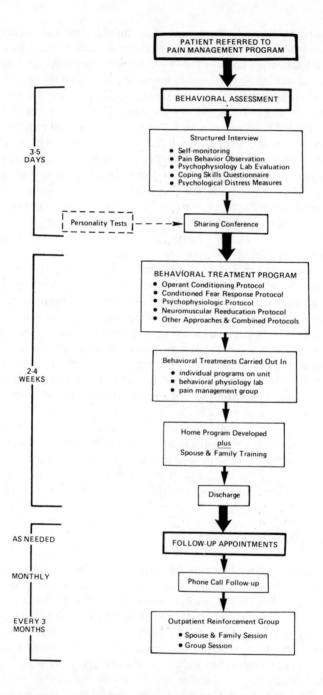

Figure 1. Flow chart illustrating the pain management program emphasizing the behavioral aspects including behavioral assessment and treatment

analyses, a pain-coping skills questionnaire, and standardized measures of psychological distress. Specialized psychological tests such as personality tests, intelligence tests, and neuropsychological tests are also requested for some patients. Finally, the assessment information collected is integrated to arrive at the selection of appropriate behavioral treatment procedures.

Each of the assessment procedures will be considered in detail. A brief description of the assessment technique will be provided, and applications to chronic pain patients will be described. Research important to understanding the assessment technique will also be cited.

Structured Interview

Behavioral assessment begins with an interview that provides the patient with an opportunity to describe his or her presenting problem. The major goals in the interview are to pinpoint presenting problems, identify probable controlling variables, and select tentative targets for behavioral treatment efforts. We use a structured behavioral interview for this

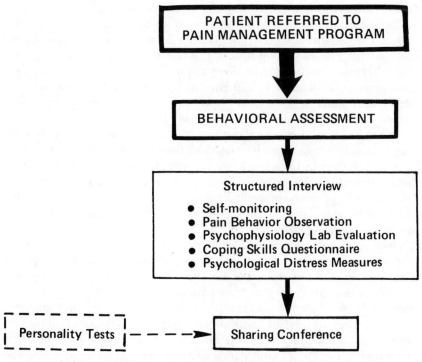

Figure 2.   Flow chart illustrating the behavioral assessment of the chronic pain patient

purpose. The Appendix presents an interview schedule that we use for this initial interview. Structured behavioral interviews are widely used in behavioral assessment and are known to yield more reliable data than unstructured interviews (6).

We begin the interview by asking patients to describe various characteristics of their pain. Patients are asked to localize their pain on a pain map (7). This consists of an outline of the human body on which the patient is asked to shade in those areas where pain is experienced. Patients are then asked to rate their pain using a 0 to 10 scale on which 0 = no pain and 10 = pain as bad as it can be (1). In order to assess the quality of pain, patients are asked what their pain feels like, and the description they provide is written down. To provide a more quantifiable measure of the quality of pain, the Adjective Checklist of the McGill Pain Questionnaire (8) is also administered. The duration of pain is a key factor in behavioral analysis (9). Two questions are particularly important. First, how many hours a day does the patient have pain? Patients having intermittent pain—lasting from 10 minutes to several hours—exhibit behavioral patterns very different from patients who report consistent pain throughout the day. Second, we ask patients when their pain first began. The duration of time since onset of the pain is an important factor. Patients who have had pain for years have had many more learning opportunities in which to associate pain with certain social environmental antecedents and consequences (9). In our research we have found that patients who have long histories of constant daily pain differ markedly in terms of response to behaviorally oriented, multidisciplinary pain management. Patients who had continuous daily pain for two years or longer were much less likely to respond to treatment than patients who had constant pain for less than two years (10).

We routinely ask patients about factors that increase or decrease their pain. Patients whose pain is related to tissue pathology typically show increases in pain in response to movement (1) and in response to other factors that might be expected to increase or decrease nociception (9). Operant pain patients, however, often are unable to identify factors that either increase or alleviate their pain, stating that "My pain never seems to change; nothing helps."

Given that the major focus of a behavioral interview is on behavior, it may seem unusual to the reader that our interview begins with patients' descriptions of their pain. We do this for several reasons. First, the patient's report and complaints of pain are very important behaviors in their own right. Patients who complain bitterly of severe pain sometimes receive operations or pain medications regardless of the fact that they do not display pain behaviorally. Furthermore, spouse and family members often take the patient's complaints of pain very seriously and respond with assistance or sympathy to these expressions alone. An initial focus on pain in the interview is also helpful in making the patient more comfortable with the whole process of behavioral assessment. Chronic pain patients are often initially resistant to behavioral and psychological assessment efforts. Asking them to begin by discussing their pain conveys to them that they are being taken seriously and that their pain complaints are a major focus of assessment and treatment. As they become more comfortable with the interview, they are more open to discussing behavioral and psychological problems that may be related to the pain complaints.

The second major section of the structured interview focuses on the patient's current patterns of pain and well behavior. Patients are asked about their living situation and difficulties they may have with activities around the house and outside the home. Their work and disability status are explored. Particularly important is determining whether there is a pending workmen's compensation/disability claim or pending lawsuit. If so, there are strong disincentives for improvements in pain behavior. We also ask approximately how much time they spend up and out of the reclining position (uptime) each day. Usually by this point in the structured interview, the interviewer has developed a basic understanding of patterns of well behavior. An individual coping well with chronic pain is usually able to stay involved in light housekeeping or social activities and often is able to work at physically nondemanding jobs or be engaged in volunteer work. These individuals typically spend 12 to 14 hours a day up and out of bed and are involved with their families. Patients who are coping poorly, in contrast, usually report that they are unable to do any housekeeping or light work and that they are virtually restricted by pain to their home. These individuals have extremely low levels of uptime (usually less than six hours a day), are unable to work and support themselves by means of disability/compensation payments.

One of the most important aspects of the structured behavioral interview is identifying potential reinforcing consequences for pain behavior. In many patients, these consequences play an extremely important role in maintaining excessive pain behavior and a sedentary and dependent lifestyle. To identify potential reinforcers for pain behavior, we try to determine whether powerful reinforcers have become contingent on pain behavior. For example, many patients rest in bed, take pain medications, use moist heat, or receive attention from their family or spouse only when their pain becomes extreme. When they are having less pain and seem to be functioning well, none of these positive consequences occur. When positive consequences become contingent on excessive pain behavior, there is a strong likelihood that these consequences can reinforce and maintain excessive pain behavior even when the tissue pathology basis for that behavior is minimal.

Another important issue is the degree to which the patient's pain behavior is observable to others. Those who send out overt and frequent signals that they are having pain are more likely to elicit solicitous responses from others. We use several techniques in the initial interview to evaluate the level of pain behavior. For example, we ask the patient to walk from their bed to the hall and back; we ask them to recline in their bed and then stand up; and, finally, we ask them to sit in an upright chair. During each of these activities, the interviewer notes whether there is any guarding, rubbing, bracing, grimacing, or sighing exhibited. Patients with chronic pain also often have "pain paraphernalia" that communicates to others that they are having pain. These paraphernalia include canes and walkers, transcutaneous nerve stimulator (TNS) units, back braces, wheelchairs, and the like. We ask about the degree to which they use these devices and also observe their use during the interview.

The next major section of the structured interview deals with the cognitive and affective responses. We find that it is particularly important to determine the patient's understanding of what is causing the pain and what the future trajectory of their pain problem is likely to be. We ask individuals what they have been told *by their doctors* about their pain and its future course, and then ask them what *they think* is causing the pain and what they think is its likely future course. In some cases, there is a marked discrepancy between what the doctor has told the patient and what the patient believes. Some, for example, are convinced that they have an undiagnosed cancer or other disease such as multiple sclerosis. Social and cultural factors play an important role in determining beliefs about pain. Those with certain religious backgrounds are sometimes convinced that their chronic pain is a punishment for sins they have committed, and this belief is reinforced by contact with family and religious leaders. Patients often have family members who suffered from pain that was only relieved once thay had chiropractic treatment or engaged in various superstitious behaviors. There is growing recognition that patients' beliefs about their own pain play an extremely important role in their willingness to accept treatment and to adhere to treatment once they have left the hospital (11).

A particularly important issue is the degree to which the individual accepts the behavioral model of pain management as a legitimate one. Most patients ascribe to a medical model of their pain. Some are convinced that the only way they will improve is if a surgical procedure can be done to remove the cause of the pain or "kill the nerve that is causing it." Still others have not accepted the chronicity of their pain and are willing only to work on treatments that promise total elimination of pain. Most require some education about behavioral pain management and its goals before they will accept this approach as a valid one. Nursing interventions (See Chapter 23) are particularly useful in helping to answer patients' questions and help them develop more realistic expectations about treatment.

As part of the structured interview, we attempt to determine whether patients exhibit particular cognitive errors or distortions. Cognitive distortions are considered by Beck (12) to be essential elements in the production and maintenance of depression. Beck claims that patients who are depressed demonstrate a cognitive triad consisting of a negative view of themselves, their world (experience), and their future. These negative views give rise to the depressive-negative-sad affect. In the interview situation, cognitive distortions can often be easily detected by analyzing patients' self-statements. These statements reflect cognitive errors such as: 1) overgeneralization—assuming that the outcome of one experience applies to the same or other similar experiences in the future; 2) catastrophizing—anticipating that an experience will invariably lead to a catastrophic outcome; 3) personalization—taking excessive personal responsibility for negative events or interpreting such events as having a personal meaning; 4) selective abstraction—selectively attending to negative aspects of these experiences. These and other cognitive distortions are noted by the interviewer and are considered to be prime factors related to depressed affect in chronic pain patients. Cognitive therapy designed to correct these distortions and replace them with more rational analyses and interpretations of daily events can benefit many depressed chronic pain patients (11).

The patient's education level and apparent intelligence level are also noted during the interview. Individuals having limited formal education often require additional assistance in behavioral assessment and treatment efforts. Patients with a low level of intelligence may also be inappropriate for certain behavioral treatment protocols.

Symptoms of affective disturbance are also noted during the initial structured interview. Methods for assessing affective disorders are discussed in other chapters of this volume and will not be discussed in detail here.

The final section of the structured interview focuses on physiologic factors involved in the patient's pain. Particularly important are indications of psychophysiologic responses that either precede, accompany, or follow periods of intense pain. We routinely ask about symptoms of muscle tension such as bruxism, muscle contraction headaches, and muscle spasm. Observations of movement patterns during the early part of the interview provide some indication of the degree of generalized tension. Patients having excessively high levels of muscle tension usually show guarded, pain-avoidant posturing when asked to walk or move about. We also ask about increases in autonomic nervous system activity associated with increases in pain. Heart rate speeding, increases in blood pressure, excessive sweating, and a nervous-panicky feeling may occur during severe pain episodes. This pattern of arousal is particularly frequent in individuals who have shorter histories of pain or whose pain is episodic. Techniques to decrease arousal, such as relaxation training, often help patients who show this pattern.

The end result of the structured interview is a selection of tentative targets for assessment and treatment efforts. Commonly, several behavioral targets can be specified, and treatment of these target behaviors is likely to lead to therapeutic improvement. The interviewer summarizes these tentative targets at the end of the interview and outlines the assessment process that will follow. The detailed assessments of these target behaviors are important because they provide opportunities to validate, modify, and adjust our understanding of the patient's behavioral problems before starting treatment. We now discuss the more detailed measurement procedures used for this purpose.

Self-Monitoring

In self-monitoring, the patient takes on the role of an observer. He or she records particular aspects of a behavior and its surrounding circumstances. Depending on the results of the initial interview, we use one of two self-monitoring procedures: daily activity diaries or a pain–tension diary form.

The daily activity diary format was developed by Fordyce (9). This diary consists of a single sheet on which the patient makes hourly entries of time spent in three categories: standing or walking, sitting, and reclining. In addition, patients are asked to indicate the type and amount of medication they take and to rate their pain on a 0 to 10 scale hourly. The forms we use are identical to those described by Fordyce (9). We have found that most patients are capable of keeping these daily activity diaries and that the information gathered during a three- to five-day baseline phase can be very useful in treatment planning. For example, daily activity diary recordings may reveal that there is a very low level of uptime, suggesting that there are likely to be major strength and endurance deficits. These patients usually require an intensive physical therapy and reconditioning program. Another common pattern is that individuals push themselves to continue with an activity such as sitting until their pain becomes intolerable and only then rest or take pain medication. This suggests a need to learn to pace activity using an activity–rest cycling procedure. Distortions in patients' estimates of their own behavior can also readily be identified with these diaries. For example, depressed individuals significantly underestimate their activity level on interview, while diary recordings indicate they are much more active than they initially reported.

The pain–tension diary format is described in Chapter 19. This simple recording procedure requires patients to rate their pain level on a 100 millimeter visual analogue scale at four points of time each day (breakfast, lunch, dinner, and bedtime). They are also asked to rate their subjective tension level using four visual analogue scales at the same time points. The pain–tension diary format is particularly useful when the structured interview has suggested that emotional stress or tension contributes significantly to pain. By reviewing ratings of pain and tension over several days, the clinician can begin to determine the degree to which these variables are correlated. Patients are also asked to record on the pain–tension diary various events that occur during their day. We often find that events that the patient may not consider stressful—for example, a telephone call from their spouse—are associated with an increase in subjective tension and an increase in pain.

Pain Behavior Observation

We have developed a direct observation method for recording pain behaviors in chronic pain patients (1) and utilize a standard pain behavior sampling method in our program (13). We have carried out a series of studies on this standard pain behavior observation procedure (1), and the results of these studies have supported its reliability and validity. The procedure possesses good interobserver reliability, sensitivity to treatment effects, construct validity, and discriminant validity (1).

We use our observation procedure to take a standard behavior sample from each patient, usually within 24 hours of the time that the structured interview has been carried out. The observation itself takes 10 minutes and is carried out by an undergraduate assistant. In the session, patients are asked to sit, walk, stand, and recline for one to two minutes each. A videotape of the session is made. Other than asking the patient to move from one position to another, the assistant does not converse with the patient. Trained observers subsequently score the videotape behavior sample to record the occurrence of five particular behaviors:

1. *Guarding:* abnormally stiff, interrupted, or rigid movement while moving from one position to another.
2. *Bracing:* a stationary position in which a fully extended limb supports and maintains an abnormal distribution of weight.
3. *Rubbing:* touching, rubbing, or holding the affected area of pain for a minimum of three seconds.
4. *Grimacing:* obvious facial expression of pain which may include furrowed brow, narrowed eyes, tightened lips, corners of mouth pulled back, and clenched teeth.
5. *Sighing:* obvious exhalation of air usually accompanied by shoulders first rising and then falling.

Prior to scoring, each patient's videotape is dubbed with a signal to denote a series of 20-second observe followed by 10-second record phases. Observers then watch the videotape during each the 20-second observe phase, and then during the 10-second record phase note the occurrence or nonoccurrence of each behavior category. Reliability checks are carried out by having two independent observers observe 20 to 30 percent of the behavior samples independently and simultaneously. Observer retraining sessions are carried out monthly to ensure that observers adhere to proper use of the recording system.

To quantify the pain behavior observations, scores are derived for each pain behavior category by adding the total frequency of occurrence of that category for the entire behavior sample. A total pain behavior score is also computed by summing the frequency of all the coding categories.

Data gathered from the pain behavior observation system are useful in several ways. First, the patient's level of pain behavior pretreatment can be examined. This is done by comparing an individual patient's pain behavior scores to those of our normative population. We find that some patients show extreme levels of pain behavior compared to other patients. Clearly these patients are sending more signals to others that they are experiencing pain. Second, pain behavior observations can be used to study the effects of movement. Patients who have a significant tissue pathology basis for their pain would be expected to consistently show pain behavior when asked to walk or move from one position to another. Separate scores can be computed for observation intervals in which the patients are asked to move, and for those intervals when the patient was not involved in movement. Patients who show excessive pain behavior typically show high levels of pain behavior not only during movement but also when they are not moving. A third application of the observation system is to evaluate treatment effects. To do this, we carry out a second observation immediately prior to discharge and compare the results of the pretreatment to the posttreatment pattern.

The pain behavior observation system we have described has many advantages. We find it is relatively simple and provides an objective and reliable measure of pain behavior. This system is now being used at several major chronic pain treatment facilities and is being applied to a wide variety of chronic pain patients.

Psychophysiologic Laboratory Evaluations

With the advent of portable physiologic monitoring devices has come an increasing interest in the use of these devices to evaluate psychophysiologic responses in pain patients. We have a well-equipped psychophysiologic laboratory that enables us to study, in controlled laboratory conditions, the effects of different stimuli on physiologic responses related to pain in our patients. We use this assessment strategy when information from the structured interview suggests that there is a psychophysiologic or neuromuscular basis for the patient's pain complaints. Separate protocols to evaluate psychophysiologic and neuromuscular factors are used.

The psychophysiologic assessment protocol involves examining patients' responses under conditions of rest and stress. Since most of our patients have muscularly based pain problems, physiological responsiveness to these different conditions is assessed using surface electromyography. Electrodes are placed over muscles believed to be involved in the patient's pain problem. For example, a patient suffering from myofascial (temperomandibular joint) pain syndrome will have electrodes attached to the masseter muscle groups. Readings of EMG activity are then taken as subjects are exposed to the following conditions: 1) rest—the patient is asked to sit quietly for five minutes; 2) mental arithmetic—the patient is asked to count backwards by sevens from 100; 3) self-relaxation—the patient is asked to try to relax as deeply as possible; 4) stressful imagery—the patient is asked to imagine confronting a stressful situation; and 5) a final rest period. Additional stressors that may be particularly salient, for example, chewing gum in a temporomandibular joint pain patient, may also be introduced in these sessions. To ensure reliability of EMG readings, a series of successive one-minute readings is taken under each condition.

An analysis of the profile of psychophysiologic responding under stress and rest conditions can be quite useful to assessment. Resting levels of muscle activity may be found to be excessive, suggesting that excessive tension may contribute to pain phenomenon. In many individuals, abnormal physiological responding is not evident until the patient is stressed, at which times inappropriate and excessive responding is noted. Finally, patients who tend to deny the stress-related nature of their symptoms often are more willing to accept a psychophysiologic explanation of their pain after they have gone through such an assessment procedure and been informed of the results obtained.

Pain problems having a neuromuscular basis can also be evaluated in a psychophysiology laboratory. Electromyographic measures can be taken from several muscle groups to study muscle activity during static and dynamic movement. We often use this approach to evaluate lumbar paraspinal muscle activity in patients complaining of low back pain. The protocol used has previously been described by Wolf and colleagues (14). This assessment protocol involves placement of electrodes bilaterally on both sides of the lumbar spine. Integrated electromyographic activity is then recorded under the following conditions: quiet standing, forward flexion, extension, and lateral rotation with the pelvis stabilized. Measures of EMG activity are taken during three repetitions of each of these activities. Previous research carried out with normals (15) has indicated that symmetrical activity occurs in the lumbar paraspinal musculature during standing, flexion, and extension. During rotational movements to the right, the left paraspinal musculature increases in activity relative to the right, and this pattern is reversed during rotation to the left. In individuals complaining of low back pain, however, abnormal patterns are often evident (14). Patients, for example, may display asymmetrical patterns of muscle activity during quiet standing with excessive elevations on one side of the spine. Muscle activity during movement may also be abnormal with inappropriate increases in left or right paraspinal musculature during rotational movements. Furthermore, these abnormal muscle responses may be highly correlated with reports of pain. Training low back pain patients to produce more normal patterns of muscle activity using EMG biofeedback has been found to alleviate and, in some cases, eliminate low back pain (14). Similar approaches can be used to study other pain problems having a musculoskeletal basis, for example, chronic cervical pain following a whiplash injury.

Coping Skills Questionnaire

Most patients who have experienced pain for some time have developed ways to tolerate, minimize, or reduce their pain. These pain coping strategies include involvement in distracting activities, focusing on pleasant events or imagery, reductions in activity level, attempting to ignore pain, and calming self-statements. Coping strategies adopted and used over prolonged time periods may significantly affect functioning. Patients who develop effective coping strategies may manage their pain well and lead active lives. Patients who rely on ineffective coping strategies may be more seriously impaired by pain and lead very sedentary and restricted lives. Methods for teaching patients to alter maladaptive behavioral and psychological coping strategies are widely used in pain management programs (11). Systematic evaluation of patients' pain coping strategies before treatment provides one means of evaluating the patient's strengths and weaknesses in coping skills.

We have developed a coping strategies questionnaire that evaluates both the extent to which subjects use different pain coping strategies and the overall effectiveness of the strategies (2). The coping strategies included in the questionnaire were selected on the basis of a review of relevant laboratory and clinical studies. The questionnaire measures the extent to which patients use each of six different cognitive coping strategies and two behavioral coping strategies when they feel pain. Each strategy is measured by a different subscale, each of which has six items. Subscales as well as typical items are listed in Table 1. Subjects rate each item using a seven-point scale to indicate how often they use that strategy when they experience pain. They are also asked to make two ratings of the overall effectiveness of coping strategies using two seven-point scales: 1) to measure the amount of control they feel over pain, and 2) to measure how much they are able to decrease pain.

In a recently published study (2), we administered the coping strategy questionnaire to a sample of 61 chronic low back pain patients. An analysis of the relative frequency of strategies indicated that patients most frequently utilized praying and hoping and coping self-statements and rarely tended to use reinterpretation of pain sensations. A statistical analysis was also carried out to determine how coping strategies were related to one another, and three factors emerged from this analysis. The first factor accounted for 35 percent of the variance in questionnaire

Table 1.   Coping Strategies Questionnaire

Scale	Sample Item
Cognitive Strategies	
1. Diverting attention	I replay in my mind pleasant experiences in the past.
2. Reinterpreting pain sensations	I don't think of it as pain but rather as a dull or warm feeling.
3. Coping self-statements	No matter how bad it gets, I know I can handle it.
4. Ignoring sensations	I don't pay any attention to it.
5. Praying or hoping	I rely on my faith in God.
6. Catastrophizing	I feel my life isn't worth living
Behavioral Strategies	
1. Increased behavioral activities	I try to be around other people.
2. Pain behavior	I take pain medication.

responses and was labeled cognitive coping and suppression. Individuals high on this factor reported making a conscious cognitive effort to reinforce their attempts to overcome pain and also made active attempts to suppress pain by ignoring pain sensations and reinterpreting them. The second factor, helplessness, accounted for 21 percent of the variance. Individuals high on this factor reported having a poor ability to deal with pain. The third factor, diverting attention and praying, accounted for 12 percent of the variance. Individuals high on this factor endorse items on the diverting attention and praying or hoping subscales. Statistical analyses also indicated that different coping strategies had different effects on patients' functional adaptation to pain. Patients who scored high on Factor 1, cognitive coping and suppression, were less likely to be depressed and have severe pain, but had a higher level of functional impairment than patients scoring low on this factor. Patients scoring high on Factor 2, helplessness, were significantly more depressed and more anxious than individuals scoring low on this factor. Patients who scored high on Factor 3, diverting attention and praying, had higher levels of pain and were more impaired functionally than patients scoring low on this factor. One significant aspect of this research is that the coping strategies were highly predictive of adjustment to chronic pain even after controlling for medical status variables and somatization.

We routinely administer the coping strategies questionnaire to all our patients, and we compute scores on the subscales as well as factor scores. Patients are compared to a normative sample of chronic pain patients to determine the degree to which they are high or low on any particular scale or factor. Ratings of the effectiveness of coping strategies are also examined closely. Patients who rate their ability to control or decrease pain as exceedingly low are often quite depressed, and benefit from training in pain coping strategies that provide them with a sense of mastery and improved control over their pain.

Psychological Distress Measures

Chronic pain patients often report that they feel depressed, anxious, and have a variety of symptoms of psychological distress. To evaluate symptoms of psychological distress in a standardized fashion, we use objective psychological test instruments. We have found two instruments to be particularly useful: The Symptom Checklist 90-R and the Beck Depression Inventory.

The Symptom Checklist 90-R (SCL-90R) is a 90-item self-report inventory developed and refined by Derogatis (16). Each item on this inventory is rated by the patient using a five-point scale of distress ranging from 0 = not at all to 4 = extremely. The SCL-90R measures nine primary symptom dimensions: 1) somatization; 2) obsessive-compulsive; 3) interpersonal sensitivity; 4) depression; 5) anxiety; 6) hostility; 7) phobic anxiety; 8) paranoid ideation; and 9) psychoticism. Three global indices of stress can also be computed that provide a good index of the patient's overall level of psychological distress. The SCL-90R has several advantages for use with chronic pain patients. First, in contrast to many other psychological tests, it is brief and well tolerated by patients. Second, it has previously been shown to be reliable and valid when used with medical populations. Third, it provides a measure of current psychological symptom status and is sensitive to fluctuations in these symptoms over time. Thus, it can be easily administered at different points during the period of treatment to provide an index of patients' progress. Finally, the questionnaire is standardized and normative profile forms are available for nonpsychiatric and psychiatric patients.

The Beck Depression Inventory (BDI) provides a good index of general severity of depression (12). The BDI is a 21-item questionnaire in which every item is written to reflect a different specific manifestation of depression. Each item consists of four or five statements ranked according to reported symptom severity. The patient responds to an item by checking the one statement that most closely matches his or her present state. Their response is scored from 0 to 4. The reliability and validity of the BDI has been examined in a number of studies. We have selected it for use in assessment because: 1) it is considered one of the best self-report measures of severity of general depression; 2) it is short; 3) it samples a broad range of symptoms of depression; and 4) the results obtained correlate well with psychiatric diagnoses of depression.

Special Psychological Tests

In some cases, we refer patients for additional psychological testing of a more specialized nature. This testing is requested only when we feel that it will contribute significantly to the assessment information already gathered. Consultations are requested in 10 to 20 percent of the patients evaluated in the Pain Management Program. Specialized tests requested include personality tests, intelligence tests, and neuropsychological tests.

The most commonly used instrument for the assessment of personality patterns in chronic pain patients is the Minnesota Multiphasic Personality Inventory (MMPI) (17).

Descriptive research using the MMPI (17) indicates that low back pain patients are likely to have elevations on the "neurotic triad," the hypochondriasis (Hs), hysteria (Hy), and depression (D scales). Research studies have also compared MMPI profiles in patients having "organic pain" to those having "functional" pain or few physical findings. These studies have generally shown that elevations on the neurotic triad characterize those patients with functional pain. A final group of research studies has examined the degree to which MMPI scores predict response of patients to medical or surgical treatment. Some studies have found that MMPI scores are predictive of treatment outcome whereas others have not.

A major problem with MMPI research on chronic pain is that it has relied almost exclusively on statistical comparisons conducted using large groups of chronic pain patients (18). By averaging data from fairly heterogeneous groups of patients, the impression has been given that chronic pain patients are similar in terms of personality. Recent MMPI studies, however, clearly indicate that chronic pain patients are not a homogeneous group (18). Homogeneous subgroups of patients, however, can be identified on the basis of MMPI scores. Bradley and his colleagues (18) used a multivariate hierarchical clustering procedure to identify three homogeneous MMPI subgroups. The first had an essentially normal profile, the second had elevations on scales Hs, D, and Hy, and the third had elevations on almost all clinical scales. Subsequent studies by other investigators have confirmed and replicated these findings and also have indicated that there are different behavioral and affective correlates for each of these profiles. Patients in the profile subgroup having elevations on almost all scales have significantly more pain and pain behavior problems than patients in the other subgroups. Patients with the essentially normal MMPI profiles have significantly less pain and fewer pain-related behavioral problems than patients in the other groups. Taken together, these results suggest that the MMPI is potentially quite useful in the assessment of personality in chronic pain patients.

On a practical level, there are problems in using the MMPI. It is a very long instrument and patients are often resistant to filling it out. Since the MMPI was developed for use with psychiatric patients, many of the items are designed to measure serious symptoms of psychopathology. When confronted with these items, chronic pain patients often become angry and feel that they are being given the message that their pain is imaginary or "in the head."

Intelligence tests and neuropsychological tests are often useful in the evaluation of pain syndromes. Patients with chronic pain can present significant intellectual and cognitive deficits that must be considered in treatment planning. These deficits may be severe enough, in fact, that they constitute the patient's primary problem. For example, an elderly patient experiencing dementia may be embarrassed by the cognitive slippage occurring and find that chronic pain provides a legitimate excuse for participating in activities that he or she is incapable of doing. In other cases, cognitive deficits are secondary to a high intake of narcotics or severe depression. Intelligence testing is useful in evaluating the patient's resources for vocational retraining. Unfortunately, many patients with chronic pain have limited formal education, a below average intelligence level, and have few options for further education and training.

MATCHING TREATMENT TO THE PATIENT

At this point in assessment, the data collected are integrated and used to select a treatment that best meets the patient's needs. Figure 3 displays the basic elements in behavioral treatment programs used in our Pain Management Program. In selecting a treatment protocol for a particular patient and determining how the patient is likely to respond to the treatment process, several issues need to be addressed. These include: 1) assessing the patient's motivation; 2) assessing the patient's skills and resources; 3) determining which treatment procedures should be used; and 4) conducting a sharing conference.

Assessing the Patient's Motivation

Motivation is a key issue in working with chronic pain patients. Some patients appear to be helpless, dependent individuals who are unable to be actively involved in treatment. Other patients with pain are clearly already making major efforts to cope with their pain and are open to learning new approaches. One useful index of motivation is the patient's response to initial assessment efforts. The assessment methods described above require the individual to actively participate in data collection. The

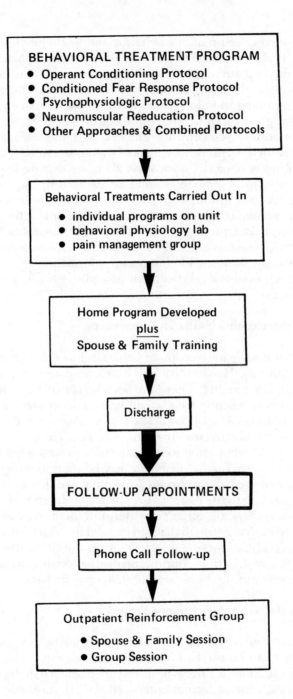

Figure 3.   Flow chart illustrating the basic elements of the behavioral treatment program

patient is asked to self-monitor behavior and to complete several questionnaires. Performance on these tasks provides an important behavior sample, indicating the degree to which the individual is able to work independently and follow through with assignments. Patients who are unable or unwilling to follow through with these assessment efforts are probably not good candidates for protocols that require a great deal of self-administered or self-control treatment. In these cases, a behavioral protocol that involves greater degrees of therapist and staff involvement would be a better choice. Conclusions about motivation level based on initial response to assessment should be made with caution, however. Those who may fail to follow through with assessment tasks may do so because they cannot comprehend the instructions or lack the skills necessary to complete the questionnaires. Alternate explanations for a failure to comply with assessment efforts should be explored because these explanations may also provide important information for making decisions about what behavioral treatment procedures are best suited to the patient's needs.

Assessing the Patient's Skills and Resources

A second major issue in selection of behavioral treatment is the patient's skills and resources. Many individuals have a long history of adequate or even superior functioning. They have been successful in home and work settings, and only recently have begun to experience significant disruptions in function because of pain. The patient's spouse and family members may also be valuable resources in treatment. The spouse, for example, may be highly motivated to assist the patient with a home program following discharge. Family members may be more than willing to become better educated about chronic pain and make changes in their own ways of responding to the patient's pain behavior. Interviews with spouse and family members are often very useful in identifying available and potentially reinforcing stimuli that can be used in the patient's treatment. They can provide important information on the degree to which one could expect any behavioral improvements that occur during treatment to be maintained in the home setting following discharge.

Selecting a Behavioral Treatment Protocol

As can be seen in Figure 3, there are four major behavioral treatment protocols that can be used with chronic pain patients. The indications and contraindications for these protocols are discussed in detail in Chapter 19. Several general factors enter into the selection of a particular protocol for a given patient. First, and most critical, is the information derived from assessment efforts. Patients whose pain appears to be related to operant factors are routinely placed on the operant conditioning protocol, whereas those who have a psychophysiologic basis for pain (for example, a stress-related migraine headache patient) are placed on the psychophysiologic protocol. Second, we usually try to select a treatment protocol which best fits into the patient's style of perceiving and solving problems. Thus, if a patient has a history of striving for self-control and is highly reinforced by mastering problems, the selection of a protocol that emphasizes behavioral self-control is indicated. Alternatively, if a patient has a long history of being dependent on family or friends for problem-solving, then a protocol that involves a greater involvement of staff and family in treatment, such as the operant conditioning protocol, would be used. A third factor in selection of a treatment approach is empirical validation of that approach for patients with similar problems. The available research data may indicate that a particular protocol is more likely to work with one type of patient than another.

An important final step in matching treatment to the patient is a sharing conference (19) held at some point early in the treatment process. In this conference, the patient is provided with a brief review of assessment information gathered and a behavioral formulation of their problems. In this conference, efforts are made to outline the details of treatment and link them to assessment information.

The sharing conference, basically, serves to help the patient better understand the behavioral approach to pain management. The patient is encouraged to question critically the rationale for specific treatments and to ask for information about the treatment procedures. The sharing conference provides a format in which the patient's willingness to accept a behavioral formulation and to start particular treatments can be assessed. Every attempt is made to avoid the use of jargon and to describe behavioral treatment procedures in terms that the patient understands.

In the sharing conference, patients are given an overview of the entire treatment process (see Figure 3). They are told, for example, that their behavioral treatment programs will be carried out either in an individual program on the unit, in the behavioral physiology laboratory, and/or in a pain management group that meets daily. They are also told that, prior to discharge, a home program will be developed that is designed to help them continue their treatment after discharge. The patient is encouraged at the time of the sharing conference to have their spouse and family visit and attend treatment sessions. The nature of follow-up appointments is also described. Patients are told about telephone follow-up calls and are informed that they will be invited after discharge to the Outpatient Reinforcement Group session that meets every three months. The inpatient phase of treatment is thus presented as the first step in the treatment process, and the importance of continuing treatment once the patient has returned to home is emphasized from the start.

REFERENCES

1. Keefe FJ, Block AR: Development of an observation method for assessing pain behavior in chronic low back pain. Behavior Therapy 13:363–375, 1982
2. Rosenstiel AK, Keefe FJ: The use of coping strategies in chronic low back pain patients: relationship to patient characteristics and current adjustment. Pain 17:33–44, 1983
3. Andrasik F, Blanchard EB, Arena JG, et al: Psychophysiology of recurrent headache: methodological series and new empirical findings. Behavior Therapy 13:407–429, 1982
4. Tursky B, Jamner LD, Friedman R: The pain perception profile: a psychophysical approach to the assessment of pain report. Behavior Therapy 13:430–437, 1982
5. Keefe FJ: Behavioral assessment and treatment of chronic pain. J Consult Clin Psychol 50:896–911, 1982
6. Thomas EJ: Bias and therapist influence in behavioral assessment. J Behav Ther Exp Psychiatry 4:107–111, 1973
7. Keele KD: The pain chart. Lancet 2:6–8, 1948
8. Melzark R: The McGill Pain Questionnaire: major properties and scoring methods. Pain 1:227–229, 1975
9. Fordyce WE: Behavioral Methods for Chronic Pain and Illness. St. Louis, CV Mosby, 1973
10. Keefe FJ, Block AR, Williams RB, et al: Behavioral treatment of chronic pain: clinical outcome and individual differences in pain relief. Pain 11:221–231, 1981
11. Turk D, Meichenbaum D, Genest M: Pain and Behavioral Medicine: A Cognitive Approach. New York, Guilford, 1983
12. Beck AT, Rush AJ, Shaw BF, et al: Cognitive Therapy of Depression. New York, Guilford, 1979
13. Keefe FJ, Crisson JE, Snipes MT: Observational methods for assessing pain: a practical guide, in Applications in Behavioral Medicine and Health Psychology: A Clinician's Sourcebook. Edited by Blumenthal JA, McKee DC. Sarasota, Florida, Professional Resource Exchange, 1986
14. Wolf SL, Nacht M, Kelly JL: EMG feedback training during dynamic movement for low back pain patients. Behavior Therapy 13:395–406, 1982
15. Wolf SL, Basmajian JV, Russe CTC, et al: Normative data on low back mobility and activity levels: implications for neuromuscular reeducation. Am J Phys Med 58:217–229, 1979
16. Derogatis LR: SCL-90-R Administration, Scoring and Procedures Manual II. Towson, Maryland, Clinical Psychometric Research, 1983
17. Keefe FJ, Brown C, Scott DS, et al: Behavioral assessment of chronic pain, Assessment Strategies in Behavioral Medicine. Edited by Keefe FJ, Blumenthal JA. New York, Grune and Stratton, 1982
18. Bradley LA, Prokop CK, Margolis R, et al: Multivariate analysis of the MMPI profiles of low back pain patients. J Behav Med 1:253–272, 1978
19. Keefe FJ, Kopel SA, Gordon SB: A Practical Guide to Behavioral Assessment. New York, Springer, 1978

APPENDIX

Name _____ Age _____

PAIN DESCRIPTION

1. Pain Location _____ (local?) _____ (diffuse?) _____

2. 0–10 Pain Ratings _____ present 3. Quality of Pain *(pts. in words)*

   _____ lowest   _____

   _____ highest   _____

4. Duration of Pain—How many hours per day? _____

   How long ago did pain start? _____

   How long has pain been constant all day long? _____

5. ↑ Pain _____

6. ↓ Pain _____

BEHAVIORAL RESPONSE

1. Living situation—who lives at home _____

   age and occupation of spouse _____

2. What do you have trouble doing? ____ light housekeeping ____ heavy housekeeping

   _____ social activities _____ work outside home

3. What do you do for work? _____

4. Receiving disability? _____   Pending disability/lawsuit? _____

5. Daily uptime _____

6. Reinforcers for pain behavior: _____ bedrest PRN, _____ Pain meds PRN,

   _____ moist heat PRN, _____ family/spouse attention PRN

   _____ does family/spouse ignore you?

7. Ask patient to walk 5m _____ Gd _____ Rb _____ BRC _____ GR _____ SI

8. Ask patient to move from standing to reclining _____ Gd _____ Rb _____

   BRC _____ GR _____ SI

9. Ask patient to sit up _____ Gd _____ Rb _____ BRC _____ GR _____ SI

10. Other overt pain behaviors? _____ Cane/Walker, _____ TENS, _____ Brace,

    _____ Hot pack/heating pad, _____ Special bed, chairs, recliner,

    _____ Wheelchair

COGNITIVE-AFFECTIVE RESPONSE

Expectations 1. What do your doctors say is causing pain? _____

   2. What do doctors think will happen in the future with your pain? _____

_____

3. What do *you* think is causing pain? _____

4. What do *you* think will happen in the future? _____

Cognitive Errors   _____ Overgeneralization _____ Selective abstraction

                  _____ Excessive responsibility ____Assuming temporal ____causality

                  _____ Self references _____ Catastrophizing

                  _____ Dichotomous thinking

Education and IQ 1. How far have you gotten in school? _____

                  2. IQ estimate _____

Affective 1. Sleep problems? _____ Onset _____, AM waking _____, Naps? _____

      2. Energy level poor? _____

      3. Δ Wt. _____

      4. Crying spells _____

      5. Appear anxious _____ Depressed _____

      6. Self-described mood _____

PSYCHOPHYSIOLOGIC RESPONSE

1. Evidence of Tissue Pathology: _____

_____

_____

2. Muscle tension? _____ ,   Bruxism _____ ,   Headaches _____ ,

Excessive guarding _____ , Limitations of movement _____ ,

Muscle spasm _____

3. In response to pain, any ANS activity? _____

TREATMENT COURSE

1. *Present*: What is the tx plan?: _____   TENS   _____

2. *Past*   Pain meds   _____

_____   PT   _____

                                 Nerve blocks   _____

What do you hope to get from tx?:   BFB/PMR   _____

_____   Brace   _____

Key:

5 m	=	5 meter walk	TENS	=	transcutaneous nerve stimulator
Gd	=	guarding	ANS	=	autonomic nervous system
Rb	=	rubbing	PT	=	physical therapy
BRC	=	bracing	BFB	=	biofeedback
GR	=	grimacing	PMR	=	progressive muscle relaxation
SI	=	sighing			

Management

Chapter 18

Psychotropic Drugs in Chronic Pain

Randal D. France, M.D.
K. Ranga Rama Krishnan, M.D.

In this chapter, the clinical use of psychotropic drugs in the chronic pain states will be examined. As detailed in earlier chapters, pain states produced by whatever the etiological cause (physical, psychological, or combination of the two) have a significant emotional component. Psychotropic drugs have been suggested as having analgesic properties that are independent of their effect on mood or behavior. It is, therefore, not surprising that psychoactive drugs have become one of the main therapeutic interventions in chronic pain syndromes. Possible mechanism of action, review of clinical studies, and therapeutic usage of the psychotropic drugs including antidepressants, monoamine precursors, neuroleptics, lithium, anticonvulsants, and minor tranquilizers will be presented.

ANTIDEPRESSANTS

Antidepressants were reported to be effective in chronic pain states more than 20 years ago (1–3). Paoli and colleagues (2) first used antidepressants for chronic pain. Since these early reports, antidepressants have been extensively used in the chronic pain population. There are few animal studies and well designed controlled clinical studies evaluating the effectiveness of antidepressants in chronic pain. Three recent reviews (4–6) on the clinical use of antidepressants in chronic pain syndromes support the use of these agents in various pain states, but the mechanism of action remains unclear.

Mechanism of Action

The antidepressant drugs may be effective in pain by their antidepressant activity or direct analgesic action.

Antidepressant Activity

In pain states in which there is the coexistence of depression, patients obtain relief from both the depression and pain when using antidepressants, heterocyclic antidepressants (HCA), or monoamine oxidase inhibitors (MAOIs) (7–15). Bradley demonstrated resolution of depression and pain when the depression preceded the onset of pain. When pain preceded the onset of depression, the treatment was only effective in alleviating the depression and not the pain (16). Antidepressants are effective in depressed patients with pain complaints (17, 18).

The biological basis of depression has been attributed to dysfunction in central neurotransmitter systems (catecholamines and indoleamines). Antidepressants (HCAs and MAOIs) alter neurotransmitter metabolites, receptor sensitivity, receptor uptake blockade, and firing rates of neu-

323

rons. Which of these effects is responsible for the antidepressant effect is unknown (19). The generic term heterocyclic antidepressants is used in this chapter to include both the imipramine-like tricyclic antidepressants (TCAs) and a newer generation of antidepressants that have a different ring structure from the TCAs.

Analgesic Action

As noted above, in some studies the analgesic effects of antidepressants have been related to the antidepressant activity. However, in six clinical studies (20–25), pain relief occurred without a parallel effect on depression in chronic pain. In three other studies (26–28), chronic pain patients without clinical evidence of depression obtained pain relief using antidepressants. These studies suggest that antidepressants may have analgesic properties in addition to their antidepressant activity. Evidence for analgesic activity of antidepressants is supported by the observation of antidepressants having direct analgesic properties (29, 30). The analgesic activity of the antidepressant was not attenuated by naloxone but was significantly reduced by reserpine (which depletes CNS monoamines) (29). However, this has not been shown in other studies (31–33). Chapman and Butler showed doxepin having no effect on experimentally induced pain in humans (34). The cause for the conflicting results is unclear at present. From a review of the studies, it does not appear to be related to dose of drug, animal types, drug, or model of pain relief in the various studies. Most of the studies have been based on animal experimentation using the acute pain model and may not be reflective of the biochemical changes in the chronic pain state and effects of antidepressants on these alterations.

In summary, the mechanism of action of antidepressants is uncertain in chronic pain states. It is unclear whether the analgesic efficacy of antidepressants is due to its antidepressant or a direct analgesic effect. There is conflicting evidence for antidepressants having analgesic activity.

Review of Clinical Studies

In the following section, we will review the efficacy of antidepressants in patients with pain from arthritis, headaches, facial pain, postherpetic neuralgia, diabetic neuropathy, back pain, pain of mixed etiologies, and pain as a symptom of depression.

Arthritis. Kuipers (35) was the first to suggest antidepressants for pain control in arthritis (Table 1). He showed that imipramine at 20–40 mg per day was 60–70 percent effective in reducing pain levels in an uncontrolled study. McDonald-Scott (26) reported on the use of imipramine in 22 selected patients without psychiatric illness having rheu-

Table 1. Antidepressants for Arthritis

Author of Study	Controlled Study	N	Type of Drug	Dose (mg/day)	Efficacy of Pain Relief (%)*
McDonald-Scott (26)	yes	22	imipramine	75	69
Gringas (27)	yes	55	imipramine	75	52
Tyber (8)	no	56	amitriptyline	75	79
Regalado (37)	no	41	clomipramine	10–25	57
Ganvir (38)	yes	49	clomipramine	25	0
Kuipers (35)	no	28	imipramine	20–40	60–70
Glick (39)	yes	11	imipramine	75	p
Thorpe (40)	yes	19	dibenzepine	240	p

p = drug significantly more effective than placebo
* = percentage of patients reporting pain relief

matoid arthritis, osteoarthritis, or ankylosing spondylitis. In a double blind crossover trial using 75 mg per day versus a placebo, he found that a significant number of patients preferred imipramine to placebo. With 55 similar patients in a multicenter study, Gringas (27) found significant improvement in pain, stiffness, and grip strength using 75 mg of imipramine per day as compared to a placebo in a double blind crossover study. In this study, patients with clinical signs of depression were excluded. The latter two studies showed pain relief in arthritic patients with an antidepressant in the absence of depression.

Haydu and colleagues (36) showed a decrease in the rheumatoid factor in nonarthritic psychotic patients using 150 mg of imipramine per day. But MacNeil and Dick (9), in a double blind trial using 75 mg of imipramine per day, failed to show a change in the level of rheumatoid factor in 20 rheumatoid arthritic patients who were free of psychiatric illness. Regalado (37) suggested the addition of a small dose of clomipramine to analgesic therapy in chronic pain patients to modify the pain threshold and reduce the dose of analgesics. In an uncontrolled study of 41 joint pain patients, he showed that 57 percent of patients felt better when clomipramine (10–25 mg per day) was added to their standard analgesic drugs. There appeared to be little difference between the 10 or 25 mg dose of clomipramine in effectiveness.

In an uncontrolled study of 56 patients with monoarticular shoulder pain, Tyber (8) used 75 mg of amitriptyline and lithium carbonate (serum lithium level was between 0.5 to 1.0 meq/l). Sixty-six percent of this sample had clinical evidence of depression and one-third had calcium deposits in the shoulder joint confirmed by radiographic examination. Forty-four patients (79 percent) showed a marked clinical improvement. In addition, there was a decrease or disappearance of the calcification in the shoulder joint by radiographic re-examination after treatment.

The efficacy of antidepressants in arthritis has been proven in four controlled studies (26, 27, 39, 40), but one controlled study (38) failed to show any effect (Table 1). The effect of antidepressants through analgesic or antidepressant action in arthritis is unclear. There is the need for further studies controlling for the presence or absence of depression before any statement can be made.

Headaches.   Antidepressants have been used for various categories of headaches, including migraine, tension, mixed vascular and tension, and psychogenic (Table 2). Anthony and Lance (47) studied the effects of phenelzine 45 mg daily in 25 patients with migraine headaches refractory to other medical treatments. Twenty out of 25 patients had greater than 50 percent reduction in headache symptoms. There was no correlation between plasma 5-HT platelet activity and response of the patients. Couch and colleagues (23) studied the effects of amitriptyline (100 mg per day) versus a placebo in 100 migraine patients. He found amitriptyline significantly more effective than placebo in reducing both the frequency and duration of migraine headaches. In nondepressed patients with severe migraine and depressed patients having less severe headaches, amitriptyline was more effective than in depressed patients with severe migraines. The prophylactic effects of the drug occurred within the first month of treatment and were independent of the drug's antidepressant activity. Gomersall and Stuart (28) demonstrated that 16 out of 20 patients had fewer migraine attacks when treated with amitriptyline (10–60 mg per day) as compared to a placebo in a double blind controlled study using crossover design. The patients were free of depression. Amitriptyline was most effective in attacks without a specific cause and least effective in migraine headaches brought about by fatigue.

Carasso and colleagues (46), in a single blind study, compared the effects of clomipramine (20–75 mg daily) and amitriptyline (30–100 mg daily) in patients suffering from chronic tension headaches. Ten out of 15 patients (66 percent) in the clomipramine group, and 7 out of 13 (54 percent) in the amitriptyline group, had a reduction in their tension headaches. The difference in effect between the two drugs was not significant.

Lance and Curran (21) compared the effects of various drugs with a placebo in 280 chronic tension headache patients. Patients treated with

Table 2. Antidepressants for Headaches

Author of Study	Controlled Study	N	Type of Drug	Dose (mg/day)	Efficacy of Pain Relief (%)*
Gomersall and Stuart (28)	yes	16	amitriptyline	10–60	80
Couch (23)	yes	100	amitriptyline	100	55.3
Lance and Curran (21)	yes	280	amitriptyline imipramine	30–75 30–75	amitriptyline > imipramine
Okasha (15)	yes	80	doxepin amitriptyline	30–50 30–150	p (doxepin > amitriptyline or diazepam)
Diamond (41)	yes	56	amitriptyline	10–25	p
Couch (22)	no	110	amitriptyline	75	72
Noone (42)	no	8	clomipramine	30	100
Mahloudji (43)	no	12	amitriptyline	30–40	100
Dalessio (44)	no	100	amitriptyline	75–100	64
Sherwin (12)	no	14	amitriptyline perphenazine	100–200 8–64	70
Morland (45)	yes	14	doxepin	100	p
Carasso (46)	no	15 13	clomipramine amitriptyline	20–75 30–110	66 54
Anthony (47)	no	25	phenelzine	45	80
Paulson (48)	no	14	imipramine	75	0

p = drug significantly better than placebo
* = percentage of patients reporting pain relief

30 to 75 mg of amitriptyline per day showed significant improvement in the relief of the headache as compared to those treated with the placebo. In addition, amitriptyline was more effective than diazepam, bellergal, chlordiazepoxide, and methysergide. Most patients did not show signs of depression. It appears that the effect of amitriptyline was independent of the occurrence of depression in these patients.

Paulson (48), in a study of 14 patients with posttraumatic headaches, excluding depression and personality disorders, found imipramine 75 mg daily no more effective than placebo. This report is limited by its small subject size.

Okasha (15) compared the efficacy of doxepin (30–50 mg per day), amitriptyline (30–50 mg per day), and diazepam (6–10 mg per day), and a placebo in 80 patients with psychogenic headache. In this double blind trial, doxepin and amitriptyline were more effective than diazepam in promoting headache relief. All three active drugs were superior to the placebo. After two months of treatment only the doxepin was significantly effective in relief of headache, depression, and anxiety. Morland and colleagues (45) studied the effects of doxepin (100 mg daily) in 14 chronic headache patients in a double blind crossover trial. They found a significant reduction in the severity and analgesic use in the doxepin period as compared to the placebo. There have been more controlled studies of antidepressants in the treatment of chronic headaches than other pain syndromes. Six controlled studies (15, 21, 23, 28, 41, 45) have demonstrated a positive effect of antidepressants in the control of tension headaches, and no study has shown a lack of effect.

Facial Pain. Lascelles (11) treated 40 patients with facial pain of various etiologies using phenelzine (45 mg. daily) for one month in a double blind placebo crossover study (Table 3). Improvement in depression of facial pain was more significant in the phenelzine period as compared to the placebo.

In a double blind study, Feinmann and colleagues (25) compared dothiepin (heterocyclic antidepressant not available in the U.S.) to

Table 3. Antidepressants for Facial Pain

Author of Study	Controlled Study	N	Type of Drug	Dose (mg/day)	Efficacy of Pain Relief (%)*
Lascelles (11)	yes	40	phenelzine	45	75
Feinmann (25)	yes	93	dothiepin	150	71
Gessel (49)	no	8	amitriptyline	100	50
Carasso (46)	no	9	clomipramine	20–75	44
		9	amitriptyline	30–110	38
Moore (50)	no	100	amitriptyline	?	71
			chlordiazepoxide	?	

* = percentage of patients reporting pain relief

placebo in 150 patients with psychogenic facial pain. In the dothiepin group, 71 percent of patients achieved pain relief as compared with 47 percent in the placebo group. At one year follow-up in the dothiepin group, 68 out of 84 patients (81 percent) were pain free. Although the dothiepin was effective at relieving the facial pain, it was no more superior to placebo in lessening the depressive symptoms. The psychiatric symptoms present in patients with psychogenic pain disappeared when the pain symptoms abated and did not recur as the drug treatment was stopped. Carasso and colleagues (46) treated 17 patients with trigeminal neuralgia with either clomipramine (20–75 mg per day) or amitriptyline (30–110 mg per day). Four out of 9 patients (44 percent) receiving clomipramine and 3 out of 8 (38 percent) receiving amitriptyline reported a moderate to marked improvement in the pain.

In three uncontrolled studies (46, 49, 50), antidepressants were effective in reducing both pain level and psychological symptoms. However, one study (46) showed minimal therapeutic effects. In the controlled studies, Lascelles (11) showed a decrease in pain and psychological symptoms when using an MAO inhibitor, whereas Feinmann (25) showed that dothiepin was effective at reducing only the pain and not the level of depression.

Two controlled studies (11, 25) showed antidepressants to be significantly more effective than placebo in facial pain syndromes. Three case studies all showed a positive effect. The role of antidepressants in these pain patients is promising, but further studies should be done, especially with the new generation of antidepressants similar to the study by Feinmann and colleagues (25).

Postherpetic Neuralgia.   Woodforde and colleagues (7) demonstrated a decrease in postherpetic pain in 11 out of 14 patients (70 percent) using amitriptyline (100 mg daily) (Table 4). In this group, all 14 patients had complaints of depressive symptoms. Taub, in 2 uncontrolled studies (51, 52), found 5 patients experiencing a decrease in pain using 75–100 mg of amitriptyline plus a low dose neuroleptic, and 14 out of 17 consecutive patients (82 percent) with postherpetic pain responding to 75 mg of amitriptyline daily plus fluphenazine 3 mg daily. He observed a pain decrease on the fourth or fifth day of drug treatment with continual improvement over one month. Clarke (53), using amitriptyline 75 mg per day and perphenazine 6 mg per day, showed pain relief in 54 percent of patients. Carasso and colleagues (46) compared the effects of clomipramine (20–75 mg daily) and amitriptyline (30–110 mg daily) in 21 patients with postherpetic neuralgia. Five out of 10 patients (50 percent) responded to amitriptyline, and 3 out of 11 patients (27 percent) responded to clomipramine. In a controlled study, Watson and colleagues (20) showed amitriptyline (25–137.5 mg per day) superior to placebo in 16 out of 24 patients (66 percent). There was no correlation

Table 4. Antidepressants for Postherpetic Neuralgia

Author of Study	Controlled Study	N	Type of Drug	Dose (mg/day)	Efficacy of Pain Relief (%)*
Watson (20)	yes	24	amitriptyline	25–137.5	66
Woodforde (7)	no	14	amitriptyline	100	79
Taub (51)	no	5	amitriptyline neuroleptic	25–100 ?	100
Taub (52)	no	17	amitriptyline fluphenazine	75 3	82
Clarke (53)	no	120	amitriptyline perphenazine	75 6	54
Hatangdi (54)	no	34	nortriptyline anticonvulsants	50–100	79
Weis (55)	no	9	amitriptyline perphenazine	6	89
Carasso (46)	no	21	clomipramine amitriptyline	20–75 30–110	27 50

* = percentage of patients reporting pain relief

between pain relief and improvement in depressive symptoms in the study. In patients with a good response, the mean combined blood plasma level for amitriptyline (67 ng/ml) and nortriptyline (38 ng/mg) was 105 ng/ml.

In the use of antidepressants for postherpetic neuralgia, there are various uncontrolled studies (7, 51–55) showing benefit. In five of the studies, the authors used a combination of an antidepressant with a neuroleptic (51–53, 55) or anticonvulsant (54). One study reported using only an antidepressant (7). It is unclear whether the combination of antidepressants with a neuroleptic is more effective than the antidepressant alone. It appears that the effects of the medications are only symptomatic and require long-term use of drugs to sustain pain relief. If this is indeed the case, a controlled study looking at the effectiveness of the combination versus an antidepressant is important, since the risk of tardive dyskinesia in long-term neuroleptic use is certainly present. It should be noted that other risk factors for tardive dyskinesia are present in these pain patients, such as depression, dementia, advanced age, and other medical illnesses.

Watson and colleagues (20) showed that the effectiveness of amitriptyline occurred when blood levels of both amitriptyline and nortriptyline were below the lower end of the therapeutic range reported for antidepressant effect. Lower drug blood levels were noted in the poor responders. This may indicate a "therapeutic window" effect. Further studies are needed.

Diabetic Neuropathy. Davis and colleagues (56) were the first to report the successful use of amitriptyline (75 mg daily) with fluphenazine in eight patients with diabetic neuropathy (Table 5). They reported pain relief occurring within the first five days of drug treatment. Turkington (10), in a controlled study of 59 patients with painful diabetic neuropathy, compared the effectiveness of amitriptyline (100 mg daily), imipramine (100 mg daily), and diazepam (15 mg daily). Patients treated with either of the tricyclics reported complete relief of pain and patients treated with diazepam showed no improvement. The relief of pain occurred with lessening of the depressive symptoms. The authors concluded that leg pains are a manifestation of a depression rather than the effects of diabetes mellitus.

Kvinesdal and colleagues (57) used imipramine at a fixed dose of 100 mg per day in a double blind crossover study with 12 patients suffering from painful diabetic neuropathy. Seven of the 12 patients (58 percent) had a positive response to imipramine, and 0 out of 12 (0 percent) patients responded to placebo. The range of plasma blood levels for imipramine and desipramine in responders was 100–120 ng/ml and 60 ng/ml for nonresponders.

In two controlled studies (10, 57), antidepressants were shown to be superior to placebo in controlling painful diabetic neuropathy. As has been shown in other denervation pain syndromes (i.e., postherpetic neuralgia) the pain relief in diabetic neuropathy was reported to occur in

Table 5. Antidepressants for Painful Diabetic Neuropathy

Author of Study	Controlled Study	N	Type of Drug	Dose (mg/day)	Efficacy of Pain Relief (%)*
Davis (56)	no	8	amitriptyline fluphenazine	75	100
Turkington (10)	yes	59	amitriptyline imipramine diazepam	100 100 15	100 100 0
Kvinesdal (57)	yes	12	imipramine	100	58

* = percentage of patients reporting pain relief

the first several days of drug treatment. In addition, the assayed drug blood levels required for pain relief in postherpetic neuralgia (20) and painful diabetic neuropathy (57) were less than the therapeutic drug level for treatment of depression. Massey and Riley (58) postulated that perhaps antidepressants are effective in painful peripheral neuropathies by affecting neuronal or axonal transmission, and recommended a trial of antidepressants in other conditions that produce painful peripheral neuropathies.

Back Pain. Jenkins and colleagues (59) studied the effect of imipramine (75 mg daily) in 44 chronic low back pain patients (Table 6). In this double blind study no statistical difference was found between the group treated with imipramine and a placebo in the assessment of pain, stiffness, straight leg raise, back flexion, and depression. However, in a double blind study comparing the effects of doxepin (2.5 mg per kg) versus placebo, Hameroff and colleagues (13) found significant improvement in the drug group compared to the placebo group. Improvement was seen in lessening of pain, depression, muscle tension, and insomnia. Similarly, Alcoff and colleagues (60), in a double blind study, compared imipramine (150 mg daily) versus a placebo in 60 chronic low back pain patients. In the imipramine group, 10 out of 21 patients (50 percent) responded. It should be noted that the responders to drug treatment had more positive physical findings on physical examination than nonresponders.

Table 6. Antidepressants for Back Pain

Author of Study	Controlled Study	N	Type of Drug	Dose (mg/day)	Efficacy of Pain Relief (%)*
Jenkins (59)	yes	44	imipramine	75	0
Hameroff (13)	yes	27	doxepin	2.5 mg/kg	p
Alcoff (60)	yes	60	imipramine	150	p
Sternbach (61)	yes	11	reserpine	0.5 to 1.5	0
		2	L-tryptophan	7–10 gm/day	0
		5	5-hydroxy-tryptophan	1.5–3 gm/day	0
		9	clomipramine	150	p
		9	amitriptyline	150	0

p = drug significantly more effective than placebo
* = percentage of patients reporting pain relief

Sternbach and colleagues (61) studied patients suffering from disc disease with demonstrable physical disease underlying their pain complaints. Eleven patients received 0.5–1.5 mg of reserpine for three days and then switched to placebo. There was no significant difference between the reserpine and placebo period. Five patients received 5-hydroxytryptophan (5-HT) (1.5–3.0 grams per day) and 2 patients received L-tryptophan (L-TP) (7–10 grams per day) for 10 days. The drugs were blindly switched to placebo after a 10-day washout period. There was no difference between 5-HT and L-TP and placebo. Nine patients received clomipramine (150 mg daily), amitriptyline (150 mg daily), or placebo in a double blind crossover study. Patients during the clomipramine period reported significantly less pain than during the placebo period. Amitriptyline did not cause a significant decrease in pain when compared to placebo in decreasing pain complaints.

In chronic low back pain, the evidence for efficacy of antidepressants in relieving pain is unclear. The serotonergic hypothesis detailed by Sternbach (61) has little substantial clinical support. The difficulty in evaluating the drug treatment effects in chronic low back pain lies in the multiple etiological causes of chronic low back pain: arachnoiditis, muscle strain, nerve damage, and postoperative effects on the back.

Pain of Mixed Etiologies. Since the early report by Paoli (2) using imipramine in various painful states, the authors have presented case studies describing the effectiveness of antidepressants in chronic pain due to musculoskeletal and neurological disorders (Table 7). Merskey and Hester (62) reported 28 out of 30 patients (93 percent) with chronic pain caused by lesions of the nervous system responding to a combination of antidepressants and phenothiazine. The effectiveness of the drug is related to the direct analgesic activity on the central nervous system. The authors' conclusions were based on the fact that only one of the patients had a primary depression while the remaining patients had depression secondary to their pain. Kocher (63) treated 103 chronic pain patients with musculoskeletal or neuropathic pain using a combination of antidepressants and phenothiazine. Eighty-two percent of patients showed a marked improvement. In a large series of studies, Blumer and Heilbronn (72) found antidepressant therapy effective in 89 percent of chronic pain patients. Evans and colleagues (64) failed to show any difference in pain control in 22 depressed hospitalized elderly patients with chronic illness using doxepin (150 mg per day) versus a placebo. Johansson and von Knorring (65) studied 32 patients with pain states due to both organic and psychogenic causes. In this double blind controlled study, zimelidine (serotonergic uptake inhibitor) produced significantly greater pain relief than placebo. The pain relief occurred independent of the changes in depression.

Montastruc and colleagues (69) evaluated the analgesic effects of clomipramine in chronic pain patients with deafferentation pain syndrome and the relationship between the analgesic action and plasma level of the drug. Twenty out of 30 patients (67 percent) reported significant pain relief with treatment. The treatment consisted of giving clomipramine 100 mg intravenously for 10 days followed by 150 mg daily by month. Beneficial effect was seen on the fourth day of intravenous

Table 7. Antidepressants for Pain of Mixed Etiologies

Author of Study	Controlled Study	N	Type of Drug	Dose (mg/day)	Efficacy of Pain Relief (%)*
Merskey (62)	no	30	various HCAs + phenothiazine		93
Kocher (63)	no	130	various HCAs phenothiazine		82
Clarke (53)	no	110	amitriptyline perphenazine	75 2	34
Evans (64)	yes	22	doxepin	150	0
Johansson (65)	yes	32	zimelidine	200	*p*
Pilowsky (66)	yes	32	amitriptyline	150	0
Singh (18)	no	60	imipramine amitriptyline chlordiazepoxide		*p* *p* 0
Duthie (67)	no	12	amitriptyline trifluoperazine	75	67
Magni (68)	no	12	amitriptyline	75	75
Montastruc (69)	no	30	clomipramine	150	67
Castaigne (70)	no	30	clomipramine	50–200	93
Langohr (71)	no	82	clomipramine + neuroleptic neuroleptic	75–150	68 45
Langohr (71)	yes	48	clomipramine	150	*p*
Blumer (72)	no	349	various HCAs		89

p = drug is significantly more effective than placebo or other comparison drug
* = percentage of patients reporting pain relief

treatment. The study indicated a "therapeutic window" of plasma between 20 and 85 ng/ml.

Pilowsky and colleagues (66) in a double blind crossover study failed to demonstrate pain reduction in 32 patients using amitriptyline as compared with a placebo. These patients had no organic cause for their pain. It is difficult to assess the effectiveness of antidepressants in this group of studies. The control studies of Johansson and von Knorring (65) and Langohr (71) are the only studies showing any significant drug effect. The drug study by Pilowsky and colleagues (66), however, did not support an antidepressant effect in the mixed population of chronic pain patients. Clearly, further studies need to be done. The use of a controlled study design and a specific pain diagnosis would help to clear the ambiguity found in these studies.

Pain as a Symptom of Depression. Lindsay and Wyckoff (73) showed that 96 of 116 patients (83 percent) obtained significant pain relief with an antidepressant when pain and depression coexisted (Table 8). Ward and colleagues (14) demonstrated that doxepin (150 mg daily) was effective in reducing pain complaints and depression in 16 unipolar depressed patients with pain. High anxiety levels (measured by a self-reporting instrument) were significantly associated with high urinary 3-methoxy-4-hydroxyphenylethylamine glycol (MHPG, metabolite of central nervous system norepinephrine metabolism) and pain relief with treatment (74). Raft and colleagues (17) studied 29 patients having a major depression with pain complaints in a double blind comparison of phenelzine (1.5 mg/kg), amitriptyline (3.5 mg/kg), and placebo. Phenelzine proved to be significantly more effective than amitriptyline and placebo. When the phenelzine was more effective than amitriptyline, the platelet MAO inhibition was 90 percent, and when phenelzine showed greater relief than placebo, platelet MAO activity was 80 percent.

It appears that antidepressants, both heterocyclic and MAOIs, are effective in alleviating the pain and depressive symptoms in patients with

Table 8. Antidepressants for Pain as a Symptom of Depression

Author of Study	Controlled Study	N	Type of Drug	Dose (mg/day)	Efficacy of Pain Relief (%)*
Raft (17)	yes	23	phenelzine	1.5 mg/kg	p*
			amitriptyline	3.5 mg/kg	p
Ward (14)	yes	16	doxepin	150	p
Lindsay (73)	no	116	various HCAs		83

p = drug more effective than placebo
* = phenelzine more effective than amitriptyline

depression. In these two studies (14, 17), there was a significant degree of depression as measured by rating instruments and standard criteria for depression. The primary diagnosis was depression, with pain being a symptom of depression. It is not surprising that the drugs were effective. What needs further study is whether MAOI inhibitors are superior to heterocyclic antidepressants as shown by Raft and colleagues (17), or whether the newer generation of heterocyclic antidepressants, such as trazodone, is more effective than the imipramine-like antidepressants.

Summary of Clinical Studies

The antidepressants are effective therapeutic agents in certain chronic pain states: headaches, diabetic neuropathy, arthritis, facial pain, and depression (Table 9). Less clear is the role of antidepressants in postherpetic neuralgia, back pain, and pain from mixed etiologies. Further controlled studies are needed. In the studies comparing the relative effectiveness of various antidepressant drugs (10, 15, 17, 18, 21, 25), there is no single antidepressant that is most effective for chronic pain. Some have advocated the use of antidepressants in combination with phenothiazines (12, 14, 37, 52, 55, 57, 62, 63, 71), antiepileptic drugs (54), lithium (8), or minor tranquilizers (50). However, these are case studies and the effectiveness of antidepressants in combination with

Table 9. Summary of Antidepressant Efficacy in Chronic Pain Syndromes

	Uncontrolled Studies		Controlled Studies	
Clinical Syndromes	No Effect	Effect*	No Effect	Effect
Arthritis		4	1	4
Postherpetic neuralgia		7		1
Diabetic neuropathy				2
Headache	1	7		6
Facial pain	1	2		2
Back pain			2	2
Mixed etiologies	1	9	2	2
Pain in depression		1		2

*greater than 50 percent response rate

these other agents is not known. With the potential for development of tardive dyskinesia with long-term use of neuroleptics and lack of superior effect over antidepressants alone, neuroleptic use in chronic pain patients should be limited.

Six studies (13, 14, 20, 57, 66, 69) reported the drug blood levels of the antidepressants. In three studies (20, 57, 69) in which the antidepressants clearly had a therapeutic effect on the pain level, the mean plasma blood levels were lower than the therapeutic plasma drug levels for depression. One study had technical problems, making it difficult to interpret the results (14). The study (66) in which the results were equivocal reported no significant findings between clinical response and drug blood levels.

The dose range of antidepressants most frequently used in these studies is approximately 50–100 mg of imipramine-like heterocyclic antidepressants. Except for clinical experience, it is unknown why this dose range, which is lower than that seen in the treatment of primary depression, appears to be effective.

The antidepressants most frequently used in these studies are doxepin, amitriptyline, imipramine, and clomipramine. These drugs have more serontonergic uptake inhibition than the other commercially available heterocyclic antidepressants. Of interest is the application of the new generation of antidepressant agents (trazodone, fluoxetine, iprindole, and maprotiline), which have more specific profiles than the imipramine-like agents.

Treatment

The two main types of antidepressants, heterocyclic antidepressants (HCAs) and monoamine oxidase inhibitors (MAOIs), used to treat chronic pain will be described (Table 10). This section will focus on the application of these drugs in chronic pain states. Considering the use of these drugs in the treatment of affective disorders, the reader is advised to consult other references (19, 75).

Heterocyclic Antidepressants

Choice of Drug. As mentioned earlier, there is no one HCA that has been shown to be superior in relieving pain. Despite the fact that doxepin, amitriptyline, imipramine, and clomipramine have commonly been used in clinical studies, there is no clear indication these agents are superior to other drugs such as desipramine, nortriptyline, trimipramine, amoxapine, or trazodone. To date, drug selection is based on matching the side-effect profile of each agent with each individual patient's need. Insomnia is a common symptom in all chronic pain disorders. It is often useful to consider the more sedating agents, such as

Table 10.   Antidepressant Drugs: Dose Range in Major Depression and
Chronic Pain

Drug		Therapeutic Dose Range (mg)	
		Depression Usual Daily Dose (Extreme Daily Dose)	Pain Usual Daily Dose (Extreme Daily Dose)
Generic	Trade		
imipramine	Tofranil Janimine	100–200 (30–300)	50–100* (10–150)
desipramine	Norpramin Pertofrane	100–300 (25–300)	50–75* (25–100)
amitriptyline	Elavil Endep	75–200 (50–300)	25–100* (10–150)
nortriptyline	Aventyl Pamelor	75–150 (20–150)	25–100* (10–100)
doxepin	Sinequan Adapin	75–150 (25–300)	25–100* (10–200)
protriptyline	Vivactyl	15–40 (10–60)	no data
trazodone	Desyrel	150–250 (50–600)	50–200 + (50–400)
amoxapine	Asendin	200–300 (50–600)	100–200 + (50–300)
maprotiline	Ludiomil	100–250 (25–300)	50–100 + (25–200)
phenelzine	Nardil	15–60 (15–90)	15–45* (15–60)
isocarboxazid	Marplan	10–40 (10–60)	10–40* (10–60)
tranylcypromine	Parnate	20–30 (10–40)	10–20* (10–40)
alprazolam	Xanax	1.0–4.0 (limited data)	.5–3.0 + (limited data)

Table 10. Antidepressant Drugs: Dose Range in Major Depression and Chronic Pain *(Continued)*

Drug		Therapeutic Dose Range (mg)	
		Depression Usual Daily Dose (Extreme Daily	Pain Usual Daily Dose (Extreme Daily
Generic	Trade	Dose)	Dose)
clomipramine**	Anafranil		25–50* (10–75)
trimipramine	Surmontil	75–150 (25–300)	50–100+ (25–150)
zimelidine***		100–200 (50–300)	50–100* (50–300)

   * Based on controlled clinical studies
  +Based on case reports, clinical experience
 ** Not commercially available in U.S.A.
*** Off the market

amitriptyline, doxepin, trazodone, trimipramine, or amoxapine (Table 11). It should be noted that these sedating HCAs also have potent anticholinergic activity. In the elderly, medically ill, and in combination with narcotics or other agents having potent anticholinergic activity, caution must be exercised when using these drugs. A drug with adequate sedating properties with little or no clinical anticholinergic activity is trazodone.

Dose of HCA. In a chronic pain patient with no accompanying major psychiatric illness, such as primary or secondary major depression, it is best to initiate treatment with 25–50 mg one to two hours before bedtime. The dose is then increased by 25 mg every three to four days until a therapeutic response is obtained, or the total dose of 100 mg is reached. Usually patients will begin to develop side effects at a range of 75–100 mg daily. The usual and extreme dose ranges for each of the antidepressants in chronic pain states are listed in Table 10. As noted earlier, the therapeutic response in pain patients occurs within the first five days of drug treatment and continues over the next month of treatment. Improvement in sleep usually occurs in the first two to three days of drug treatment. If the drug is progressed too rapidly, oversedation surely will occur. In patients showing a positive response to the drug, pain intensity will diminish but the character and location will not change. With ex-

Table 11. Relative Potency of Antidepressants in Sedative, Anticholinergic Activity

Drug	Sedative Effects	Anticholinergic Activity
imipramine	+ + +	+ + +
desipramine	+	+
clomipramine	+ + + +	+ +
amitriptyline	+ + + +	+ + + +
nortriptyline	+ + +	+ +
protriptyline	+	+ + +
trazodone	+ + +	+
doxepin	+ + + +	+ + +
trimipramine	+ + + +	+ + +
amoxapine	+ +	+
maprotiline	+ +	+ +

+   weak
+ +   mild
+ + +   moderate
+ + + +   strong

This table has been adapted from the following sources: Baldessarini RJ: Biomedical Aspects of Depression. Washington, DC, American Psychiatric Press, 1983; Baldessarini RJ: Drugs and the treatment of psychiatric disorders, in The Pharmalogical Basis of Therapeutics. Edited by Goodman AG, Goodman LS, Gilman A. New York, Macmillan, 1980; and American Medical Association: Drug Evaluation, fifth edition. Chicago, American Medical Association, Division of Drugs, 1983.

tended treatment, the pain will either disappear or diminish to tolerable levels, but location of the pain remains unchanged. This is seen in chronic pain states caused by neuropathy, neuralgia, and arthritis. In several pain syndromes including myofascial pain syndrome, tension headaches, and psychogenic pain, a positive response to drug treatment will produce a diminution of the pain and reduction in the number of pain sites.

If there is no response to the drug at the usual dose ranges for one week, the dose is increased gradually by 25 mg every three to four days if there is no medical contraindication or toxic effect. Due to the long plasma half-life of these agents, a single dose one hour before bedtime is satisfactory. After three weeks of treatment without a therapeutic response and good patient compliance to medication intake, a positive response is unlikely. It is best to discontinue the medication and to use another agent.

For patients who have had significant psychiatric illness—that is, major affective disorder—the starting dose and dose range is similar to that used in primary depression. When pain is a symptom of primary depression, the relief of pain does not occur within the first week of treatment, like that observed in other chronic pain states responding to antidepressants. In these patients with primary depression the neurovegetative signs of depression resolve before the cognitive, emotional, and pain aspects of depression do.

Lower doses and slow rates of increase are necessary in patients over the age of 60. This especially applies to the patient with postherpetic neuralgia, since these patients tend to be older. The response to drug treatment in a chronic pain patient with accompanying dementia is limited. Screening for dementia in chronic pain is important. Lack of drug response may be based on a dementia process as opposed to inadequate dose or selection of antidepressant medication.

Preadministration Evaluation. After determining the potential usefulness of HCAs, the physician should discuss the expected benefits and possible adverse effects of the medications. This is important in chronic pain patients since they usually have a past experience with multiple medications with little or no effect. This open approach adds to patient compliance with the drug treatment and other parts of a multi-disciplinary treatment. A careful drug history should be recorded to determine which drugs the patient is currently taking. Chronic pain patients usually are taking numerous prescribed medications at the time of their initial evaluation. Any potential drug interfering or causing a toxic reaction with an HCA should be discontinued if medically feasible. Blood counts, liver functions, and EKGs, especially in the elderly, should be performed. Patients with a history of cardiovascular disease, liver disease, and senility should be carefully assessed, and careful monitoring of drug treatment is necessary.

Maintenance. Once a clinical response is obtained most patients require treatment for extended periods (months to years). In patients for whom the pain is a symptom of depression or other self-limiting psychiatric illness, the medications can be tapered and discontinued in the usual manner. After the first six months of treatment, a gradual tapering of the medication should be tried, watching for relapse of pain and depression. In some patients, medications may need to be continued for years at a maintenance level (50–75 percent of the original therapeutic dose of the drug). If antidepressants are discontinued, a withdrawal syndrome may occur (76). The symptoms include somatic distress, gastrointestinal disturbance, anxiety, agitation, and sleep disturbance. These withdrawal symptoms are prevented by gradual tapering of the antidepressant. If the withdrawal syndrome develops after abrupt withdrawal of antidepressants, reinstitution of the antidepressant or treatment with atropine (0.8 mg every four hours, orally) will abate the reaction.

Side Effects.   The side effects seen with HCAs include anticholinergic effects, hypersensitivity reactions, cardiovascular complications, weight gain, and central nervous system problems (77). The anticholinergic side effects are the most common ones seen in chronic pain patients (Table 11). If a patient is bothered by the anticholinergic effects, then changing to an HCA with less anticholinergic activity is desirable (trazodone, desipramine). The advantage of trazodone over desipramine is that the former is more sedating, in addition to its lack of anticholinergic activity. The side effects are intensified if HCAs are used in combination with narcotic analgesics, especially dry mouth, constipation, postural hypotension, urinary retention, paralytic ileus, and peripheral edema. The peripheral edema is also enhanced when it is used in combination with nonsteroidal anti-inflammatory drugs. If the peripheral edema is acute and painful, then several days of diuretic therapy is indicated. If the peripheral edema occurs in a milder form, it can be controlled by a low sodium diet. Extrapyramidal reactions are commonly reported by chronic pain patients on antidepressants as compared to the low incidence seen in antidepressant-treated patients with major depression.

The hypersensitivity reactions (cholestatic jaundice, skin reactions, and agranulocytosis) are uncommon in pain patients. Pain patients are at no greater risk from the cardiovascular side effects of HCAs than are non-pain patients. However, caution should be used when HCAs are combined with narcotic analgesics (especially methadone). The combination can produce significant orthostatic hypotension. It should also be noted that methadone has a particularly long half-life as compared to other narcotics; and when it is combined with the long activity effects of HCAs, the duration of toxic reactions can last up to several days.

Heterocyclic antidepressants potentiate the sedating properties of alcohol, anxiolytics, and narcotics. Nonsteroidal anti-inflammatory drugs can also be sedating, and this effect intensified when combined with antidepressants. Little is known about the long-term use of HCAs, but no reports of adverse effects with long-term maintenance therapy have been received. Unfortunately, HCAs often produce significant weight gain. In some patients the therapeutic effects of the drug occur at the dose producing the weight gain. A trial of HCAs associated with little or no weight gain is warranted (trazodone).

Monoamine Oxidase Inhibitors

Choice of Drug. The monoamine oxidase inhibitor most commonly used in chronic pain states is phenelzine.

Dose of Drug. Phenelzine is usually started at 15 mg per day and increased by 15 mg every two to three days. The drug is given in equally divided doses during the day. Phenelzine has been known to produce insomnia when given close to bedtime. The drug is increased initially to a total dose of 45 mg per day. If there is no response within the first week, then the drug should be cautiously increased to 60–75 mg per day. On occasion, the patient may develop significant side effects after the first week at therapeutic levels of the MAOIs. If this occurs, a decrease in phenelzine by 15 mg each day until the reaction subsides is warranted. The drug is then gradually increased by 15 mg every two to three days to the desired therapeutic level. Raft and colleagues (17) found that phenelzine was effective in relieving pain as a symptom of depression when platelet MAO inhibition was 80 percent. This may be a useful marker for the therapeutic level.

Preadministration Evaluation. Education of the patient concerning the tyramine-free diet and avoidance of certain medications (meperidine, sympathomimetic amines, HCAs) should be done. Laboratory evaluation for MAOIs should be similar to that for HCAs.

Maintenance. There are no data as to the maintenance level of MAOIs, including pain states. Clinical experience suggests that the maintenance level is the same as the initial dose.

Side Effects. The most common side effects seen in chronic pain patients using MAOIs include dizziness, nausea, drowsiness, and weight gain. The most serious side effect is the hypertensive crisis that occurs with the combination of an MAOI and certain food and drugs. The hypertensive crisis is treated with intravenous injection of 2–5 mg of phentolamine. If phentolamine is not available, chlorpromazine 50–100 mg intramuscularly can be used. The combination of an MAOI and meperidine can cause a hyperpyrexic reaction (78).

MONOAMINE PRECURSORS

The importance of monoamine neurotransmitters in the central nervous system regulating nociceptive control has been described in the preceding section. Alterations in monoamine metabolism may also account for depressive illness in some patients (79, 80). Depression may, therefore, be associated with a relative lack of monoamine neurotransmitters. A similar explanation of altered monoamine function has been postulated for the development of chronic pain as noted in the preceding section. A serotonergic deficiency has been implicated in the pathogenesis of depression (80) and chronic pain (61).

Mechanism of Action

A review of the literature reveals that tryptophan has no therapeutic effect on unipolar or bipolar depressed patients (81). However, tryptophan may potentiate the action of heterocyclic antidepressants, and tryptophan's usefulness in mildly depressed unipolar outpatients is unknown. It appears that depression is a biochemically heterogeneous disease (82). Therefore, a subgroup of depressed patients may readily respond to tryptophan treatment. Tryptophan, by its antidepressant activity, may be as effective in chronic pain states through their therapeutic effects on depressive illness. Further work in classifying depression and chronic pain biochemically with respect to deficiency in biogenic amines and therapeutic response to drugs altering specific biogenic amines needs to be done.

Tryptophan (2 grams per day) compared to placebo in a double blind study produces an elevation in the pain tolerance threshold level, but without increasing the perceptual pain threshold level in humans (83). This effect was also demonstrated in patients with chronic facial pain (84). Tryptophan (3 grams per day) compared to placebo significantly decreased facial pain and increased the pain tolerance threshold in 30 patients in a double blind study. There was no effect on changes in anxiety and depression between the placebo and the tryptophan groups. From these studies it appears that tryptophan may have antinociceptive activity by elevating the pain tolerance threshold.

It has been postulated that tryptophan may have anti-inflammatory activity similar in effect to the anti-inflammatory drugs. Anti-inflammatory drugs displace bound tryptophan from plasma proteins and increase free tryptophan in plasma (85, 86). This effect has also been observed in pregnancy (85), and rheumatic conditions often improved during pregnancy (87). In animal models, L-tryptophan decreases the inflammatory response to clinically induced inflammation, similar to the effects of anti-inflammatory drugs (88, 89). It is postulated that anti-inflammatory drugs act by displacing tryptophan and other peptides from binding sites on serum protein. The free peptides protect the connective tissue from effects of inflammation (85). In addition, it has been observed that nonsteroidal anti-inflammatory drugs possess some antidepressant effect (86, 90). Broadhurst (86) reported that some patients with rheumatoid disease show a decrease in symptoms and a fall in erythrocyte sedimentation rate when treated with L-tryptophan. These observations await further testing in a large sample of patients suffering from rheumatoid disease using a controlled study. It is interesting to speculate on whether these chronic pain states associated with an inflammatory process would respond therapeutically to tryptophan. In summary, the mechanism of action of L-tryptophan in chronic pain syndromes may be due to: 1) antidepressant activity, 2) direct analgesic activity, and 3) anti-inflammatory effects in some chronic pain syndromes.

Review of Studies

Tryptophan, 2–4 grams daily, was as effective as methysergide in 16 patients with migraine headaches in a noncontrolled study (91). Kangassiemi and colleagues (92), in a double blind study, compared the effects of tryptophan (2 grams daily) to levoleucine in eight migraine headache patients. Four of eight patients report a significant decrease in the frequency and severity of their headaches. Migraine headache patients have a low free plasma tryptophan level as compared to normals. It was noted that tryptophan treatment produced a rise in cerebrospinal fluid tryptophan, free plasma tryptophan, and total plasma tryptophan.

Hosobuchi (93) has described the reversal of opiate tolerance in chronic pain patients who developed tolerance to opioid drugs after long-term use. The dose of L-tryptophan was 4 grams daily for two to nine weeks. Electrical stimulation of the periaqueductal and periventricular grey matter results in a reduction of severe intractable pain. However, in some patients receiving central grey stimulation, tolerance to the antinociceptive effects develop. Hosobuchi (94) reported a reversal of this tolerance in five patients using 3 grams of L-tryptophan daily. King (95) reported the effects of L-tryptophan in chronic pain patients who had undergone dorsal rhizotomy and cordotomy. In five patients, a regression of sensory deficit and recurrence of pain developed after the surgical procedure. Treatment with L-tryptophan (2 grams daily) for one month caused a decrease in pain and expansion of the sensory deficit originally produced by the rhizotomy or cordotomy. The authors believed this effect was due to neuropharmacological manipulation of monoamine neurotransmitter systems. DeBenedittis and colleagues (96), in a pilot study, used 5-hydroxytryptophan (5-HTP) in patients having central deafferentation pain syndromes. In addition, they assayed plasma and cerebrospinal fluid (CSF), 5-hydroxyindoleacetic acid (5-HIAA), beta-endorphins, and plasma serotonin (5-HT) pre- and postdrug treatment with 300–800 mg per 5-HTP. They reported significant diminution of pain complaints in all seven patients. There was a significant increase in plasma 5-HT and CSF 5-HIAA comparing pre- and posttreatment levels with drug treatment. Interestingly, there was no change in beta-endorphins measured in plasma and CSF. As noted earlier, Sternbach and colleagues (61) treated five chronic low back pain patients with 5-hydroxytryptophan (1.5–3.0 grams daily) and two patients with similar pain conditions using L-tryptophan (7–10 grams daily). They found no significant difference in reduction of pain when compared to a placebo treatment period.

Treatment

Choice of Drug. Precusor treatment can occur with the use of either L-tryptophan or 5-hydroxytryptophan (5-HTP), the intermediate metabolite of L-tryptophan. 5-HTP is rapidly decarboxylated in the brain to form serotonin (5-HT) using moderate doses (10–20 mg/kg) (97). L-tryptophan is used for the treatment of insomnia at doses ranging from 1 to 5 grams at bedtime. Recent studies (98, 99) report that L-tryptophan works best for patients with mild sleep disturbance and less well for patients with chronic insomnia. Sleep disturbance often occurs in patients with chronic pain with or without the occurrence of depression. L-tryptophan can be effective in symptomatically treating the insomnia that occurs in chronic pain patients.

Dose. In the few clinical studies using L-tryptophan in chronic pain patients, the daily oral dose ranges from 2–4 grams. The dose range of L-tryptophan used in the treatment of depression varies from 2–18 grams daily (81). Doses of L-tryptophan above 7 grams do not appear to increase the formation of serotonin to any significant extent (100). It appears that doses up to 7 grams daily do not lead to enzyme induction (100). The dose of 5-HTP to treat depression is 200 mg daily (101).

Preadministration Evaluation. Tryptophan can be safely used in most patients. The metabolism of L-tryptophan occurs in the liver (98 percent) (100). Patients with severe liver dysfunction may need close monitoring of drug effects.

Maintenance. Tryptophan has been administered to patients over an extended period of time without adverse effects. Chronic administration of L-tryptophan may lead to depletion of vitamin B_6 since the metabolism of L-tryptophan is B_6-dependent (100). It is advisable to give L-tryptophan with pyridoxine to minimize the accumulation of L-tryptophan metabolite side effects. Nausea, vomiting, and diarrhea are the most common side effects reported with the use of L-tryptophan. Some patients also report a euphoria, itching, and urinary changes.

NEUROLEPTICS

Neuroleptics possess a variety of peripheral and central nervous system effects. Their actions on the adrenergic and dopaminergic system have led investigators to suspect neuroleptics of potentiating analgesic drugs and/or possessing analgesic properties of their own. Courvoisier and colleagues (102) were the first to demonstrate chlorpromazine-enhancing analgesic drugs.

Mechanism of Action

Lasagna and DeKornfeld (103) showed methotrimeprazine (15 mg) to be equally as effective as 10 mg of morphine in the control of postoperative pain. Montilla and colleagues (104) confirmed this finding with a similar dose-response relationship between methotrimeprazine and morphine in postherpetic pain and pain from fractures, herpes zoster, and pleurisy. They noted, however, that methotrimeprazine produced greater sedation than morphine at the same analgesic level which was attained by each drug. Bloomfield and colleagues (105) found similar results in various chronic pain states. Moore and Dundee (106), using an experimental pain model (acute pain), found some phenothiazines having mild analgesic properties but not others. They postulated the analgesic action of the neuroleptic drugs was secondary to the adrenolytic action of these drugs. Neuroleptic drugs potentiate agents producing general anesthesia and, when injected locally, have local analgesic action on peripheral nerves (70).

Maltbie and colleagues (107–109) theorized that haloperidol may have analgesic activity for several reasons: isometric similarity of haloperidol to meperidine, analgesic effects of haloperidol in cancer pain, and effectiveness in the withdrawal of narcotic drugs. They further suggested that the dopamine blockade and direct opiate receptor antagonist action of haloperidol may explain the analgesic effects of the drug.

Review of Clinical Studies

The following review of clinical studies will include the use of neuroleptic agents used alone or in combination with an antidepressant in various chronic pain states (headaches, thalamic pain syndrome, facial pain, postherpetic neuralgia, diabetic neuropathy, and pain as a symptom in psychotic illness) (Tables 12 and 13). In addition, there will be a brief discussion of neuroleptics used as analgesic potentiators.

Headaches. Polliack (110) reported the successful treatment of seven chronic headache patients with the use of trifluoperazine 1 mg and diclophenac sodium. Hakkarainen (111) studied 50 patients with chronic tension headaches in a double blind crossover study comparing fluphenazine 1 mg daily with a placebo. The duration of the headaches decreased and the severity of the pain was reduced significantly with fluphenazine treatment as compared to the placebo. Thirty-six out of the 50 patients considered fluphenazine superior to the placebo in relieving

Table 12. Neuroleptics in Chronic Pain Syndromes

Clinical Syndrome and Author	Controlled Study	N	Type of Drug	Dose (mg/day)	Efficacy of Pain Relief (%)*
Headaches					
Polliack (110)	yes	50	fluphenazine	1	70
Hakkarainen (111)	no	7	trifluoperazine	1	100
Thalamic syndrome					
Margolis (112)	no	1	chlorpromazine	400	100
Facial pain					
Raft (113)	no	12	haloperidol	2–6	65–85
Postherpetic neuralgia					
Faber (114)	no	30	chlorprothixene	200	96
Nathan (115)	no	30	chlorprothixene	100	43
Taub (52)	no	17	fluphenazine + amitriptyline	3 75	82
Weis (55)	no	9	perphenazine + amitriptyline	6 75	89

* = percentage of patients reporting pain relief

their headaches. Two of the 50 patients discontinued the fluphenazine because of extrapyramidal side effects.

Thalamic Pain Syndrome. Margolis and Gianascol (112) found chlorpromazine 400 mg daily to be effective in reducing the pain associated with thalamic pain syndrome. This was in contrast to earlier reports showing no effect from chlorpromazine on thalamic pain syndrome in dose ranges from 50 to 150 mg daily. Miley and colleagues (119) used apomorphine, a dopamine receptor agonist, to treat two patients with thalamic pain syndrome. One patient had a 40 percent reduction of pain with oral apomorphine (5 mg/kg) daily for 10 days. The effects were not reversed with 0.2 mg intravenous naloxone. With this meager amount of clinical data and somewhat conflicting pharmacological approaches to the management of thalamic pain syndrome with neuroleptic agents, treatment is on a trial-and-error basis.

Facial Pain. Raft and colleagues (113) treated 18 patients with chronic facial pain (10 with myofascial pain syndrome, 6 with neuropathic pain, and 2 with atypical facial pain) using haloperidol (2–6 mg daily) plus behavior modification. Four patients discontinued the treatment. Two were lost to follow-up. The remaining 12 patients reported 65–85 percent improvement. All of the patients had previously failed at behavioral modification, hypnosis, and biofeedback. It appeared that the addition of haloperidol was a significant factor in promoting pain relief.

Postherpetic Neuralgia. Farber and Burks (114) reported on 30 patients with moderate to severe postherpetic neuralgia who were treated successfully with chlorprothixene 200 mg daily for 4 to 10 days. Twenty-nine out of 30 patients (96 percent) had a positive response. Eleven patients experienced pain relief within 24 hours of drug treatment, and 27 patients experienced pain relief within 72 hours. Nathan (115) used chlorprothixene 100 mg daily and found only one-third of patients with postherpetic neuralgia responding to treatment. The author observed

Table 13. Neuroleptics in Chronic Pain Syndromes

Clinical Syndrome and Author	Controlled Study	N	Type of Drug	Dose (mg/day)	Efficacy of Pain Relief (%)*
Diabetic neuropathy					
Davis (56)	no	8	fluphenazine + amitriptyline	3 75	100
Gade (116)	no	1	fluphenazine	5	100
Pain as a symptom of psychotic disorder					
Schubert (117)	no	1	chlorpromazine	400	100
Mixed etiologies					
Merskey (62)	no	30	neuroleptic + antidepressant		93
Kocher (63)	no	103	neuroleptic + antidepressant		92
Duthie (67)	no	12	trifluoperazine + amitriptyline	3 75	66
Daw (118)	no	1	haloperidol	50	100

* = percentage of patients reporting pain relief

frequent side effects (mostly sedation) with the use of chlorprothixene and was not able to use the 200 mg dose used by Farber and Burks. Weis and colleagues (55) used a fixed dose of amitriptyline 75 mg and perphenazine 6 mg daily in nine patients with postherpetic neuralgia and found the combination effective in 89 percent of cases. Similarly, Taub (52) using amitriptyline 75 mg and fluphenazine 3 mg daily in 17 consecutive cases of postherpetic neuralgia, reported 82 percent effectiveness in pain relief.

Due to the lack of controlled studies, there is no indication that the combination of an antidepressant and neuroleptic is superior to either the antidepressant or neuroleptic alone. While chlorprothixene may be effective, the high incidence of side effects limits its usefulness.

Painful Diabetic Neuropathy. As described earlier in the section on antidepressants, Davis and colleagues (56) used fluphenazine 3 mg and amitriptyline 75 mg daily in eight patients with painful diabetic neuropathy. All patients reported pain relief with this combination. Gade (116) described a case of diabetic neuropathic cachexia with severely painful neuropathy. A combination of amitriptyline 25 mg and fluphenazine 5 mg daily produced effective pain relief and improvement in mental status. There is a lack of controlled studies to evaluate the therapeutic role of neuroleptics in painful diabetic neuropathy.

Mixed Etiologies. Merskey and Hester (62) used a combination of antidepressants and neuroleptic drugs in the treatment of 30 patients with chronic pain from organic lesions. Pain relief occurred in 28 out of 30 patients. Kocher (63), using a similar combination, reported on the successful treatment of 82 out of 103 patients with persistent neuropathic and musculoskeletal pain. Duthie (67) used a fixed dose of trifluoperazine 3 mg and amitriptyline 75 mg daily to treat 12 patients with chronic pain from organic lesions. Eight out of 12 patients had a positive response. The authors reported that there was little effect in the patients' mood with successful treatment. Daw and Cohen-Cole (118) used haloperidol 50 mg per day to successfully treat a patient with chronic pain secondary to radiation neuropathy. As described earlier, Langohr (71) demonstrated that the combination of clomipramine and a neuroleptic was significantly more effective than a neuroleptic alone in the treatment of chronic pain from mono- and polyneuropathies. This was not a controlled study and the dose and type of neuroleptic was not controlled.

Pain as a Symptom of a Psychotic Disorder. Schubert (117) reported the successful treatment of a patient, who had various nondelusional pain complaints that were associated with a psychotic break, using chlorpromazine 400 mg daily. As the patient's thinking became less disorganized, he had fewer complaints of acute pain.

Potentiation of Opioid Analgesics. As mentioned earlier, several authors (103, 104) showed methotrimeprazine 15 mg to be equianalgesic to morphine 15 mg in acute pain. However, the increased tolerance to pain may be secondary to the sedating properties of the phenothiazine tested (104). Keats (120) found no analgesic activity or potentiating of meperidine analgesia with promethazine. Houde (121) compared single dose morphine, chlorpromazine, placebo, and a combination of morphine and chlorpromazine. He found no analgesic effect or enhancement of morphine with chlorpromazine. McGee and Alexander (122) reviewed controlled studies using phenothiazines as an analgesic or potentiator of analgesics. They found promethazine, promazine, and propiomazine possessing no analgesic or potentiating properties, with the exception of methotrimeprazine. It has no addictive properties and can cause less respiratory depression than meperidine. In patients with narcotic hypersensitivity or compromised pulmonary function, methotrimeprazine may be useful. Limiting its usefulness is its potential for causing sedation and hypotension.

In summary, there is only one controlled study evaluating the effectiveness of phenothiazines in chronic pain (Table 14). It is interesting to note in a review of the literature that there are fewer case studies reporting on phenothiazines in chronic pain syndromes than there are case studies reporting on antidepressants. The combination of a phenothiazine and an antidepressant has been extensively used in clinical practice

Table 14. Summary of Neuroleptics Efficacy in Chronic Pain Syndromes

Clinical Syndrome	Uncontrolled Studies		Controlled Studies	
	No Effect	Effect*	No Effect	Effect
Headache		1		1
Thalamic pain	1	1		
Facial pain		1		
Postherpetic neuralgia		4		
Diabetic neuropathy		2		
Pain as a symptom of psychiatric disorder		1		
Mixed etiologies		4		

* = greater than 50%

for the treatment of chronic pain (123). However, this practice is based only on case studies or clinical experience. No controlled studies to date have been performed to evaluate whether the phenothiazine alone or a combination of a phenothiazine and an antidepressant is more effective. The effectiveness of neuroleptics as an analgesic or as a potentiator of analgesic drugs has not been confirmed by controlled studies, with the exception of methotrimeprazine. There are interesting case reports on the use of haloperidol in cancer pain, and narcotic potentiation, but there are no controlled studies to confirm this observation.

Treatment

Choice of Drug. With the lack of controlled studies, there are no specific guidelines for the choice of neuroleptics in chronic pain. The choice of drugs mainly depends upon the side effect profile of the drug. For patients with insomnia or restlessness, chlorpromazine or thioridazine may be useful. For patients requiring a daytime schedule for drug administration, or sedating drugs not indicated, haloperidol, fluphenazine, perphenazine, or trifluoperazine may be useful. Methotrimeprazine may be useful in acute pain states in which the effects of sedation and hypotension can be safely monitored and managed. The usefulness of this agent in chronic pain states is unknown. Neuroleptics do not produce addiction or physical dependency.

Dose of Drug. From a review of the case studies, the dose range of the piperazine phenothiazines (fluphenazine, perphenazine, and trifluperazine) was between 1 and 6 mg per day. The dose range is below the maintenance antipsychotic dose for these drugs. Chlorpromazine (aliphatics, phenothiazines) is reported to be effective in the 400 mg dose range. This dose is in the antipsychotic maintenance dose range for phenothiazine. The dose reported for haloperidol varies from 2 to 50 mg daily. Methotrimeprazine 10 to 20 mg intramuscularly is equal in analgesic potency to 10 mg intramuscularly of morphine. Methotrimeprazine can be given orally at a maintenance dose level of 20 to 30 mg per day. A majority of the daily dose can be given one to two hours before bedtime to take advantage of the drug's sedating properties.

Preadministration Evaluation. In addition to the routine check of physical health and physical examination, signs of parkinsonism, movement disorders, and liver disease should be assessed. Laboratory studies should include liver test, urinalysis, complete blood count, and, in older patients, an electrocardiogram.

Maintenance. With the lack of proven clinical efficacy in chronic pain states and potential risk for tardive dyskinesia, neuroleptics have questionable value for long-term use in chronic pain states (124).

Side Effects. Neuroleptics produce a variety of side effects. Sedation is common with chlorpromazine and less common with piperazine phenothiazines and haloperidol. Tolerance to the sedating effects may occur with continual use. Extrapyramidal reactions (pseudo-parkinsonism, akathesia, dystonia, and dyskinesia) are less common with chlorpromazine but increase with the use of piperazine phenothiazines and haloperidol. All neuroleptics lower the seizure threshold. Chlorpromazine and thioridazine have hypotensive effects, whereas haloperidol and piperazine phenothiazines have less effect on blood pressure. It should be noted that neuroleptics have anticholinergic activity and potentiate the anticholinergic effects of atropine-like drugs. Significant weight gain can occur with the use of neuroleptics, which is an undesirable side effect in most chronic pain states of musculoskeletal origin. Neuroleptics inhibit the metabolism of heterocyclic antidepressants. Abrupt discontinuation of the neuroleptic may produce insomnia and muscle discomfort.

MINOR TRANQUILIZERS

Benzodiazepines are given to chronic pain patients to decrease anxiety, insomnia, and muscle tension. These agents are also frequently given in acute pain states, especially after minor surgery, after injury to musculoskeletal systems in order to decrease muscle spasm or strain, and so on. These drugs are commonly given preoperatively or preprocedure to decrease the anticipatory anxiety and discomfort in patients.

Mechanism of Action

Benzodiazepines cause a release of gamma-amino-butyric acid (GABA) and inhibit the presynaptic release of serotonin and, to some degree, norepinephrine (125, 126). Mantegazza and colleagues (127) showed that muscinal, a potential GABA receptor agonist, antagonizes both morphine and beta-endorphin analgesia, and that various inhibitors of GABA uptake decrease the analgesic effects of morphine. They concluded, in an animal pain model, that activation of the brain GABA receptors reduces morphine analgesia. If the serotonergic hypothesis of chronic pain is valid, then the use of benzodiazepines is not justified. Recently, alprazolam has been introduced as a benzodiazepine that is a GABA agonist, but that also reverses the norepinephrine suppression by reserpine. There is also evidence the drug may have some use as an antidepressant.

Chapman and Feather (128) studied the effects of oral diazepam (10 mg) on an experimental pain paradigm in humans. They reported that diazepam is effective in reducing the emotional reactivity to pain but does not alter the sensory-discriminative aspects of pain. Diazepam decreases the transitional anxiety associated with pain. Control of anxiety and reactivity to the pain increases the patient's ability to tolerate pain without affecting this pain sensation.

Gracely and colleagues (129), using an experimental pain model of electrical stimulation, demonstrated that diazepam significantly lowers the affective response to pain stimulus, but not the sensory descriptors of the pain. In acute pain states, benzodiazepines appear to increase a patient's ability to endure painful episodes by decreasing the reactivity to the pain without modifying the pain threshold.

Review of Clinical Studies

There are a few clinical studies evaluating the effectiveness of benzodiazepines in chronic pain syndromes. Lasagna suggested the short-term use of benzodiazepines for gastrointestinal disorders associated with anxiety and acute muscle spasms caused by intervertebral disc disease (130). Turkington (10) compared diazepam with amitriptyline and imipramine in a double blind controlled study in 59 patients with painful diabetic neuropathy. The antidepressants were superior to the benzodiazepines. Lance and Curren (21), in a study of 280 patients with chronic tension headaches, found amitriptyline 30 to 75 mg daily and imipramine 30 to 75 mg daily superior to diazepam 15 mg daily and chlordiazepoxide 30 mg daily. Okashi and colleagues (15) found doxepin 50 mg and amitriptyline 50 mg superior to diazepam 10 mg daily in the treatment of psychogenic pain. Singh and colleagues (18) compared the effects of imipramine (75–100 mg daily), imipramine (50–150 mg daily), and chlordiazepoxide (30–150 mg daily) in patients presenting to a psychiatric clinic with pain complaints. Sixteen of the 20 patients responded to the antidepressants and 2 of the 20 responded to the chlordiazepoxide. Patients treated with antidepressants as compared to minor tranquilizers had significantly greater improvement in nervousness, anxiety, palpitation, insomnia, and fatigue. From these studies, it appears that antidepressants provide greater therapeutic benefit to the chronic pain patient than minor tranquilizers. In addition, antidepressants do not cause addiction, whereas long-term use of benzodiazepines are associated with dependency and withdrawal syndromes on abrupt discontinuation of the drug. In the elderly patient cognitive impairment may occur, especially with long-acting benzodiazepines. Hendler and colleagues (131) found significantly greater cognitive impairment in nonelderly chronic pain patients taking benzodiazepines than in those taking narcotics alone. With the occurrence of cognitive impairment, addiction, and questionable therapeutic value, the use of benzodiazepines in chronic pain should be limited.

Treatment

The doses, initial and maintenance, are similar to those usually recommended for anxiety. Mild tranquilizers are sedating and potentiate the sedating effects of alcohol and other CNS depressants. Minor tranquilizers have little or no autonomic side effects. Tolerance to the therapeutic effects may occur in three to four weeks of continuous use. The potential for drug abuse and addiction occurs with minor tranquilizers. Withdrawal symptoms similar to those seen with sedative hypnotics may occur with the abrupt discontinuation of minor tranquilizers.

LITHIUM

The effectiveness of lithium in bipolar illness is well documented. It is also thought to be effective in acute depression, chronic alcoholism, aggressive behavior, hyperthyroidism, and neutropenia (132). Ekbom (133, 134) was the first to use lithium in cluster headaches based on the cyclic nature of cluster headaches such as bipolar illness. The initial observation has been confirmed by other authors (135–137).

Mechanism of Action

In addition to the cyclic nature of chronic cluster headaches noted by Ekbom (134), Graham (138) observed that the behavior of patients with cluster headaches may consist of running, screaming, pacing, head banging, and other bizarre actions that may resemble patients in a manic episode. The similarity of clinical manifestations of chronic cluster headaches to bipolar illness may suggest a common psychopathological dysfunction responsive to lithium. Kudrow (139) suggested that lithium may act centrally to decrease excessive autonomic activity associated with chronic cluster headaches. Lithium's action on the central nervous system is complex and an explanation for its therapeutic role in bipolar illness and other conditions (cluster headaches) is unknown. Lithium carbonate (135, 140) has been shown to have mild analgesic properties in humans, but use in chronic pain states is limited to cluster headaches.

Review of Clinical Studies

Cluster Headaches. Kudrow (139) studied the effects of lithium in 32 patients with cluster headaches. Four patients discontinued treatment secondary to side effects. Of the 28 remaining patients, 27 had marked improvement (96 percent) and beneficial effects were maintained at follow-up at eight months. The serum lithium was maintained between 0.5 to 1.2 meq/l. Twenty-five percent of the patients had mild side effects. The improvement with lithium occurred within the first week of treatment. Lithium did not prevent the precipitation of alcohol-induced cluster headaches. Mathew (141) reported on the effects of lithium in 31 patients with chronic cluster headaches. Eighty percent of patients showed improvement with the serum level between 0.5 to 1.2 meq/l. Improvement was maintained at six-month follow-up and no evidence of tolerance was seen. Fifty-five percent of patients had mild side effects including tremor, nausea, diarrhea, and lethargy. One patient had to discontinue treatment secondary to side effects.

Other Chronic Pain States

As previously mentioned, Tyber (8) used amitriptyline 75 mg daily and therapeutic doses of lithium that resulted in relief of pain in patients with the painful shoulder syndrome. The evidence for the effectiveness of lithium in cluster headaches is quite interesting even though there are no controlled studies to date. The authors (139, 141) report beneficial effects of lithium in chronic sufferers of cluster headaches who had previously failed multiple medical treatment. Lopez-Ibor and Lopez-Ibor (142) found lithium salts to be effective in two patients with recurrent psychological symptoms (recurrent depression and mania) plus pain symptoms related to arthritis, paresthesia, and headache.

Treatment

Choice of Drug. Lithium carbonate was the preparation of lithium used in the above-mentioned studies.

Dose of Drug. In the studies of cluster headaches and painful shoulder syndrome, the oral dose of lithium was adjusted to achieve a serum lithium level between 0.5 and 1.2 meq/l. Kudrow (139) observed greater improvement in the treatment of patients with cluster headaches as the serum lithium level progressed from subtherapeutic ranges (less than 0.5 meq/l to 0.8 meq/l). The same mean dose of oral lithium was between 700 and 900 mg per day. Treatment is initiated with lithium carbonate 300 mg twice a day. After two to three days, the lithium level is checked. If the level is out of therapeutic range, increasing the lithium by 300 mg every two to three days is recommended. Increase the lithium dose until after the serum lithium level is obtained. Increasing lithium to achieve serum levels of 0.8 to 0.9 meq/l is desirable, and side effects should be observed over a period of one to two weeks. If side effects develop, decreasing lithium by 300 mg and observing for changes in therapeutic effects and side effects is warranted. Each 300 mg dose of lithium raises the serum level by approximately 0.25 meq/l. The serum lithium level is obtained 12 hours after the last dose of lithium (A.M. sample before the first dose of lithium).

Preadministration Evaluation. Patients should be screened for goiter, kidney disease, cardiovascular disease, brain damage, diuretic use, diarrhea, excessive sweating, and low salt diets. Laboratory tests include blood chemistries with creatinine, urinalysis, electrocardiogram, and thyroid panel.

Maintenance. It appears that there is no development of tolerance to the therapeutic effectiveness of lithium in cluster headaches. Maintenance lithium level is between 0.5 and 1.0 meq/l. The determinations of serum lithium should be done once a week until a stable lithium dose is achieved. After stabilizing the lithium level, serum lithium levels should be performed every two to three months. There should be six-month checks on thyroid panel, blood chemistry with blood urea nitrogen (BUN), and creatinine.

Side Effects. The most common side effects of lithium in patients with cluster headaches include tremor, gastrointestinal upset, and lethargy. The tremor is not affected by any parkinsonian drug but does respond to propranolol 10 mg four times per day. The side effects can occasionally be controlled by decreasing the dose of lithium. In addition, lithium may produce polydypsia, polyuria, weight gain, extrapyramidal reactions, granulocytosis, and dermatological changes.

ANTICONVULSANTS

Anticonvulsants have been reported to be effective in chronic pain states for 40 years. Bergouignon (143) was the first to report the successful use of diphenylhydantoin (DPH) in the treatment of three patients with neuralgia. Twenty years later, Blom (144) reported on the efficacy of carbamazepine in patients with trigeminal neuralgia. Carbamazepine is now the treatment of choice for trigeminal neuralgia. The effectiveness of diphenylhydantoin (20 percent) is much lower than the reported effectiveness of carbamazepine (at least 70 percent) (145, 146). Recently clonazepam has been reported to be effective in cranial neuralgias (147). There is strong clinical evidence that anticonvulsants are effective in specific chronic pain states. The following discussion will address the use of certain anticonvulsants in specific pain states.

Mechanism of Action

The use of anticonvulsants in chronic pain is limited to neurogenic pain in which pain is produced by a dysfunction of the nervous system. Since the drugs are effective anticonvulsants, the pathophysiology of neurogenic pain and epilepsy may be similar. Loeser and Ward (148) proposed that seizure-like activities result when there is a loss of incoming sensory messages (deafferentation pain syndromes). This hypothesis is based on the evidence showing deafferentation producing hyperactivity in the postsynaptic parts of the central nervous system. This hyperactivity of deafferentation and epilepsy share similar pathophysiological mechanisms, and it follows that anticonvulsant drugs should be effective.

Lesions in the nervous system that interfere with the normal sensory inputs result in a state of increased excitability in pain-transmitting neurons (149). Diphenylhydantoin has a direct "stabilizing" effect on nerve membranes by decreasing the inward sodium movement during the action potential (150, 151) and preventing inward calcium movement during the action potential (151). This produces a decrease in the repetitive firing of neurons. If the pain caused by neurogenic pain disorder is dependent upon neural membrane instability producing abnormal hyperexcitability of pain transmitting cells, then anticonvulsants may act by stabilizing the membrane. This mechanism of action may explain the effectiveness of diphenylhydantoin but carbamazepine only has a similar effect on the neural membrane at high concentrations (152, 153). Therefore, the clinical effectiveness of carbamazepine is not likely to be based upon its stabilizing action on neural membrane. Carbamazepine, within therapeutic doses, produces more pronounced reduction of repetitive discharges than diphenylhydantoin in second-order trigeminal neurons following stimulation of the maxillary nerves (154). This observation is consistent with the clinical effectiveness of carbamazepine as compared to diphenylhydantoin in the treatment of shooting pains of trigeminal neuralgia, as noted above.

Carbamazepine is becoming one of the prime drugs in the treatment of temporal lobe epilepsy. It has been observed that the behavioral and mood disturbances associated with temporal lobe epilepsy improved as the improvement in the seizure disorder occurred with carbamazepine (155). Investigators believed that carbamazepine may have psychotropic activity apart from the anticonvulsant effects (156). Carbamazepine is chemically and pharmacologically similar to the imipramine-type antidepressants. Carbamazepine is noted to have greater temporal lobe and limbic anticonvulsant effects than other anticonvulsant agents.

The temporal lobe-limbic system axis is thought to be involved in the regulation of affect. These rationales led to the use of carbamazepine in the treatment of affective disorders. Carbamazepine blocks the reuptake of norepinephrine in a way similar to the imipramine-type of antidepressants, and also has been shown to block the stimulation-induced release of norepinephrine (156). Carbamazepine also has been shown to potentiate certain opiate-induced behaviors in animal studies (156). These preliminary studies of the activity of carbamazepine point to several mechanisms of action. The effectiveness of carbamazepine in pain states may be due to: 1) psychotropic activity similar to the antidepressant, and 2) anticonvulsant action.

Clonazepam, a benzodiazepine, recently has been used for the treatment of seizure disorders in certain neurogenic pain syndromes. Benzodiazepine stimulates the inhibitory neurotransmitter, gamma-aminobutyric acid (GABA). This pharmacological effect is thought to be responsible for the decreased firing of normal and epileptic neurons in the central nervous system. As noted earlier, benzodiazepines, used as anxiolytic drugs, have not been shown to be effective in chronic pain states. It would appear that therapeutic effectiveness of clonazepam in chronic pain is related more to its anticonvulsant activity than to its anxiolytic properties.

Review of Clinical Studies

Trigeminal Neuralgia. Borgouignon (143, 157) was the first to report the usefulness of diphenylhydantoin (DPH) in facial neuralgia. These earlier reports were followed by case studies (157, 159, 160–163) showing that 56 to 100 percent of patients with trigeminal neuralgia had good to excellent pain relief using DPH (Table 15). The mean daily dose of DPH was 300 mg. Pain relief with DPH occurred within the first 48 hours of drug treatment. Pain relief continued as long as the patients were maintained on the drug (163); but Jensen (159) reported that 20 out of 59 patients were pain free after DPH was discontinued after a successful drug trial. In 37 patients, pain returned after DPH was discontinued.

Initially, Blom (144) reported that carbamazepine was effective in patients with trigeminal neuralgia. The effect was noted within 24 hours of drug treatment, and pain returned within 48 hours after the drug was stopped. Eighty-one percent of the patients were pain free after six months of treatment. Lloyd-Smith and Sachdev (165) found that low dose carbamazepine (100–400 mg daily) was effective in 46 patients with trigeminal neuralgia in long-term follow-up.

In a double blind placebo crossover study, Rockliff and Davis (166) found carbamazepine (400–600 mg per day) significantly more effective than placebo in trigeminal neuralgia. The effectiveness of carbamazepine in trigeminal neuralgia was documented in two controlled studies (167, 168). Taylor and colleagues (169) reported on the long-term (up to 16 years) use of carbamazepine. The drug was effective at pain reduction in 69 percent of cases of trigeminal neuralgia. In long-term follow-up, 19 patients developed resistance to drug effect 2 months to 10 years after treatment. Of the remaining 80 patients, the drug was effective for 49 out of 80 patients for 1 to 4 years, and for 31 out of 80 patients for 5 to 16 years. The range of plasma carbamazepine level was 2.5 to 8.5 μg/ml.

Caccia (147) treated seven patients with trigeminal neuralgia using clonazepam 4 mg daily for one month. Six out of seven patients had good to excellent pain relief. Initially, patients complained of marked

Table 15. Anticonvulstants for Trigeminal Neuralgia

Author of Study	Controlled Study	N	Type of Drug	Dose (mg/day)	Efficacy of Pain Relief (%)*
Iannone (162)	no	5	DPH		100
Jensen (159)	no	59	DPH		96
Crue (161)	no	56	DPH	300	70
Lindblom (163)	no	30	DPH		56
Bergouignon (157)	no	17	DPH	300	94
Lamberts (158)	no	30	DPH	300	96
Braham (160)	no	20	DPH	300	70
Blom (144)	no	40	carbamazepine	0–1400	81
Lloyd–Smith (165)	no	100	carbamazepine	100–800	72
Spillane (164)	no	52	carbamazepine	400–600	82
Tomson (170)	no	6	carbamazepine	400–1600	100
Rockliff (166)	yes	9	carbamazepine	400–600	p
Nicol (167)	yes	44	carbamazepine	400–600	p
Caccia (147)	no	7	clonazepam	4	85
Killiam (168)	yes	30	carbamazepine	400–1000	70
Taylor (169)	no	143	carbamazepine	200–600	69
Smirne (171)	no	14	clonazepam	1.5–6	64

p   = drug is significantly more effective than placebo or other comparison drug
DPH = diphenylhydantoin
*   = percentage of patients reporting pain relief

sedation but this diminished with treatment. Smirne and Scarlato (171) found clonazepam (1.5 to 6 mg daily) to be effective in 9 out of 14 patients (64 percent) with trigeminal neuralgia, and 4 out of 6 patients with other types of cranial neuralgias. Baclofen, which is not an anticonvulsant but facilitates gamma aminobutyric acid transmission, has also been used in chronic pain states. Baclofen has similar action on the trigeminal nucleus to carbamazepine and DPH (172). This suggests that baclofen would be effective in trigeminal neuralgia. Fromm and colleagues (172) evaluated the effects of baclofen in 10 patients with trigeminal neuralgia in a double blind placebo crossover study. Daily doses of 60 to 80 mg were used. Seven of 10 patients reported a significant reduction in the frequency of the pain episodes. There were no serious side effects with treatment. The results indicate that baclofen is a useful drug in the management of trigeminal neuralgia.

Painful Diabetic Neuropathy. Ellenberg (173) studied the effects of DPH in 60 patients with painful diabetic neuropathy. Good to excellent results were achieved in 41 out of 60 patients (68 percent) (Table 16). No adverse effects were noted during treatment. Improvement in pain was noticed within 48 hours of drug treatment and continued improvement occurred over the next four days. If the patient did not have any initial drug response within three days, no improvement was seen with prolonged treatment. Chadda and Mathur (174) demonstrated that DPH was significantly more effective at pain relief in 45 patients with diabetic neuropathy as compared to placebo.

In an open design study, Chakrabarti and Samantaray (175) showed that carbamazepine was effective in 49 out of 50 patients with diabetic neuropathy. Rull and colleagues (176) examined the effects of carbamazepine compared to placebo in a double blind crossover study in 30

Table 16. Anticonvulstants for Diabetic Neuropathy

Author of Study	Controlled Study	N	Type of Drug	Dose (mg/day)	Efficacy of Pain Relief (%)*
Ellenberg (173)	no	60	DPH	300–400	68
Chadda (174)	yes	45	DPH	300	p
Chakrabarti (175)	no	54	carbamazepine	variable	90
Rull (176)	yes	30	carbamazepine	600	p

p = drug is significantly more effective than placebo or other comparison drug
DPH = diphenylhydantoin
* = percentage of patients reporting pain relief

patients with painful diabetic neuropathy. Twenty-eight out of 30 patients had a positive response to 600 mg of carbamazepine daily as compared to placebo. In two patients, carbamazepine had to be discontinued secondary to side effects. Somnolence and dizziness occurred in nearly one-half of the patients, but the side effects diminished after one week of treatment.

Central Pain. Chronic pain due to Wallenberg syndrome (177) and thalamic pain syndrome (178) has been shown to diminish with DPH (Table 17). Gibson and White (179) reported carbamazepine (500–800 mg daily) to be effective in neurogenic pain in paraplegic patients. The lancinating pain seen in these patients is similar to that reported in trigeminal neuralgia.

Migraine Headaches. Various case reports demonstrate the benefit of DPH in treating migraine headaches (180–183). Some authors have stated that electroencephalographic patterns associated with migraine attacks predict a favorable response to DPH (180, 182, 184). However, clinical evidence to support this notion is weak (149).

Other Chronic Painful Conditions. Hallaq and Harris (185) reported the successful use of DPH in patients with postherpetic neuralgia. However, clinical experience does not support the use of DPH in postherpetic neuralgia due to the lack of effect (149). In six patients with postherpetic neuralgia, Killiam and Fromm (168) found carbamazepine more effective than placebo in a double blind study. Raskin and colleagues (186) reported a reduction in the pain syndrome in some patients who undergo lumbar sympathectomy using carbamazepine in 7 out of 9 patients. Ekbom (187, 188) described the successful treatment of lightning pain secondary to tabes dorsalis using carbamazepine 400–800 mg daily. The pain relief occurred within 72 hours of drug treatment. Martin (189) reported on the use of carbamazepine or clonazepam in the relief

Table 17. Anticonvulsants for Central Pain

Author of Study	Controlled Study	N	Type of Drug	Dose (mg/day)	Efficacy of Pain Relief (%)*
Cantor (178)	no	2	DPH	150–?	100
Mladinich (177)	no	1	DPH	300	100
Gibson (179)	no	2	carbamazepine	500–800	100

DPH = diphenylhydantoin
* = percentage of patients reporting pain relief

of lightning pain following laminectomy for lumbar disc disease in 14 patients. Dunsker and Mayfield (190) successfully treated five patients with flashing pain due to various injuries to the spinal cord using 200 to 800 mg daily of carbamazepine.

Hatangdi (191) treated patients with postherpetic neuralgia using carbamazepine (600–800 mg daily) and nortriptyline (50–100 mg daily). The blood level of carbamazepine was maintained between 8 and 12 μg/ml. When patients had to stop drug treatment, the paroxysms of pain quickly returned. In some patients, the medication was discontinued after three to six months of treatment without a return of symptoms. In some patients, drug treatment had to be maintained. Sixty percent of patients complained of side effects during the first two weeks of treatment. Most of the patients with side effects had serum carbamazepine levels over 8 mcg/ml. Gerson and colleagues (192) evaluated the effects of carbamazepine (up to 1000 mg daily) and clomipramine (75 mg daily) in 16 patients with postherpetic neuralgia. All patients received considerable relief of pain in an eight-week trial of drug treatment.

A summary of the clinical studies on the use of diphenylhydantoin shows it has been successfully tried in neuralgia, migraine headaches, phantom limb, diabetes neuralgia, trigeminal neuralgia, and glossopharyngeal neuralgia (193). Recently, it has also been reported to be effective in case studies in thalamic syndrome, postherpetic neuralgia, and postsympathetic neuralgia (194). These findings are based on anecdotal or case reports with one controlled study. Since the first report on the successful use of carbamazepine in the treatment of trigeminal neuralgia (144), others have reported on the effectiveness of carbamazepine and trigeminal neuralgia in both case studies (165, 169, 195) and double blind controlled studies (167, 168, 196). The effectiveness of carbamazepine is achieved with the blood level of carbamazepine in the therapeutic range reported for anticonvulsant activity (167, 197). Clonazepam also appears to be effective in neurogenic pain but these observations are based only on noncontrolled studies, and the extent of the drug's effectiveness is awaiting the outcome of controlled studies. Although based on limited studies, baclofen has been shown to be effective in neurogenic pain syndromes. The lack of controlled studies makes it difficult to assess the effectiveness of anticonvulsants in chronic pain syndromes of neuropathic origin. However, due to the lack of effectiveness of other medical treatments and the severity of these pain disorders, these agents should be tried in neurogenic pain syndromes.

Treatment

Choice of Drug. Carbamazepine is the drug of choice in the treatment of trigeminal neuralgia, with approximately 70 percent of patients having positive therapeutic effects. However, the high incidence of side effects precludes the use of the drug in approximately 20 to 30 percent of patients benefiting from the drug. This makes the overall effectiveness of carbamazepine in patients with trigeminal neuralgia approximately 50 percent (198). If a patient is unable to tolerate or has no response to carbamazepine, then a trial of diphenylhydantoin may be indicated. It must be kept in mind that the response to diphenylhydantoin is limited (positive response in 20 percent of patients). Clonazepam or baclofen may be tried if there is no response or limited response to carbamazepine or diphenylhydantoin.

Dose of Drug. Carbamazepine is started at 100 mg twice daily, then increased by 100 mg every two to three days until side effects develop or a level of 600–800 mg is achieved. After a week of observation and no pain relief or intolerable side effects, the dose may be increased 100–200 mg per day every three to four days until therapeutic effects or side effects appear. The maximum total dose is 1800 mg daily. Doses above this level rarely are beneficial. The usual dose range is between 200–1600 mg per day. The therapeutic serum carbamazepine level is between 8–12 mcg/ml. It should be noted that carbamazepine is a gastric irritant and needs to be taken with food.

Diphenylhydantoin is started at 300 mg per day and blood level is checked in three weeks. The therapeutic blood level is 15–20 mcg/ml. Clonazepam is started at 0.5 mg three times per day, and increased by 0.5 to 1 mg every three to four days until a total dose of 6 mg per day is achieved. Baclofen is initiated at 5 mg three to four times per day and increased by 5 to 10 mg every two to three days until a total daily dose of 60 to 80 mg is achieved. The total daily dose is dependent upon the development of intolerable side effects or desired therapeutic effects.

Preadministration Precaution. In addition to a complete history and physical examination, laboratory studies should include a complete blood count and liver studies. The patient should be advised as to the frequent occurrence of side effects with carbamazepine. If the white blood cell count is below 4,000, it is recommended by some not to give carbamazepine (196).

Maintenance. From the various studies described above, it appears that in some patients carbamazepine can be discontinued after three to six months of treatment whereas with other patients, treatment is maintained. After a maintenance level of the drug is established, complete blood count and liver panel should be done monthly for the first year, then three to four times per year thereafter. The anticonvulsant drugs and baclofen should be tapered to prevent withdrawal symptoms.

Side Effects. At least 25 percent of patients who have a positive response to carbamazepine in terms of pain relief have to discontinue the drug due to intolerable side effects. Side effects include disorientation, gastric irritation, ataxia, nausea, anticholinergic activity, orthostatic hypotension, slurred speech, lethargy, and dizziness. Transitory decrease in white cells can occur within the first several months of treatment. Agranulocytosis and aplastic anemia may also develop during any phase of treatment (196). Bone marrow suppression, while it does occur with carbamazepine therapy, does not appear to the extent of withholding the medication in patients suffering from trigeminal neuralgia or other "shooting" pain disorders (196). Side effects due to clonazepam include sedation, but tolerance does develop with continual use. Baclofen may produce drowsiness, nausea, and vomiting. Abnormal liver functions have been reported with long-term treatment using carbamazepine.

SUMMARY

Psychotropic drugs and anticonvulsants are widely used in the treatment of chronic pain syndromes. We have reviewed the rationale, various clinical studies (both controlled and uncontrolled studies), indications, and utility of these drugs in the management of chronic pain. We have also provided a guide for the use of these drugs.

REFERENCES

1. Saunders C: The treatment of intractable pain in terminal cancer. Proceedings of the Royal Society of Medicine 56:295–297, 1963
2. Paoli F, Darcourt G, Cossa P: Note preliminaire sur l'action de l'imipramine don les etats douloureaux. Rev Neurol (Paris) 102:503–504, 1960
3. Bourel M, Sabourand O, Gouffault I, et al: Results obtained with Tofranil in the treatment of certain painful states. L'Ovest Medical 15:99, 1962
4. Butler S: Antidepressants in chronic pain therapy, in Advances in Pain Research and Therapy, vol. 7. Edited by Benedetti C, Chapman CR, Moricca G. New York, Raven Press, 1984
5. France RD, Houpt JL, Ellinwood EH: Therapeutic effects of antidepressants in chronic pain. Gen Hosp Psychiatriy 6:55–63, 1984
6. Walsh TD: Antidepressants in chronic pain. Clin Neuropharmacol 6:271–295, 1983
7. Woodforde JM, Dwyer B, McEwen BW, et al: Treatment of postherpetic neuralgia. Med J Aust 2:869–872, 1965
8. Tyber MA: Treatment of the painful shoulder syndrome with amitriptyline and lithium carbonate. Can Med Assoc J 111:137–140, 1974
9. MacNeil AL, Dick WC: Imipramine and rheumatoid factor. J Int Med Res 4:23–27, 1976
10. Turkington RW: Depression masquerading as diabetic neuropathy. JAMA 243:1147–1150, 1980
11. Lascelles RG: Atypical facial pain and depression. Br J Psychiatry 112:651–659, 1966

12. Sherwin D: New method for treating "headaches." Am J Psychiatry 136:1181–1183, 1979
13. Hameroff SR, Cork RC, Scherer K, et al: Doxepin effects on chronic pain, depression and plasma opioids. J Clin Psychiatry 43:22–26, 1982
14. Ward GN, Bloom VL, Friedel RO: The effectiveness of tricyclic antidepressants in the treatment of coexisting pain and depression. Pain 7:331–341, 1979
15. Okasha A, Ghaleb HA, Sadek A: A double-blind trial for the clinical management of psychogenic headache. Br J Psychiatry 122:181–182, 1973
16. Bradley JJ: Severe localized pain associated with the depressive syndrome. Br J Psychiatry 109:741–745, 1963
17. Raft D, Davidson J, Wasik J, et al: Relationship between response to phenelzine and MAO inhibition in a clinical trial of phenelzine, amitriptyline and placebo. Neuropsychobiology 7:122–126, 1981
18. Singh G, Verma HC: Drug treatment of chronic intractable pain in patients referred to psychiatry clinic. Journal of the Indian Medical Association 56:341–345, 1971
19. Baldessarini RJ: Biomedical Aspects of Depression. Washington, DC, American Psychiatric Press, Inc, 1983
20. Watson CP, Evans RJ, Reed K, et al: Amitriptyline versus placebo in postherpetic neuralgia. Neurology 32:671–673, 1982
21. Lance JW, Curran DA: Treatment of chronic tension headache. Lancet 1:1236–1239, 1964
22. Couch JR, Ziegler DK, Hassanein R: Amitriptyline in the prophylaxis of migraine. Neurology 26:121–127, 1976
23. Couch JR, Hassanein RS: Amitriptyline in migraine prophylaxis. Arch Neurol 36:695–699, 1979
24. Johansson F, Knorring LV, Sedvall G, et al: Changes in endorphins and 5-hydroxyindoleacetic acid in cerebrospinal fluid as a result of treatment with a serotonin reuptake inhibitor (zimelidine) in chronic pain patients. Psychiatry Res 2:167–172, 1980
25. Feinmann C, Harris M, Cawley R: Psychogenic facial pain: presentation and treatment. Br Med J 288:436–438, 1984
26. McDonald-Scott WA: The relief of pain with an antidepressant in arthritis. The Practitioner 202:802–807, 1969
27. Gringas M: A clinical trial of Tofranil in rheumatic pain in general practice. J Int Med Res 4:41–49, 1976
28. Gomersall JD, Stuart A: Amitriptyline in migraine prophylaxis. J Neurol Neurosurg Psychiary 36:684–690, 1973
29. Spiegel K, Kalb R, Pasternak GW: Analgesic activity of tricyclic antidepressants. Ann Neurol 13:462–465, 1983
30. Goldstein FJ, Malseed RT: Differential effects of tricyclic antidepressants and morphine analgesics.
31. Spencer PSJ: Some aspects of the pharmacology of analgesia. J Int Med Res 4:1–14, 1976
32. Malseed RT, Goldstein FJ: Enhancement of morphine analgesics by tricyclic antidepressants. Neuropharmacology 18:827–829, 1979
33. Botney M, Fields HL: Amitriptyline potentiates morphine analgesics by a

direct action on the central nervous system. Ann Neurol 13:160–164, 1982

34. Chapman CR, Butler SH: Effects of doxepin on perception of laboratory-induced pain in man. Pain 5:253–262, 1978

35. Kuipers RK: Imipramine in the treatment of rheumatic patients. Acta Rheumatoid Scandinavica 8:45, 1962

36. Haydu GG, Goldschmidt L, Drymiotis AD: Effects of imipramine on the rheumatoid factor titre of psychotic patients with depressive symptomatology. Ann Rheum Dis 33:273–275, 1974

37. Regalado RG: Clomipramine (Anafranil) and musculoskeletal pain in general practice. J Int Med Res 5:72–77, 1977

38. Ganvir P, Beaumont G, Seldrup J: A comparative trial of clomipramine and placebo: an adjunctive therapy in arthralgia. Int Med Res 8:60–66, 1980

39. Glick EN, Fowler PD: Imipramine in chronic arthritis. Pharmacology and Medicine 1:94–96, 1979

40. Thorpe P, Marchant-Williams R: The role of an antidepressant, dibenzepin (Noveril), in the relief of pain in chronic arthritic states. Med J Aust 1:264–266, 1974

41. Diamond S, Baltes BJ: Chronic tension headaches: treated with amitriptyline—a double-blind study. Headache 11:110–116, 1971

42. Noone JF: Psychotropic drugs and migraine. J Int Med Res 5:66–71, 1977

43. Mahloudji M: Prevention of migraine. Br Med J 1:182–183, 1969

44. Dalessio DJ: Chronic pain syndrome and disordered corticol inhibition effects of tricyclic compounds. Diseases of the Nervous System 28:325–328, 1967

45. Morland TJ, Storli OV, Mogstad TE: Doxepin in the treatment of mixed vascular and tension headaches. Headache 19:382–383, 1979

46. Carasso RL, Yehuda S: Clomipramine and amitriptyline in the treatment of severe pain. Int J Neurosci 9:191–194, 1979

47. Anthony M, Lance JW: Monoamine oxidase inhibition in the treatment of migraine. Arch Neurol 21:263–268, 1969

48. Paulson G: Treatment of post-traumatic headache with imipramine. Am J Psychiatry 119:368, 1962

49. Gessel AH: Electromyographic biofeedback and tricyclic anti-depressants in myofascial pain-dysfunction syndrome: psychological predictors of outcome. J Am Dent Assoc 91:1048–1052, 1975

50. Moore DS, Nally FF: Atypical facial pain: an analysis of 100 patients with discussion. Journal of the Canadian Dental Association 7:396–401, 1975

51. Taub A: Relief of postherpetic neuralgia with psychotropic drugs. J Neurosurg 39:235–239, 1973

52. Taub A, Collins WF: Observations on the treatment of denervation dysesthesia with psychotropic drugs: postherpetic neuralgia, anesthesia dolorosa, peripheral neuropathy, in Advances in Neurology, vol 4. Edited by Bonica JJ. New York, Raven Press, 1974

53. Clarke IMC: Amitriptyline and perphenazine in chronic pain. Anaesthesia 36:210–212, 1981

54. Hatangdi VS, Boas RA, Richard EG: Postherpetic neuralgia: management with antiepileptic and tricyclic drugs, in Advances in Pain Research. Edited by Bonica JJ, Albe-Fessard D. New York, Raven Press, 1976

55. Weis O, Sriwatanakul K, Weintraub M: Treatment of postherpetic neuralgia annd acute herpetic pain with amitriptyline and perphenazine. S Afr Med J 62:274–275, 1982

56. Davis JL, Lewis SB, Gerick JE, et al: Peripheral diabetic neuropathy treated with amitriptyline and fluphenazine. JAMA 238:2291–2292, 1977

57. Kvinesdal B, Molin J, Froland A, et al: Imipramine treatment of painful diabetic neuropathy. JAMA 251:1727–1730, 1984

58. Massey EW, Riley TL: Tricyclic antidepressants for peripheral neuropathy. JAMA 243:1133, 1980

59. Jenkins DG, Ebbutt AF, Evans CD: Tofranil in the treatment of low back pain. J Int Med Res 4:28–40, 1976

60. Alcoff J, Jones E, Rust P, et al: A trial of imipramine for chronic low back pain. J Fam Pract 14:841–846, 1982

61. Sternbach RA, Janowsky DS, Huey LY, et al: Effects of altering brain serotonin activity on human chronic pain, in Advances in Pain Research and Therapy, vol 1. New York, Raven Press, 1976

62. Merskey H, Hester RA: The treatment of chronic pain with psychotropic drugs. Postgrad Med J 48:594–598, 1972

63. Kocher R: The use of psychotropic drugs in the treatment of chronic, severe pains. Eur Neurol 14:458–464, 1976

64. Evans W, Gensler F, Blackwell B, et al: The effects of anti-depressant drugs on pain relief and mood in the chronically ill. Psychosomatics 14:214–219, 1973

65. Johansson F, von Knorring L: A double-blind controlled study of a serotonin uptake inhibitor (zimelidine) versus placebo in chronic pain patients. Pain 7:69–78, 1979

66. Pilowsky I, Hallett EC, Bassett DL, et al: A controlled study of amitriptyline in the treatment of chronic pain. Pain 14:169–179, 1982

67. Duthie AM: The use of phenothiazines and tricyclic anti-depressants in the treatment of intractable pain. S Afr Med J 51:246–247, 1977

68. Magni G, Bertolini C de, Bodi G: Treatment of perineal neuralgia with antidepressants. Journal of the Royal Society of Medicine 75:214–215, 1982

69. Montastruc JL, Tran MA, Blanc M, et al: Measurement of plasma level of clomipramine in the treatment of chronic pain. Clin Neuropharmacol 8:78–82, 1985

70. Castaigne P, Laplane D, Morales R: Traitement par la clomipramine des douleurs des neuropathies peripheriques. Nouvelle Presse Medicale (Paris), 8:843–845, 1979

71. Langohr HD, Stahr M, Petruch F: An open and double-blind crossover study on the efficacy of clomipramine (Anafranil) in patients with mono- and polyneuropathies. Eur Neurol 21:309–317, 1982

72. Blumer D, Heilbronn M: Antidepressant treatment for chronic pain: treatment outcome of 1,000 patients with the pain-prone disorder. Psychiatric Annals 14:796–800, 1984

73. Lindsay PG, Wyckoff M: The depression-pain syndrome and its response to antidepressants. Psychosomatics 22:571–577, 1981

74. Ward NG, Bloom VL, Fawcett J, et al: Urinary 3-methoxy-4-hydroxy-

phenethylene glycol in the prediction of pain and depression relief with doxepin: preliminary findings. J Nerv Ment Dis 171:55–58, 1983

75. Baldessarini RJ: Drugs and the treatment of psychiatric disorders, in The Pharmacological Basis of Therapeutics. Edited by Goodman AG, Goodman LS, Gilman A. New York, Macmillan, 1980

76. Dilsaver SC, Greden JF: Antidepressant withdrawal phenomena. Biol Psychiatry 19:237–255, 1984

77. American Medical Association: Drug Evaluation, fifth edition. Chicago, American Medical Association, Division of Drugs, 1983

78. Sjogvist F: Psychotropic drugs, II: interaction between monoamine oxidase inhibitors and other substances. Proceedings of the Royal Society of Medicine 58:967–978, 1978

79. Schildkraut JJ: The catecholamine hypothesis of affective disorders: a review of supporting evidence. Am J Psychiatry 122:509–522, 1965

80. Copper A, Shaw DM, Herzberg B, et al: Tryptophan in the treatment of depression. Lancet 2:1178–1180, 1967

81. Chouinard G, Young SN, Brodwejn J, et al: Tryptophan in the treatment of depression and mania. Adv Biol Psychiatry 10:47–66, 1983

82. Moller SE, Kirk L, Brandrup E, et al: Tryptophan availability in endogenous depression—relation to efficacy of L-tryptophan treatment. Adv Biol Psychiatry 10:30–46, 1983

83. Seltzer S, Stock R, Marcus R, et al: Alteration of human pain thresholds by nutritional manipulation and L-tryptophan supplementation. Pain 13:385–393, 1982

84. Seltzer S, Dewort D, Pollack RL, et al: The effects of dietary tryptophan on chronic maxillofacial pain and experimental pain tolerance. J Psychiatry Res 17:181–186, 1983

85. McArthur JN, Dawkins PD, Smith MJH, et al: Mode of action of anti-rheumatic drugs. Br Med J 2:677–679, 1971

86. Broadhurst AD: Tryptophan and rheumatic disease. Br Med J 2:456, 1977

87. Taylor WM: Schizophrenia, rheumatoid arthritis and tryptophan metabolism. J Clin Psychiatry 39:499–503, 1978

88. Sethi PD: L-tryptophan and inflammation. Indian J Physiol Pharmacol 18:355–357, 1974

89. Madan BR, Khanna NK: Anti-inflammatory activity of L-tryptophan and DL-tryptophan. Indian Journal of Medical Research 68:708–713, 1978

90. Aylward M, Maddock J: Plasma-tryptophan levels in depression. Lancet 1:936, 1973

91. Sicuteri F: The ingestion of serotonin precursors (L-5-hydroxytryptophan and L-tryptophan) improves migraine headache. Headache 13:19–22, 1973

92. Kangassiemi P, Falck B, Langvik VA, et al: Levotryptophan treatment in migraine. Headache 18:161–166, 1978

93. Hosobuchi Y, Lamb S, Bascom D: Tryptophan loading may reverse tolerance to opiate analgesics in humans: a preliminary report. Pain 9:161–169, 1980

94. Hosobuchi Y: Tryptophan reversal of tolerance to analgesia induced by control grey stimulation. Lancet 2:47, 1978

95. King RB: Pain and tryptophan. J Neurosurg 53:44–52, 1980
96. DeBenedittis G, DiGuilio AM, Massci R, et al: Effects of 5-hydroxytryptophan on central and deafferentation chronic pain: a preliminary clinical trial, in Advances in Pain Research and Therapy, vol 5. Edited by Bonica JJ, Lindblom U, Iggo A. New York, Raven Press, 1983
97. Gibson CJ: Control of monoamine synthesis by amino acid precursors. Adv Biol Psychiatry 10:4–18, 1983
98. Hartman E, Lindsley JG, Spinweber C: Chronic insomnia: effects of tryptophan, flurazepam, secobarbital, and placebo. Psychopharmacology 80:138–142, 1983
99. Hartman E: Effects of L-tryptophan on sleepiness and on sleep. J Psychiatr Res 17:107–113, 1983
100. Green AR, Aronson JK: The pharmacokinetics of oral L-tryptophan: effects of dose and of concomitant pyridoxine, allopurinol or nicotinamide administration. Adv Biol Psychiatry 10:67–81, 1983
101. von Praag HM, Westenberg HGM: The treatment of depression with L-5-hydroxytryptophan. Adv Biol Psychiatry 10:94–128, 1983
102. Courvoisier S, Fournel J, Ducrot R, et al: Properties pharmocodynamiques du chlorhydrate de chloro-3 (dimethyl-amino-3'propyl)-10 phenothiazine (4560 RP). Arch Int Pharmacodyn Ther 92:305–361, 1953
103. Lasagna L, DeKornfeld JJ: Methotrimeprazine: a new phenothiazine derivative with analgesic properties. JAMA 178:887–890, 1961
104. Montilla EE, Frederick W, Cass L: Analgesic effects of methotrinephrazine and morphine. Arch Intern Med 111:725–728, 1963
105. Bloomfield S, Simard-Savoie S, Bornier J, et al: Comparative analgesic activity of levomepramazine and morphine in patients with chronic pain. Can Med Assoc J 90:1156–1159, 1964
106. Moore JA, Dundee JW: Alterations to somatic pain associated with anesthesia, VII: the effects of nine phenothiazine derivatives. Br J Anaesth 33:422–431, 1961
107. Cavenar JO, Maltbie AA: Another indication of haloperidol. Psychosomatics 17:128–130, 1976
108. Maltbie AA, Cavenar JO, Sullivan JL, et al: Analgesia and haloperidol: a hypothesis. J Clin Psychiatry 40:323–326, 1979
109. Maltbie AA, Cavenar JO: Haloperidol and analgesia: case reports. Milit Med 142:946–948, 1977
110. Polliack J: Chronic recurrent headaches. S Afr Med J 56:980, 1979
111. Hakkarainen H: Brief report: fluphenazine for tension headache: double-blind study. Headache 17:216–218, 1977
112. Margolis LH, Gianascol AJ: Chlorpramazine in thalamic pain syndrome. Neurology 6:302–304, 1956
113. Raft D, Toomey T, Gregg JM: Behavior modification and haloperidol in chronic facial pain. Southern Med J 72:155–159, 1979
114. Farber GA, Burks JW: Chlorprothixene therapy for herpes zoster neuralgia. South Med J 67:808–812, 1974
115. Nathan PW: Chlorprothixene (Taractan) in post-herpetic neuralgia and other severe pain. Pain 5:367–371, 1978
116. Gade GN, Hofeldt FD, Truce GL: Diabetic neuropathic cachexia. JAMA 243:1160–1161, 1980

117. Schubert DSP, Patterson MB, Long C: Phenothiazine analgesics in a patient with psychotic symptoms. Psychosomatics 24:599–600, 1983
118. Daw JL, Cohen-Cole SA: Haloperidol analgesia. South Med J 74:364–365, 1981
119. Miley DP, Abrams AA, Atkinson JH, et al: Successful treatment of thalamic pain with apomorphine. Am J Psychiatry 135:1230–1232, 1978
120. Keats AS, Telford J, Kurosu Y: Potentiation of meperidine by promethazine. Anesthesiology 22:31–41, 1961
121. Houde RW: On assaying analgesics in man, in Pain. Edited by Knighton RS, Dumke PR. Boston, Little, Brown, 1966
122. McGee JL, Alexander MR: Phenothiazine analgesia—fact or fantasy. Am J Hosp Pharm 36:633–640, 1979
123. Reuler JB, Girard DE, Nardone DA: The chronic pain syndrome: misconceptions and management. Ann Int Med 93:588–596, 1980
124. Rubin EA, Zorumskia CF: Chronic pain and tricyclic antidepressants. Ann Int Med 94:415, 1981
125. Snyder S, Enna JJ, Young AB: Brain mechanisms associated with therapeutic actions of benzodiazepines: focus on neurotransmitters. Am J Psychiatry 134:622–642, 1977
126. King RB: Neuropharmacology of depression, anxiety, and pain. Clin Neurosurg 28:116–136, 1981
127. Mantegazza P, Tammiso R, Vicentine L, et al: The effects of GABAergic agents on opiate analgesia. Pharmacol Res Commun 12:239–247, 1980
128. Chapman CR, Feather BW: Effects of diazepam on human pain tolerance and pain sensitivity. Psychosom Med 35:330–340, 1973
129. Gracely RH, McGrath P, Dubner R: Validity and sensitivity of ratio scales of sensory and affective verbal pain descriptors: manipulation of affect by diazepam. Pain 5:19–29, 1978
130. Lasagna L: The role of benzodiazepines in nonpsychiatric medical practice. Am J Psychiatry 134:656–658, 1977
131. Hendler N, Cimini A, Terence MA, et al: A comparison of cognitive impairment due to benzodiazepines and to narcotics. Am J Psychiatry 137:828–830, 1980
132. Lewis DA: Lithium in internal medicine and psychiatry: an outline. J Clin Psychiatry 43:314–320, 1982
133. Ekbom K: Lithium vid kroniska symptom av cluster headache. Preliminart Meddelande Opuscula Medica 19:148–156, 1974
134. Ekbom K, Olivarius B: Chronic migrainous neuralgia—diagnostic and therapeutic aspects. Headache 11:97–101, 1971
135. Schou M: Lithium in the treatment of other psychiatric and non-psychiatric disorders. Arch Gen Psychiatry 36:856–859, 1979
136. Pearce JMS: Chronic migrainous neuralgia: a variant of cluster headache. Brain 103:149–159, 1980
137. Bussone G, Boiaroi A, Merati B, et al: Chronic cluster headache: response to lithium treatment. J Neurol 221:181–185, 1979
138. Graham JR: Treatment of cluster headache (workshop). Sixteenth Annual Meeting, American Association for the Study of Headache, Chicago, June, 1974
139. Kudrow L: Lithium prophylaxis for chronic cluster headache. Headache

17:15–18, 1977
140. Tosca P, Bezzi G, Cecchi M, et al: Effects of lithium salts on pain experience in depressed patients. Bibliotheca Psychiatrica (Basel) 161:134–140, 1981
141. Mathew NT: Clinical subtypes of cluster headaches and response to lithium therapy. Headache 18:26–30, 1978
142. Lopez-Ibor JJ, Lopez-Ibor JM: Indications of lithium salts in psychosomatic medicine. International Pharmacopsychiatry 5:187–189, 1970
143. Bergouignon M: Successful cures of essential facial neuralgias by sodium diphenylhydantoinate. Revue de Laryngologie Otology Rhinologie (Bordeaux) 63:34–41, 1942
144. Blom S: Tic douloureux treatment with new anticonvulsant. Arch Neurol 9:285–290, 1963
145. Hayward M: Headache and pain in the head and neck, in Persistent Pain: Modern Methods of Treatment. Edited by Lipton S. London, Academic Press, 1977
146. Budd K: Psychotropic drugs in the treatment of chronic pain. Anaesthesia 33:531–534, 1978
147. Caccia MR: Clonazepam in facial neuralgia and cluster headache. Eur Neurol 13:560–563, 1975
148. Loeser JD, Ward AA: Some effects of deafferentation on neurons of the cut spinal cord. Arch Neurol 17:629–636, 1967
149. Fields HL, Raskin NH: Anticonvulsants and pain. Clin Neuropharmacol 1:173–184, 1976
150. Glaser GH, Penry JK, Woodbury DM: Antiepileptic Drugs: Mechanism of Action. New York, Raven Press, 1980
151. Hasbani M, Pincus JH, Lee SH: Diphenylhydantoin and calcium movement in lobster nerves. Arch Neurol 31:250–254, 1974
152. Julien RM: Carbamazepine: mechanism of action, in Antiepileptic Drugs. Edited by Woodbury DM, Penry JK, Pippenger CE. New York, Raven Press, 1982
153. Rodin EA: Carbamazepine (Tegretol), in Epilepsy: Diagnosis and Management. Edited by Browne TR, Feldman RG. Boston, Little, Brown, 1983
154. Fromm GH, Killiam JM: Effect of some anticonvulsant drugs on the spinal trigeminal nucleus. Neurology 17:275–280, 1967
155. Dalby MA: Behavioral effects of carbamazepine: complex partial seizure, in Advances in Neurology, vol. 11. Edited by Penry JK, Daly DD. New York, Raven Press, 1975
156. Post RM, Uhde TW, Ballenger JC, et al: Carbamazepine, temporal lobe epilepsy, and manic-depressive illness, in Advances in Biological Psychiatry. Edited by Mendlewicz J, von Praag HM, Kaizer S. Basel, Karger 1982
157. Bergouignon M, D'Aulnay N: Effects of sodium diphenylhydantoin in essential trigeminal neuralgia. Revue D'Oto-Neuro-Ophtalmologie (Paris) 23:427–431, 1951
158. Lamberts T: Tic douloureux. Journal of the Michigan State Medical Society 158:95–96, 1959
159. Jensen HP: The treatment of trigeminal neuralgia with diphenylhydantoin. Therapiewoche 5:345, 1955
160. Braham J, Saia A: Phenytoin in the treatment of trigeminal and other neuralgias. Lancet 2:892–893, 1960

161. Crue BL Jr, Todd EM, Loeu AG: Clinical use of mephenesin carbonate (Tolseram) in trigeminal neuralgia. Bulletin of the Los Angeles Neurological Society 30:212–215, 1965
162. Ianmore A, Baker AR, Morrell F: Dilantin in the treatment of trigeminal neuralgia. Neurology 8:126–128, 1958
163. Lindblom U: Diphenylhydantoin for trigeminal neuralgia. Soensk Lakartidn 50:3186–3191, 1961
164. Spillane JD: The treatment of trigeminal neuralgia. The Practitioner 192:71–77, 1964
165. Lloyd-Smith DL, Sachdev KK: A long-term low dosage study of carbamazepine in trigeminal neuralgia. Headache 9:64–72, 1969
166. Rockliff BW, Davis EH: Controlled sequential trials of carbamazepine in trigeminal neuralgia. Arch Neurol 15:129–136, 1966
167. Nicol CF: A four-year double-blind study of carbamazepine in facial pain. Headache 9:54–57, 1969
168. Killiam JM, Fromm GH: Carbamazepine in the treatment of neuralgia: use and side effects. Arch Neurol 19:129–136, 1968
169. Taylor JC, Brauer S, Espir MLE: Long-term treatment of trigeminal neuralgia with carbamazepine. Postgrad Med J 57:16–18, 1980
170. Tomson T, Bertilsson L: Potent therapeutic effects of carbamazepine-10,11-epoxide in trigeminal neuralgia. Arch Neurol 41:598–601, 1984
171. Smirne S, Scarlato G: Clonazepam in cranial neuralgias. Med J Aust 1:93–94, 1977
172. Fromm GH, Terrence CF, Chattha AS: Baclofen in the treatment of trigeminal neuralgia: double-blind study and long-term follow-up. Ann Neurol 15:240–244, 1984
173. Ellenberg M: Treatment of diabetic neuropathy with diphenylhydantoin. NY State J Med 68:2633–2655, 1968
174. Chadda VS, Mathur MS: Double-blind study of the effects of diphenylhydantoin sodium on diabetic neuropathy. J Assoc Physicians India 26:403–406, 1978
175. Chakrabarti AK, Samantaray SK: Diabetic peripheral neuropathy: nerve conduction studies before, during and after carbamazepine therapy. Aust NZ J Med 6:565–568, 1976
176. Rull JA, Quibrera R, Gonzalez-Millan H, et al: Symptomatic treatment of peripheral diabetic neuropathy with carbamazepine (Tegretol) double-blind crossover trial. Diabetologia 5:215–218, 1969
177. Mladinich EK: Diphenylhydantoin in the Wallenberg Syndrome. JAMA 230:372–373, 1974
178. Cantor FK: Phenytoin treatment of thalamic pain. Br Med J 4:590, 1972
179. Gibson JC, White LE Jr: Denervation hyperpathia: a convulsive syndrome of the spinal cord responsive to carbamazepine therapy. J Neurosurg 35:287–290, 1971
180. Friedman AP: The migraine syndrome. Bull NY Acad Med 44:45–62, 1968
181. Jonas AD: The distinction between paroxysmal and non-paroxysmal migraine. Headache 7:79–84, 1967
182. McCullagh WH, Ingram W Jr: Headaches and hot tempers. Diseases of the Nervous System 17:279–281, 1956

183. Rowntree LG, Waggoner RW: Prevention of migraine attacks by Dilantin sodium. Diseases of the Nervous System 11:148, 1950
184. Dimsdale H: Migraine. Practitioner 198:490–494, 1967
185. Hallag IY, Harris JD: The syndrome of postherpetic neuralgia: complication and an approach to therapy. J Am Osteopath Assoc 681:1265–1268, 1968
186. Raskin NH, Levinson SA, Hoffman PM, et al: Post sympathectomy neuralgia, amelioration with diphenylhydantoin and carbamazepine. Am J Surg 128:75–78, 1974
187. Ekbom K: Tegretol, new therapy of tabetic lightning pains. Acta Medica Scandinavica 179:251–252, 1966
188. Ekbom K: Carbamazepine in the treatment of tabetic lightning pain. Arch Neurol 26:374–378, 1972
189. Martin G: Recurrent pain of a pseudotabetic variety after laminectomy for lumbar disc lesion. J Neurol Neurosurg Psychiatry 43:283–284, 1980
190. Dunsker SB, Mayfield FH: Carbamazepine in the treatment of the flashing pain syndrome. J Neurosurg 45:49–51, 1976
191. Hatangdi VS, Boas RA, Richard EG: Postherpetic neuralgia: management with antiepileptic and tricyclic drugs, in Advances in Pain Research and Therapy, vol. I. Edited by Bonica JJ, Albe-Fessard D. New York, Raven Press, 1976
192. Gerson GR, Jones RB, Luscombe DK: Studies on the concomitant use of carbamazepine and clomipramine for the relief of postherpetic neuralgia. Postgrad Med J 53:104–109, 1977
193. Bogock S: The Broad Ranges of Use of Diphenylhydantoin, vol I. New York, Dreyfus Medical Foundation, 1970
194. Bogock S: The Broad Ranges of Use of Diphenylhydantoin, vol II. New York, Dreyfus Medical Foundation, 1975
195. Loeser JD: What to do about tic douloureux. JAMA 239:1153–1155, 1978
196. Killiam JM: Carbamazepine in trigeminal neuralgia with special reference to hematopoietic side effects. Headache 9:58–63, 1969
197. Tomson T, Tybring G, Bortilison L, et al: Carbamazepine therapy in trigeminal neuralgia: clinical effects in relation to plasma concentration. Arch Neurol 37:699–703, 1980
198. Delfino U: An advance in trigeminal therapy, in Persistent Pain, vol. IV: Modern Methods of Treatment. Edited by Lipton S, Miles J. London, Grune & Stratton, 1983

Chapter 19

Behavioral Treatment of Chronic Pain: Four Pain Management Protocols

Karen M. Gil, Ph.D.
Suzanne L. Ross, M.A.
Francis J. Keefe, Ph.D.

Preparation of this chapter was supported by NIMH grant number 1 RO3 MH38407–01 (Behavioral Assessment of Chronic Low Back Pain); NIADDK grant number 1 RO1 AM35270–01 (Coping with Osteoarthritic Knee Pain); and a grant from the John D. and Catherine T. MacArthur Foundation.

There are a variety of behavioral approaches applicable to the management of chronic pain (Figure 1). In this chapter, we describe four behavioral treatment protocols we frequently employ in our pain management program. The conceptual background of each protocol is briefly described and specific elements of the baseline and treatment phases are outlined. Indications and contraindications for each protocol are also noted.

OPERANT CONDITIONING PROTOCOL

Conceptual Background

The central focus of an operant conditioning approach to chronic pain is a careful examination of the patient's behavior and socioenvironmental responses to that behavior. Patients who are candidates for this protocol display pain behaviors that do not appear to be closely linked to evidence of underlying tissue pathology. Many operant pain patients have few or no physical findings on neurologic testing and negative diagnostic studies. Thus, their pain behavior may be considered to be excessive. The pain behavior of these patients also is inconsistent. The patient may appear to be in extreme pain while walking down the hall on the pain

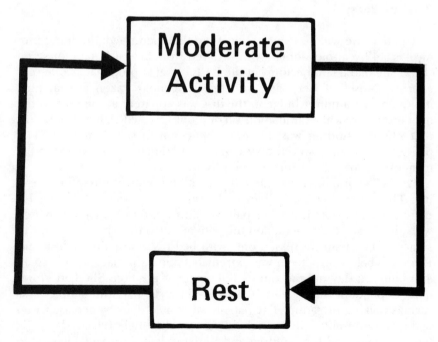

Figure 1. Activity/rest cycle

377

unit, but show little or no pain behavior when walking across the hospital grounds.

A major assumption of the operant approach is that the pain behavior displayed by these patients is controlled more by the consequences of that behavior than by underlying nociception. Patients may learn that pain behavior results in positive reinforcement such as the solicitous attention from a spouse, or provides a legitimate excuse for avoiding unwanted responsibilities. At the same time that pain behaviors are being reinforced, well behavior is usually not reinforced. Patients, for example, may notice that they are criticized or rejected when they attempt to return to work. Many operant pain patients have a long history of problems in living that date back to before pain onset.

Successful treatment of the operant pain patient involves two steps. First, an analysis of the effects of environmental and social events on pain and well behaviors is undertaken. Second, there is an attempt to change the patient's behavior by modifying the contingencies of that behavior so as to decrease the frequency of pain behavior and increase the frequency of a variety of well behaviors.

We have developed and refined an operant conditioning protocol over the past five years in our pain management program. We now describe the assessment and treatment phases of this protocol using a case example.

Baseline Phase

The patient we will be using to illustrate the operant conditioning protocol is a 42-year-old woman who suffered from low back pain for seven years. She had a laminectomy at the L4-L5 level approximately one year after the onset of her pain, and operative notes taken at that time indicated that a minor bulge in the disc was apparent at the time of the operation. Physical examination carried out revealed that the only current physical finding was moderate limitation in spinal mobility. The patient did show, however, an exaggerated "flinch" response to simple maneuvers carried out during the physical exam.

The behavioral interview carried out with this patient was quite revealing. The patient rated her pain at the time of interview at 10 on a 10-point scale and stated that her pain varied from 8 to 10. Pain increased with almost any movement, and the patient stated that she was unable to sit at all. The pain decreased only with bed rest and pain medications. Her daily behavior pattern was extremely limited, in that she only spent 45 minutes a day up and out of the reclining position. She had grown quite dependent on her family who would assist her with simple tasks such as walking or eating. The patient was visited daily by her sister who had taken over all of the household chores. She rarely ventured outside her bedroom, and her children and husband had set up a table next to her bed and ate meals there with her. Her typical day involved getting up for 20 minutes in the morning until the pain became so severe that she felt she had to lie down. At that point her husband would bring her oxycodone (Percodan), meperidine, and diazepam. She would try to ambulate again later in the day when her husband returned from work. Her intake of medication had increased substantially over the past year to the point that her referring physician referred to her as taking "whopping doses of medications."

Mrs. S. was angry and very agitated during our initial interview. She was upset because she had to wait 20 minutes to get medications from one of the unit nurses. She stated "You folks don't believe I have pain if you think I can wait so long for my medication." The patient was quite preoccupied with her physical complaints and described them in great detail. Throughout the interview, she stayed in the reclining position and appeared to be relatively comfortable. She refused to stand or walk when asked to do so, stating that this would increase her pain to intolerable levels. She denied feeling depressed or discouraged.

The patient complained of frequent muscle spasms and stated that she had fallen on several occasions because her legs gave way. There was no indication that she had injured herself during any of these falls, however. She complained of chronic feelings of fatigue and weakness which were probably secondary to her sedentary lifestyle.

Behavioral observations carried out by the nursing staff on the unit were also quite interesting. Mrs. S. had dramatic displays of pain behavior whenever she was asked to stand or walk. On one occasion when she was being assisted by a nurse to the bathroom, the telephone rang and she very quickly walked back to the telephone showing no pain behavior at all. During the baseline phase of observation, the patient made frequent demands for narcotic medications.

Mrs. S. had a difficult time keeping a pain diary during the three-day inpatient baseline phase primarily because of her high level of narcotic intake. She frequently had to be reminded to make entries in the diary, and most of the recording was carried out by the nursing staff. One interesting fact did emerge, however, and that was that the patient consistently rated her pain at 10. Because of her difficulties with the pain diary, we decided not to administer any psychological tests.

The patient refused to go through our standardized pain behavior observation. She stated that she was unable to engage in the sitting, standing, walking, and reclining required for the 10-minute videotaped observation. It was quite clear nonetheless from nurses' observations that this patient's pain behavior was quite excessive and inconsistent.

An interview with spouse and family members is often one of the most useful techniques for analyzing operant pain behavior patterns. This was certainly true in Mrs. S.'s case. Mr. S. was quite concerned about his wife and also confused by her behavior. He reported that at times she seemed to be in severe pain and at these times he was quite sympathetic. However, he also felt his wife might be playing the role of a "martyr." He was convinced that on some days she was up and around and doing things during the day when he was at work. He felt very guilty about these feelings, however, and had not admitted them to his wife. He stated that he had begun to withdraw from his wife and had stopped making attempts at trying to be affectionate. When her pain became extreme, however, he found that he was unable to keep his distance and that he would lapse back into his old pattern of bringing her medications, giving her back rubs, and comforting her. During these periods of extreme pain, his wife would become very depressed and discouraged. Mr. S. was also quite critical of his wife's sister, feeling that she "catered" to his wife. Mr. S. also reported that his wife had fewer and fewer outside interests. Her life seemed to center around discussions of her pain, visits to doctors, and requests for help from her sister or himself.

Treatment Phase

Inpatient Treatment.   Prior to initiating operant treatment procedures, it is always important to provide the patient with a rationale and general description of the treatment approach in a sharing conference. It is very helpful to have the patient's spouse and family members present for this conference. Several important facts are stressed in the sharing conference. First, the development of the patient's problems over time is summarized. We routinely use a simple diagram of the pain cycle to illustrate the sequence of behaviors and consequences involved. The diagram helps direct attention to the fact that patients have learned to associate being active with increased pain and that over time they have, therefore, become less and less active. We also tell patients that they have learned to associate increased pain with relief from pain in the form of medication or assistance from a spouse or other family member. Because these consequences are positive, they may have learned to become overly reliant on them for pain relief. The major goal of treatment is to break this pain cycle. Improvement depends on learning a new way to manage and deal with pain so that activity and involvement in a more functionally effective lifestyle is reinforced. A simple diagram of the activity–rest cycle is drawn and the basic elements of the operant treatment program are described. Patients are specifically told that nurses and members of the treatment team will try to help them become more active and functional by using praise, encouragement, and attention to reward them for progress. They are also told that complaints of pain will be listened to, but will be handled in a more matter-of-fact fashion that does not place undue attention on them.

We have found that most patients respond to this sharing conference positively. We feel the conference helps establish mutually agreeable goals and enables us to assess the patient's willingness to accept treatment interventions. A simplified version of the sharing conference can be used if narcotic intake or other factors make it difficult for the patient to understand the material discussed. Even in these cases, however, we feel the sharing conference serves an important function.

One of the most important components of the operant conditioning protocol is the activity–rest cycle (Figure 1). This consists of an hourly schedule in which patients are asked to spend a certain number of minutes up and out of the reclining position (uptime) and a certain number of minutes down and reclining (downtime). Over a period of days the amount of activity is gradually increased and the amount of rest gradually decreased. To establish initial activity levels, we typically take the average amount of time recorded on the patient's pain diary for three days of baseline and subtract 10 to 20 percent. An uptime goal for each hour is established by dividing the resulting uptime level by 16 hours (the hours in a waking day). In the case of Mrs. S., an initial activity level of five minutes per hour was attempted. To enhance compliance with this activity–rest cycle, the nursing staff initially spends time with the patient during their "uptime" each hour.

Two nurses helped Mrs. S. in the early stages of her program to reward her efforts and to ensure that she would not fall during the time she was up. Mrs. S. stated that she was unable to sit, so her five-minute uptime was spent standing by her bed. Within three hours of instituting this program, however, she stated that she was unable to tolerate five minutes out of bed each hour. A team meeting was held and the activity quota dropped to 1½ minutes per hour. She complied with this schedule, and her activity was increased to two minutes per hour on the second day. On subsequent days increases of one minute per hour per day were instituted.

Nurses and other team members make every attempt to positively reinforce patients on a frequent basis during the first few days of an operant conditioning program. To facilitate this, a simple graph of uptime is made and placed above the bed. Frequent notes are also placed in the chart to alert staff about progress. Most patients seem to enjoy the attention and develop a good working relationship with nursing staff. Within two to three days, they begin to take over many aspects of the program on their own, such as keeping diary records and getting themselves up and out of bed at the appointed time. We have found that it is helpful to use mechanical or electronic kitchen timers as aids that cue the individual when it is time for them to start their up or downtime. We use a commercially available electronic timer that emits a beeping tone when it counts down from a preset value to zero. The tone is loud enough to be heard by the patient and staff and provides a clear reminder that the uptime or downtime period has ended.

Another major component of the operant conditioning protocol is the use of a *pain cocktail*. The procedures used for this cocktail are described in detail in other chapters of this volume. The pain cocktail consists of methadone delivered in a cherry syrup base at regular time intervals. Over several days the amount of methadone is tapered until the patient is off of narcotics entirely. From a learning perspective the pain cocktail is important because it is delivered on a time-contingent schedule that breaks the association between increased pain and relief from pain (that is, delivery of narcotic medications).

A major goal of an operant conditioning program for chronic pain is to teach patients alternative and more functionally adaptive ways to manage pain. Once regular progress is made in increasing activity and decreasing intake of narcotics, we begin training in relaxation and other pain control methods. This training is carried out in our Behavioral Physiology Laboratory by technicians. The methods used are described in detail in subsequent sections of this chapter. The major emphasis of training in relaxation for operant pain patients is to teach them to use relaxation as a method to decrease excessive pain-avoidant posturing that occurs when they are active. During biofeedback sessions, technicians work during the uptime portion of the hour to teach the patient to decrease excessive and inappropriate muscle tension responses that occur during simple activities such as sitting, climbing stairs, or walking. The technicians use a great deal of verbal encouragement to reward patients for carrying out these activities in a more relaxed fashion.

A second approach to enhancing adaptive responses to pain is physical therapy. The principle of activity–rest cycling is used in almost all aspects of the physical therapy program. Patients, for example, are told to do a certain number of exercises daily and to rest upon completion of these exercises. Each day the number of exercises is gradually increased. By pairing moderate exercise with rest, patients learn that exercise does not increase pain, and they become confident that they can increase strength and mobility. In individual physical therapy sessions, rest and moist heat are also used as reinforcers, delivered after patients have completed a prescribed amount of exercise.

Mrs. S.'s overall response to the operant protocol was fairly typical. Major decreases in motor pain behaviors such as body posturing and painful facial expressions were evident within the first 10 days of the program. Mrs. S. was able to walk and even sit for brief periods of time in a much more comfortable and relaxed fashion. She generally showed good compliance with the program. Her husband stayed at a nearby hotel during the first 10 days of the program and was quite pleased and supportive of her progress. At times, however, Mrs. S. seemed to be testing the limits of the program. For instance, when her husband left, she reported increased pain and was unwilling to participate in the program for the remainder of the day. The next morning on rounds she was approached by the team and encouraged by all to start on her program once again. She did this and was able to continue making gradual increases in her activity level. Several weeks later, when a new resident joined the team, Mrs. S. tried to make arrangements with him for as-needed pain medications to be given at night. When this information was brought to the attention of the team, the basic elements of the program were again reviewed and she was encouraged to follow through. The patient's overall progress in treatment is summarized in Figure 2. As

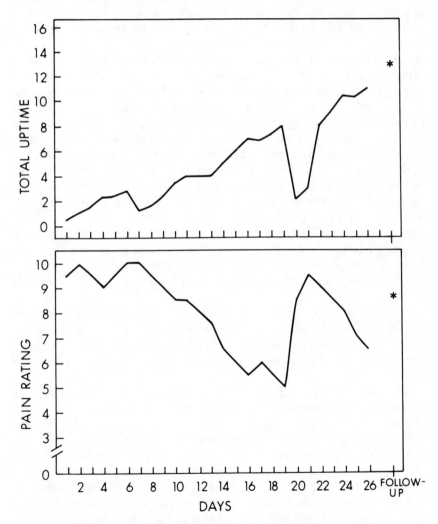

Figure 2. Graph illustrating the relationship between pain
rating and total uptime

can be seen, a gradual increase in activity was obtained at the same time narcotic medications were decreased. Pain level also decreased from 8 to 10 on a 10-point scale to a more variable pattern ranging from 5 to 8 on a 10-point scale.

Spouse Training and Home Programs. One of the most important phases in the operant protocol is spouse training. The major assumption of the operant approach is that patients do not change independent of their environment. Much of the improvement occurring on an inpatient unit may be attributable to the social reinforcement given for increased well behavior and the minimal attention given to excessive pain behavior. If progress is to continue after discharge, continued reinforcement of well behavior will need to be given by spouse and family members. We have found one of the best ways of ensuring that this occurs is to have the spouse spend two to three days toward the end of the inpatient treatment phase observing the pain management program. The spouse is required to go to treatment sessions and to become familiar with the program. The spouse is often surprised to see the level of function obtained in physical therapy or the effects that biofeedback-assisted relaxation training has on pain. Exposure to a full day of treatment also familiarizes the spouse with the activity–rest cycle. We usually encourage the spouse and patient to go out to lunch or dinner together. This may mean, for example, that the patient needs to recline during their downtime in the car on the way to the restaurant, or that during the meal they need to go out to the car for 10 or 15 minutes and recline once again. Through this experience, limitations that the activity–rest cycle places on typical daily functioning become quite apparent. The advantages of this approach, however, also become clear as the couple is able to go out and do things together (shopping, visiting, movies) that they have not done for months or years.

Members of the treatment team also encourage the spouse to increase the amount of attention given to well behaviors and decrease or minimize attention given to complaints of pain. Giving spouses an instruction sheet on the use of social reinforcement in pain management is also quite helpful.

A second sharing conference with the patient and spouse is held prior to discharge to establish each patient's *home program*. The major task is to design a home pain management program uniquely suited to the patient's needs. The session typically begins by asking the patient to summarize their progress and to describe the reasons they feel they have made progress. The spouse is also asked to comment on signs of progress that they have noticed. The therapist emphasizes that learning of new pain coping skills is a key element in progress and that continued reinforcement of these skills is needed if progress is to be maintained. A home program designed to maintain progress is then developed.

In developing home programs we use a summary sheet depicted in Table 1. This sheet displays the four basic elements of the home program: 1) the daily program; 2) the flair-up plan; 3) goals for the next two months; and 4) the don't list. A copy of the summary sheet is given to the patient and one is kept for the file. The home program developed for Mrs. S. is depicted on the summary sheet in Table 1.

Daily Program. For Mrs. S., the daily program was almost identical to her daily schedule in the hospital. She was to continue her activity–rest cycle at the same level that she had attained prior to discharge and to increase her activity level gradually (by 1 minute every 7 days over the

Table 1. Pain Management Program

Home Program Summary	Name: Mrs. S.

Daily Program	Flare-up Plan—3-Day Plan
1. Continue activity—rest cycle	1. Inform spouse that plan is being started
2. Increase activity by 1 minute every seven days	2. Decrease activity by 50%, increase rest
3. Trip out of home daily	3. Cut back, do not eliminate PT exercises
4. Walking program	4. Increase relaxation training sessions
5. All meals at table	5. Increase reading time
6. Practice relaxation—twice a day	6. Do distracting activities—cards, crossword puzzles, needlework
7. Physical therapy exercises—twice a day	7.
8. Continue to keep diary records	8.
9.	9.

Don't List	Goals for the Next Two Months
1. Avoid prolonged driving	1. Do some volunteer work
2. Avoid prolonged sitting	2. Take a college course
3. Avoid increasing narcotic intake	3. Weekends away with husband
4.	4. Out to eat
5.	5.

PROBLEMS I ANTICIPATE UPON GOING HOME: Adhering to activity–rest cycle. Will purchase a timer to help remind me of time.

NEXT OUTPATIENT REINFORCEMENT GROUP IS SCHEDULED FOR: September 13, 1985, 2–5 pm
2–3 pm   Spouse session
3–5 pm   Patient, spouse and family session

next 10 weeks). To overcome her isolation, we suggested that she take a trip out of the house—to go shopping or to visit a friend at least once each day. A walking program to be carried out with her spouse was also instituted. It was reasoned that this would not only increase her endurance but also would help give Mr. and Mrs. S. a positive goal to work on as a couple. It was suggested that the dinner table be moved out of her bedroom to the dining room and that all meals be taken in the seated position at the table. Practice with daily relaxation and physical therapy exercises were also included as part of the program. Finally, Mrs. S. was asked to continue her daily activity/pain diary and to bring the diary sheets back to her follow-up session. We have found that continued self-monitoring is very important in enhancing maintenance to the home program. The diary records are reviewed at the time of follow-up and provide a good index of progress.

Flare-Up Plan. The patient and spouse are told that a flare-up or increase in pain is likely to occur at some time following discharge. A plan is developed to deal with flare-ups, which involves modifying the daily program for a three-day period. Mrs. S. was encouraged to inform her spouse that the flare-up plan was being implemented so as to remove much of the guess-work involved on his part as to how to respond to her increased pain. Her flare-up plan involved decreasing her activity level by 50 percent and increasing the use of relaxation techniques and involvement in distracting and pleasant activities.

Development of a flare-up plan is a very important part of a behavioral program. It psychologically prepares patients for a possible relapse, and frames this experience not as a sign of failure but as a challenging task to be coped with. By dealing with increased pain in a more open fashion, patients may well be prevented from cycling to higher levels of pain that might result in further increases in narcotic medication intake and bed rest. In order to reduce the possible reinforcing effects of going on the plan, patients are instructed to adhere rigidly to the plan for three days regardless of whether an improvement in pain occurs.

Spouse and family members often report that the flare-up plan is the most helpful part of the home program. Many find that they are able to deal with increases in pain in a more calm and confident fashion. They report that they learn to view periods of increased pain as manageable events rather than as disastrous occurrences.

Goal Setting. As part of the home program, the patient and spouse are encouraged to identify goals that can be realistically met within several months of discharge. Developing this list of goals further emphasizes the importance of returning to well behaviors in social, vocational, and recreational spheres. For Mrs. S., these goals included becoming involved in volunteer work with children in the community, taking a course at a local community college, and working with house plants.

Patients often set unrealistic goals and are disappointed when they fail to achieve them. Unrealistic goals are labeled as such by the therapist, and alternative goals are discussed. One of the major goals for many individuals is improvement in marital and sexual relationships. The couple may need additional time together free from the responsibilities of home or work. Goals that foster this, such as weekend get-away trips or a regular evening out, can be built into the program.

Don't List. In this section of the home program, patients are asked to write down activities that they should avoid. For Mrs. S., these activities included prolonged driving or prolonged sitting, and also rapidly increasing narcotic intake. Listing these items on the home program sheet makes them more public so that the spouse and family are aware that there are definite limitations on activity, and that these should be considered an important part of the overall treatment program.

Preventing Relapse. Continued reinforcement of learned pain coping skills is needed if operant pain patients are to maintain progress. Several techniques are used in our program to provide this reinforcement. First, biofeedback technicians make regular telephone follow-ups on a monthly basis. Patients are typically pleased to be called and report that having the telephone follow-ups help them stay on their daily program. The telephone calls often uncover problems such as increased life stress or spouse reinforcement of pain behavior which may be making it hard for the patient to follow through with treatment recommendations. As part of each telephone call, a structured interview to assess pain and pain behavior patterns is carried out, and a report of this interview is forwarded to the behavioral psychologist who directs the program. Patients who need more intensive follow-up are then contacted.

A second effective approach to maintenance of treatment gains is the *outpatient reinforcement group.* This group meets every three months and an invitation is sent to all patients who have completed the inpatient program. This session is used to review the major components of the behavioral approach to pain management. The first hour of the group is a training session for spouses and the second two hours are for patients and spouses. All elements of the home program are reviewed in detail. Patients are also encouraged to discuss both their failures and successes in dealing with pain. The role of stress in disrupting home programs frequently is discussed.

Indications and Contraindications

The operant conditioning protocol is an effective treatment for many chronic pain patients. This protocol is indicated for certain patients only, however. First of all, there must be evidence that pain behavior is excessive or inconsistent in light of physical findings. Patients whose pain behavior appears to be closely related to underlying pathology may benefit from certain components of the operant protocol, such as the activity–rest cycling, but do not need the structure and amount of staff attention required by this protocol. A second indication for this protocol is that there is evidence that the patient has become highly dependent on spouse and family members. Patients may, for example, rely routinely on the spouse for simple activities such as bringing them food or assisting them during walking. A third indication is a progressive decline in activity over time. Patients who are spending less than four to six hours a day up and out of bed often develop an operant pain problem. A fourth indication is that patients are taking escalating doses of pain medications on an as-needed basis. The patient typically waits until pain is intolerable before taking medication, and then frequently will take two or three times the dose prescribed. Some patients deny taking narcotic medication but careful interviewing reveals that they are making frequent visits to the emergency room for "pain shots" or are developing a reliance on alcohol. A final indication for the operant protocol is that the patient is responsive to social reinforcement. Patients who do best on this protocol are those who seem to enjoy the praise, attention, and encouragement that they get from others. We find that operant pain patients are often exquisitely sensitive to social reinforcement. One reason is that many of them have such a low level of social interaction at home that any degree of positive attention is quite reinforcing.

There are several contraindications for the operant conditioning protocol. First, individuals who are involved in a pending disability decision or pending litigation do not do well with this protocol. The financial outcome of these decisions is a very important contingency that can affect behavior. Those who show dramatic reductions in pain behavior during hospitalization may well be denied disability payment or other compensation for their pain problem. We have seen only two or three patients involved in a pending litigation/disability decision who have benefited from the operant conditioning protocol. Other clinical researchers, however, have reported greater success in working with this population. Steven Fey and his colleagues (1), in fact, have developed a program that is designed to work primarily with individuals involved in pending disability claims. Patients are screened by a physician at the time of admission to the program and given an estimate of the likely outcome of their disability application. They are told that the physician will be writing up a report and rating their disability, and that performance in the program will determine to a large extent the rating given. This program has been quite effective in returning patients to work.

A second contraindication for the operant conditioning protocol is that the patient refuses treatment. There are usually several ways this happens. First, some refuse to become involved in the program unless it will provide complete pain relief. That is, they are unwilling to settle for the goal of management of pain but are seeking a complete cure. A second reason is that the individual may be unwilling to have medications placed on a time-contingent schedule. While many individuals express initial resistance, most are able to accept this aspect of the program quite well. Some become very angry, however, and request premature discharge from the program because they desire their medications on an as-needed basis. A third way of refusing treatment is evident in extremely poor compliance with important aspects of the program such as the activity–rest cycle. Some patients verbally state that they are willing to become involved in the program, but on a day-to-day basis refuse to actually carry out any of the treatment recommendations. We typically respond to this by exploring the reasons for the resistance and modifying the program if necessary. Even with this understanding approach and a great deal of social reinforcement for compliance by the nursing staff, some patients refuse to comply and are deemed inappropriate for the protocol.

A final contraindication for the operant conditioning protocol is a pronounced lack of spouse or family support for the program. In some cases, the patient's spouse may feel threatened psychologically if substantial improvements occur. For example, the husband of one patient felt extremely guilty about the fact that his wife was hurt in a boating accident in which he was the skipper. He was preoccupied with the fact that he was the cause of his wife's chronic pain. Whenever his wife attempted to try to return to activities around the home such as housework, he reacted in an extremely anxious and overly solicitous fashion. He refused to allow her to do these activities and hired a maid to help her. When she later attempted to become active around the house, he would become angry and force her to return to bed. In order to work with this patient, it was necessary to ask the husband to stay away from the hospital for several weeks until the patient had increased her activity substantially. As this occurred, her pain level decreased and her mood improved as well.

When the spouse returned for a visit and noticed the change, he was finally able to become more supportive and encouraging of her progress.

The operant conditioning approach to chronic pain was one of the first behavioral treatment methods developed for this population. Treatment programs that use operant conditioning protocols have been successful in helping many chronic pain patients who failed to respond to traditional medical and surgical approaches. The operant protocol is expensive and requires careful and systematic manipulation of contingencies such as pain medication and social reinforcement. A highly trained staff and coordinated team approach is necessary to prevent inadvertent reinforcement of maladaptive pain behaviors.

While the operant conditioning approach can help many, it is important to point out that not all chronic pain sufferers need to go through such a highly structured program. Individuals who appear to have some ability to control their own behavioral and psychological response to pain do not require an operant program. These patients have the resources to benefit from training in self-control techniques. They are best treated behaviorally using protocols that emphasize the patient's responsibility in managing and coping with pain. This emphasis on self-control is a hallmaker of the three remaining protocols described in this chapter.

PSYCHOPHYSIOLOGICAL PROTOCOL

Conceptual Background

The psychophysiological protocol emphasizes the importance of stressful environmental events in eliciting psychological and physiological responses that cause pain. Stress is presumed to induce autonomic arousal and/or heightened muscle tension, which, in turn, produces increased nociceptive input in the periphery and pain. Assessment involves comprehensive investigation of both environmental stressors and physiological responses. Patients are often unaware of the relationship between their psychological state and physiological responses. They often focus on physical symptoms and pain and may be resistant to questions about psychological factors. Yet, assessment of environmental stress is crucial to determining whether the psychophysiological model fits the patient's pain problem. Many pain problems, such as those starting with injury or disease, lead to stressful events such as frequent doctor visits, surgery, and so on. Thus, a comprehensive behavioral analysis is needed to determine the nature of the stress–pain relationship; that is, does stress *cause* the pain, or is stress a *reaction* to having chronic pain? Whenever a stress–pain relationship is evident and extreme reactivity to stress with pain is observed, the psychophysiological protocol is applicable.

In Chapter 8, the psychophysiological model was applied to the analysis of migraine headaches. In patients with migraines, stressful events can lead to physiological reactions such as cerebral vasoconstriction, release of serotonin and further decreases in blood flow, focal neurologic signs such as an aura, vasodilation of the extracranial and intracranial arteries, and sensitization of pain receptors. These physiological changes are considered responsible for much of the pain of migraine headaches. Patients often become increasingly anxious and depressed during episodes of severe migraines, which, in turn, increases pain. Other pain problems with primary psychophysiological mechanisms include muscle contraction headaches, colitis, peptic ulcer, coronary artery disease, and temporomandibular joint (TMJ) pain.

To illustrate the psychophysiological protocol, a case of a patient with TMJ pain will be presented. Extensive research has indicated that stress causes painful muscle spasms and tension in the masseter muscles in this population (2). First, research has demonstrated that psychological stress results in increased masticatory muscle activity in patients with TMJ pain 3–5). In a review of these studies, Rugh (2) concluded that there is strong evidence that a diverse population of TMJ patients respond to a variety of stressors under varying experimental conditions with heightened masticatory activity. Second, there have been numerous experimental studies which show that increased facial muscle tension and muscle spasms induced through teeth clenching, grinding, and jaw protrusion produce facial pain symptoms in normal subjects (6–8). Thus, research has demonstrated a link between muscle activity and pain under experimental conditions in normal subjects (2). Third, clinical studies of TMJ pain patients in their natural environment further support the link between stress, muscle activity, and pain (9, 10). Finally, the literature suggests that TMJ patients may be more anxious in general and hypersensitive to stressful situations (11). Therefore, the research data strongly support a psychophysiological conceptualization of TMJ pain, at least for many patients (2).

Baseline Phase

The patient, Ms. H., is a 28-year-old single woman employed as a secretary in an insurance office. Ms. H. was referred as an outpatient to the Pain Management Program by the Oral Surgery Department. She complained of left-sided facial pain and pain in her left ear. The pain began gradually two months previously. In addition to pain, Ms. H. complained of popping and clicking in her left jaw and nighttime bruxism. Although she had extensive dental work done two years earlier, no clear link was found between this dental work and her current symptoms. Her oral surgeon told her he thought her symptoms were stress-related.

Ms. H. arrived early for her initial appointment. She appeared anxious, agitated, and defensive, claiming from the start that her pain was not related to stress. Her reaction was one typical of individuals with psychophysiological pain problems; that is, they usually deny that stress plays a role. Thus, it is useful to start the interview with questions aimed at a clear description of the pain quality and location. Ratings of pain severity are also helpful. During the interview, Ms. H. rated her pain as a 4 on a 0- (no pain) to 10- (pain as bad as it can be) point scale. She reported that her pain ranged from a rating of 2 to 10 on this scale with some degree of pain constantly present. When asked what circumstances caused an increase in her pain, Ms. H. stated that her pain increased at work, although she denied that this was due to work-related stress. She also thought that eating and talking exacerbated her pain. Ms. H. obtained some pain relief through resting in bed and the application of heat to the left side of her face.

Rather than asking directly about stressful events, it is useful to ask patients like Ms. H. about *changes* in their life. Although Ms. H. insisted that she had gotten over it, she noted that her father died about one year ago. As a result, she spent more time driving her mother around, since her mother did not drive. In addition, her boyfriend of several years had recently broken up with her and this greatly limited her social activities.

Since her pain problems started, Ms. H. noticed a number of changes in her behavior. Although she had been a hyperactive child and considered herself a "hyper" adult, she noticed that she was even more restless and "keyed up" these past two months. Ms. H.'s work involved mostly secretarial duties. However, she was being considered for a promotion and thus was gradually experiencing more direct contact with insurance customers. Although she considered this challenging at first, concentrating on her work was becoming a problem and her boss had recently made some critical remarks. At home, she was less "hyper" but was still unable to relax. She had become more impatient with her mother on the telephone, especially when her mother gave her advice. Her social life was limited to outings with her church group. Although she continued to sleep throughout the night, she had occasional difficulty falling asleep. Her appetite remained good, although her diet included more soft foods since chewing hard foods exacerbated her pain.

Cognitively, Ms. H. was worried that she might not get her promotion at work if her pain continued. She was aware that this worry sometimes made her pain worse, but she didn't know what to do. She was frustrated by the inability of many specialists to find the cause of her problem.

In the interview, it was discovered that Ms. H. experienced other psychophysiological reactions when under stress. She had a long history of headaches described as tightness and pressure in the occipital and frontal regions of her head and tightness in her neck. These muscle contraction headaches were becoming more frequent and recently were occurring about twice weekly. When in college, Ms. H. was bothered by chronic stomach upset and diarrhea. After an extensive work-up, her physician decided her symptoms were psychophysiologic and she was referred to the student counseling center. At the time of our interview, Ms. H. reported infrequent stomach distress and diarrhea about once per month.

Observation during our interview revealed that Ms. H. was indeed quite tense and restless. She sat on the edge of her chair and shifted her position frequently. She also spoke quite rapidly. She rubbed the left side of her face when talking and pursed her lips together when thinking over the answers to questions.

During the baseline phase, several sources of additional data are collected as part of the psychophysiological protocol. The evaluation in the Behavioral Physiology Laboratory is a major source of baseline data. This evaluation involves assessment of relevant physiological responses. In the case of migraine headaches, the assessment would include measures of frontalis surface electromyography (EMG) and digital skin temperature. For psychophysiologic back pain, the assessment would include EMG measures of paraspinal muscle activity during stress and during static and dynamic postures.

In the case of Ms. H., a TMJ patient, EMG readings from the right and left masseter muscles were obtained under several conditions, including reclining, sitting, standing, and two stress conditions. For reclining, sitting, and standing, the patient was instructed to assume the position and the average of three one-minute trials was obtained from each position. To obtain an index of masseter activity while under stress, we use two tasks, mental arithmetic and chewing gum. First, subjects are informed that they must complete a "pop quiz" and count backwards out loud by sevens from 1,000. The technician emphasizes that the patient must count "quickly and accurately." Any hesitation or inaccurate response by the patient is followed by the technician stating: "Quickly and accurately, please begin again." Three 10-second readings of EMG activity are taken in this condition. Afterwards, the patient is instructed to relax as much as possible and readings of the patient's ability to relax on command are taken. The second stress condition is a measure of masseter activity during the chewing of gum. Three one-minute trials are obtained while the patient is chewing gum on the right side and then three trials are obtained with chewing gum on the left side. Again, measures of the patient's ability to relax after this condition are obtained.

The results of the laboratory evaluation for Ms. H. revealed bilateral masseter muscle activity elevated significantly above normal levels. Furthermore, EMG levels for the left masseter muscle were much higher than for the right masseter muscle group. These asymmetrical and elevated readings were even more evident under the stress conditions. Ms. H. was observed to have some degree of control over masseter EMG activity. When instructed, she was able to relax the tension levels somewhat.

Also, during the evaluation in the laboratory, a pre- and postevaluation self-reporting rating of pain level is obtained on a 0 to 10 scale. Ms. H. rated her initial pain level at 1 and her postevaluation pain level at 5, indicating a marked increase in pain level during the evaluation. A similar rating of tension level is obtained pre- and postevaluation on a scale in which 0 = completely calm and relaxed and 10 = "as tense and anxious as I have ever felt." Ms. H. rated her tension at 0 before the evaluation and 8 at the end of the evaluation.

A second major source of baseline information is self-monitoring data. The patient is asked to self-monitor pain levels and tension levels for one week. At four times each day (breakfast, lunch, dinner, and bedtime), the patient makes a mark on a 100-mm line to rate pain level and on a separate scale to rate tension level. The form used for these ratings (the pain–tension diary) is depicted in Figure 3. The purpose of these data is to assess the relationship between tension and pain. In the case of Ms. H., the relationship was quite obvious. Whenever her tension level was rated as high, she rated her pain level high. Lunchtime was consistently given the highest tension and pain ratings, and bedtime was usually the lowest.

Ms. H. was also asked to keep an ongoing record of the situations she was in when her pain reached a severe level. To do this, each time she felt her pain level was 8 or greater on a 10-point scale, she recorded the situation she was in, with specifics such as who she was with and what were her thoughts. She kept this record in a small notebook she carried in her pocketbook, and she was instructed to make her entries as they occurred rather than relying on recall at the end of the day. From her diary, several situations were found to be associated with high pain levels. These included: handling customer telephone calls; being criticized by her boss; thinking about her promotion; and getting telephone calls from her mother.

Other self-report measures are also completed by the patient for the psychophysiological protocol. These include measures of pain quality and severity (McGill Pain Questionnaire, pain map); an index of coping abilities (the Pain Coping Skills Questionnaire); and measures of psychological function (SCL-90R). For Ms. H., the significant results included that she had a characterological tendency to express psychological distress in indirect ways such as through the development of physical symptoms. It was also found that she had few adaptive pain coping skills.

A final source of data is obtained by the physical therapy team and includes measures of muscle strength, endurance, and flexibility. Palpation of Ms. H.'s muscles revealed tension in most of the muscles of the shoulders, upper back, neck, face, and scalp.

From the assessment of Ms. H.'s condition, it was concluded that her TMJ pain was psychophysiologic. Psychological distress, especially during work, appeared to result in increased muscle tension in several muscle groups, producing pain primarily in the left masseter region. Specific environmental stressors that triggered this psychophysiological reaction included: telephone calls with her mother and customers at work, criticism from her boss, and thoughts about her promotion. The psychophysiological protocol was considered appropriate for Ms. H.'s problem. In our opinion, she needed to learn to physically relax muscle

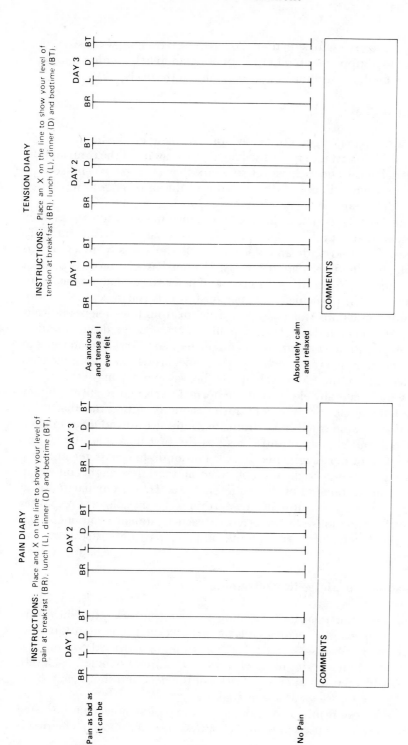

Figure 3. Pain and tension diary

activity during stressful situations. Assertiveness training was also recommended as a supplement to her treatment plan to help her learn to cope with her mother, customers, and boss more effectively (12).

Treatment Phase

There are two major goals of behavioral treatment of psychophysiologic disorders. The first is to make the patient more aware of the contribution of psychological and behavioral stressors that elicit pain. The second goal is to teach patients to directly control the physiological responses that produce pain.

In the case of Ms. H., a sharing conference was held to increase her awareness of her problem and provide a rationale for treatment. The conference started with an explanation of the stress–pain cycle. To individualize the explanation for Ms. H., her baseline records of pain and tension levels, her diary material, and her EMG evaluation data were summarized. In particular, the relationship between specific stress-related work situations (for example, criticism from boss, telephone calls from customers), and heightened pain levels was pointed out. In addition, her attention was focused also on the tendency for her pain levels to be highest at midday as compared to bedtime. Ms. H. was shown the data obtained during the EMG evaluation. She was told her masseter muscle activity was bilaterally elevated above normal levels and relatively higher in the left muscle (or masseter) during static postures, and that these elevations became even more dramatic in the stress conditions (mental arithmetic and chewing gum). This was the first time that Ms. H. was made aware of her heightened muscle tension in her masseter muscles. During the conference she was able to admit that stress might contribute to her pain. At the end of the conference, Ms. H. was familiarized with the primary goal of treatment: to control psychophysiological responses in stressful situations. An overview of each treatment component was provided. A total of 10 50-minute outpatient treatment sessions was planned.

Relaxation and Biofeedback Training

In this protocol, relaxation training and biofeedback procedures are used to help patients achieve relaxation of certain muscle groups. For Ms. H., biofeedback-assisted relaxation training was used to help her relax both left and right masseter muscles to normal symmetrical levels. Since she had tension in other muscles of the neck and shoulder, relaxation of these muscles was also a goal.

There are two primary components of the typical biofeedback-assisted relaxation training used in the psychophysiological protocol. The first is progressive muscle relaxation exercises (13). The body is divided into major muscle groups, and patients are taught a series of steps whereby they tense and relax each muscle group systematically, starting with the feet and progressing to the muscles of the face. Gradual building of tension under the person's control is emphasized. These procedures are explained in the first session in the laboratory, and the patient is given a 20-minute tape of the relaxation exercises to practice with twice daily, between sessions. Since Ms. H. was an outpatient, she was instructed to practice these exercises while reclining in a quiet room twice daily for one week. Inpatients are often seen about three times weekly. A relaxation training manual is also given to reinforce concepts explained in the first session.

During the second session, EMG biofeedback training procedures were introduced. For Ms. H., this involved placing a set of electrodes on the left and right masseter muscles. She was then supplied with biofeedback concerning her muscle activity while in a reclining position. In her case, a pulsating tone of increasing pitch signaled muscle tension, while a decreasing pitch and shutting the tone off indicated deep relaxation. Feedback was first given to Ms. H. from her left masseter muscle, while her right masseter activity was monitored. Criteria for shutting the tone off was initially set near her baseline level of left masseter activity to provide her an opportunity for immediate success. Gradually, the criteria was set progressively lower, resulting in the need for her to relax more fully to shut the tone off. At the end of the session, feedback for the right masseter muscle was given. During the second session, Ms. H. was able to demonstrate some ability to relax both left and right masseter muscle groups.

Over the next three to eight sessions, EMG feedback continued in a progressive fashion. Once Ms. H. was able to relax left and right masseter activity while reclining, EMG feedback was supplied while sitting and standing. As the patient achieved control over masseter muscle activity, training with other relevant facial, neck, and shoulder muscles was introduced. Training progressed to providing EMG feedback during actual activities of daily living such as talking and chewing food. For Ms. H., training in the laboratory also emphasized stressful situations she might confront outside the laboratory. For instance, she was given EMG feedback while imagining that she was sitting in her office talking on the telephone. In the laboratory, she actually was given a telephone receiver to talk into while practicing relaxation. Portable EMG equipment was also used to teach her to relax while walking in crowded areas of the hospital.

After eight weekly sessions, two additional sessions were scheduled, spaced one month apart to test maintenance of treatment effects. The initial EMG evaluation was repeated at the final session in order to track progress and identify any remaining problem areas. Telephone call follow-up was scheduled for three to six months after Ms. H.'s final session.

Record Keeping

Throughout treatment on the psychophysiological protocol, patients continue to keep pain and tension ratings on the pain–tension diary. This self-monitoring promotes continued awareness of the pain–tension relationship and is critical to measuring progress through treatment. Ms. H. also continued to record situations she was in when her pain level reached 8 or above. This helped her to remain aware of stressful situations that increased pain. In particular, it was found that Ms. H. experienced increased pain when dating men.

Home Program
(Refer to Figure 1).

Daily Program. Since Ms. H. was seen as an outpatient, she worked on her daily program between visits to the laboratory for biofeedback training. At first, her daily home program consisted of keeping her pain–tension records and dairy in addition to twice daily practice with her relaxation tape. After two weeks of practice with this tape, she was given a shortened version of the relaxation tape and she was instructed to practice twice daily with this tape. By the sixth session, "mini-practices" had been introduced in the laboratory and Ms. H. was instructed to include these in her daily home program. The mini-practice is a 30-second brief relaxation technique in which the patient scans the muscles of the body and relaxes any excess tension. Ms. H. was instructed to use approximately 20 mini-practices each day and to continue her twice daily practice with the relaxation tape. By the seventh and eighth sessions, daily homework assignments became more specific. Ms. H. was instructed to practice relaxation in the stressful situations she had identified during the baseline phase. She was given specific assignments to set aside 30 minutes each day where she telephoned customers at work or her parents at home, and she practiced relaxation techniques during these calls. Another assignment required her to spend five minutes thinking of her promotion while at work and practice relaxing.

A prompting strategy is used to facilitate generalization of relaxation techniques to the natural environment. A set of colored adhesive-backed dots is given to patients. They are instructed to place these dots in their natural environment and use them as cues to relax. Ms. H. placed a dot on her telephone at work and at home. She also placed one on her stenographer's pad so that she would remember to relax each time she entered her boss' office.

Thus, by the end of her outpatient laboratory visits, Ms. H.'s daily program included: a) practice with her relaxation tape twice during the day; b) 20 "mini-practices" each day; c) record keeping of pain–tension levels and a diary of stressful events; and d) practice time set aside to apply relaxation techniques in specific stressful situations.

Flare-Up Plan. Ms. H. was prepared for the possibility of relapse and given specific strategies to use to help her cope with periods of increased pain, thereby preventing cycling to higher levels of pain. Her flare-up plan involved modification of her daily program for a three-day period. She was to decrease her usual activity level by 50 percent and increase the use of her relaxation tape and mini-practices. She was encouraged to inform her mother and co-workers of her situation. Gradually, over the three days, she was to build back up to her usual daily program and resume practice of relaxation techniques in stressful situations.

Goal Setting. As part of her program, Ms. H. developed a list of goals she planned to accomplish in the several months after discharge. She planned to take an assertiveness training class at the local mental health center and begin an aerobics class to increase social contacts.

Indications and Contraindications. The psychophysiological protocol is indicated for patients whose pain problem is produced by exposure to severe emotional stress. Two sources of information from the assessment phase help determine whether this protocol is indicated. The first is evidence of a clear pain–stress relationship on the basis of interview content or observations. The second is evidence of marked physiological reactivity in response to stress.

In addition, the protocol is indicated for pain problems in which physiological target responses such as muscle activity can be easily monitored. Some psychophysiological pain problems such as abdominal pain are difficult to treat by way of this protocol, since the target abdominal responses are impossible to monitor directly.

This protocol emphasizes the application of self-management techniques in daily life, and therefore requires a certain degree of intellectual functioning and motivation. This protocol is contraindicated for patients who are not motivated to work on their own and for patients who lack the necessary intellectual skills. In addition, patients who have significant operant factors contributing to their pain problem, such as narcotic dependence and an overly solicitous spouse, may not be motivated to participate in this self-control approach. Some elderly patients with deteriorating memory or cognitive impairments may be unable to retain important instructions.

CONDITIONED FEAR RESPONSE PROTOCOL

Conceptual Background

The major premise underlying the concept of conditioned fear is that a phobic response is learned in situations that elicit anxiety. The fear response can be elicited by pain which is conceptualized as a "warning signal" of impending danger or harm. The fear response is common when there is uncertainty regarding the etiology of the pain. For example, low back pain patients with negative neurological findings may believe that there is a serious undiagnosed underlying medical condition, and they may fear that activity will produce increased pain or irreversible bodily damage. When activity repeatedly increases pain, patients quickly learn to fear and, hence, to avoid activity.

The conditioned fear response protocol is appropriate when excessive anxiety is associated with activity. Those who could potentially benefit from this protocol often display a fear response that is disproportionately greater than that which would be expected for a given activity. In these cases, anxiety is often evident when the person is asked to perform even the simplest of activities such as walking for a very brief period.

Fear is a learned response which in pain patients may be elicited by situations or activities that in the past produced increased pain. Avoidance of these situations may be either adaptive or maladaptive. For example, a low back pain patient quickly learns that lifting heavy objects produces increased pain levels, and the failure to engage in this activity is adaptive since the action could potentially produce further injury. However, this becomes dysfunctional when the avoidance response generalizes to other activities that the patient is capable of engaging in. For example, simple activities such as sitting, standing, and walking for brief periods that could be executed without producing further injury may well be avoided. Individuals suffering from chronic pain sometimes become extremely disabled by fear and limit their lives to a narrow range of activities they feel comfortable with (for example, reclining and watching television or resting in bed).

Anxiety accompanying the fear response can also produce higher levels of pain and further avoidance of activity. Subjective anxiety is accompanied by autonomic arousal, increased heart rate and blood pressure, as well as increased muscle tension. These muscular and autonomic responses often produce greater nociception, and the increased pain promotes behavioral avoidance.

The basic goal of the conditioned fear response protocol is to decrease the anxiety which is associated with a wide variety of activities. This involves training the patient to relax and then encouraging participation in simple activities (such as sitting, standing, and walking) in addition to more complex activities such as increasing involvement in vocational, recreational, and social pursuits. Our pain management program employs a multidisciplinary approach to achieve this aim. The treatment intervention involves the services of a wide variety of disciplines such as psychology, psychiatry, and physical and recreational therapy.

Baseline Phase

The patient we will be using to illustrate the conditioned fear response protocol is a 38-year-old male who developed chronic head, neck, and left arm pain following an accident in which a piece of mining equipment fell on his shoulder and pinned him against a wall. A traumatic event which produces pain such as this one often provides the setting for the development of the conditioned fear response. Mr. J., the patient, complained of extreme incapacitating pain. A neurological examination revealed an unremarkable computerized axial tomography (CAT) scan and negative myelogram. Mr. J. was preoccupied with a variety of symptoms (headaches, dizziness, and slurred speech), and he was convinced that he had a serious underlying neurological condition that had not been adequately diagnosed. He interpreted his left arm pain as a sign of an impending heart attack, and this belief greatly increased his fear and anxiety. His difficulty coping with his pain was complicated by his limited educational background that interfered with his capacity to understand medical explanations for his pain that could have decreased his fear. Overall, Mr. J. remained extremely anxious and firmly convinced that he would continue to be incapacitated by the pain and that he would become a total invalid in the future.

The behavioral interview revealed a number of problems that contributed to the patient's pain and low level of functioning. Mr. J. was unable to rate his pain (on a scale from 0–10); rather, he repeatedly stated, "I hurt all of the time." He maintained that almost any activity exacerbated his pain and believed that the only way to decrease his pain was to abandon vocational, domestic, social, and recreational pursuits. With the passage of time, the patient's daily behavior pattern had become extremely restricted. He resigned from his job after he developed severe headaches when he had returned to work. Mr. J. spent most of his time at home, where he functioned at a marginal level. He avoided housekeeping responsibilities as he feared that the chores would trigger increased pain. He isolated himself from family interactions, as he was afraid that his young children might inadvertently bump into his arm and thereby increase his pain. He withdrew from interactions with friends as he was afraid that a friend might grab his arm in a friendly gesture and potentially reinjure the arm or further exacerbate the pain. Mr. J. was irritable and angry with his wife and children and he began to fear that he might "lose control." He felt guilty about being angry with his solicitous wife who had taken over most of the household and financial responsibilities. The restricted nature of Mr. J.'s life contributed to suicidal thoughts which became evident when Mr. J. stated, "It would be better to be dead then to live with the pain." There was also an increasing dependence on alcohol and pain medications to control the anxiety and pain, and this further perpetuated the inactivity and passivity. For example, when questioned about interests and activities, Mr. J. stated, "I don't do anything." The significant reduction in activities resulting from anxiety and fear led to a severe depression.

Mr. J. primarily attributed his depression to the loss of his vocational and financial status. The patient had a ninth grade education and had pursued his former vocation as a miner for 18 years. When confronted by the suggestion to explore alternative vocational opportunities, he stated, "It is too difficult to start over at my age." Mr. J. complained of many symptoms of depression including crying spells, insomnia, decreased appetite, increased weight, a decline in libido, and memory and concentration problems.

Behavioral observations carried out using our standard observations system and by the nursing staff corresponded with Mr. J.'s self-report. In the videotaped observation, the patient displayed excessively high levels of pain behaviors even when doing simple activities that did not require use of his arm. On the treatment unit it soon become evident that Mr. J. largely refused to use the arm that had been injured in the accident. Moreover, he tended to remain in his room and failed to socialize with the other patients or to participate in unit recreational activities.

Mr. J. initially failed to comply with the pain management program. The patient was inactive, frequently requested pain medication, and viewed surgery as the only viable approach to his pain problem. Mr. J. expressed strong fears about participating in physical therapy, and he was resistant to exploring vocational possibilities with the social worker. Overall, Mr. J. appeared very anxious and depressed.

Treatment Phase

Inpatient Treatment.   It is very useful to present to the patient a conceptual framework that describes the process of conditioned fear prior to instituting the conditioned fear response protocol. Patients should be told in a sharing conference format that they have developed a fear of specific activities that they believe will exacerbate their pain. They should also be told that avoidance behaviors result from this fear, and that the avoidance response maintains and perpetuates anxiety, as it prevents them from confronting feared activities. Patients are then told that they will acquire skills that will help them to confront feared activities in a gradual manner.

Behavior therapists have found that desensitization is a highly effective intervention for the treatment of anxiety and phobic states. Desensitization is based on the principle of reciprocal inhibition (14), which states that the strength of anxiety-evoking stimuli is decreased when a response incompatible with anxiety occurs in the presence of the anxiety-evoking stimuli. Progressive relaxation (13) is the technique used to produce a deep muscle relaxation response that is incompatible with anxiety. This involves systematically tensing and relaxing various muscle groups, which decreases physiological arousal and creates the subjective feeling of relaxation. In desensitization training, progressive relaxation is used while the individual imagines or actively exposes himself or herself to anxiety-producing situations. This desensitization technique decreases anxiety that is evoked by diverse stimuli, and has a high degree of efficacy for the treatment of many types of phobias.

In our program, we instruct patients to write down feared activities and situations on index cards, which are then arranged in a hierarchy progressing from the least to the most anxiety-producing items. Progressive relaxation is used to help the patient cope with the pain and anxiety produced by the activity on a given card, while maintaining a low level of arousal. When the task on the index card is mastered, the patient moves on to the next card, which contains another activity that is somewhat more demanding. The number of activities that are successfully mastered can then be plotted on a cumulative graph, which provides a visual display of progress. The graphs become a powerful source of reinforcement since they provide a tangible display of progress. Patients are also instructed to use index cards in the home setting as they are often confronted by new activities and situations when they are discharged from the hospital.

A desensitization hierarchy of feared activities was set up for the treatment of Mr. J. Initial steps in the hierarchy were relatively simple (walking for 3 minutes, lifting the arm off a table for 10 seconds) and subsequent steps on the hierarchy were more difficult. The cumulative graph in Figure 4 displays Mr. J.'s progress in completing hierarchy items.

There are the two reasons why progressive relaxation disrupts the conditioned fear response. First, since patients remain relaxed, they maintain low muscle tension and arousal levels and reduce physiological concomitants of anxiety which increase pain. Second, progressive relaxation allows individuals to confront feared activities without high levels of anxiety, thereby breaking the link between activity and anxiety. This desensitization technique promotes exposure to, rather than avoidance of, feared activities.

Encouragement from staff enhances compliance with the desensitization program and helps patients to engage in activities that they might otherwise avoid. For example, attention and praise was used by nurses to

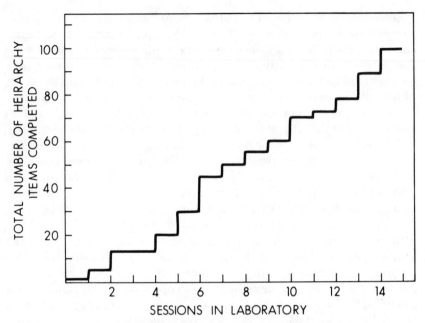

Figure 4. A cumulative graph displaying progress in completing desensitization hierarchical items

reinforce Mr. J. as he spent more time "up" and active (for example, walking, socializing, participating in recreational therapy). Physical therapy supplies a structured format that also encourages increased exposure to feared activity. A course in body mechanics helped Mr. J. to recognize that he can be active without exacerbating pain or producing bodily injury. In vivo exposure to anxiety-producing situations also takes place through participation in recreational therapy activities such as arts and crafts. By employing pain management principles—for example, the activity–rest cycle—patients recognize that they can engage in a wide variety of activities without exacerbating their pain. Successfully approaching these activities on the ward decreases the likelihood that the individual will remain in a passive and inactive role. The pain management group also provides an important setting for patients to share their experiences with chronic pain. Often there is significant disclosure about "fears," and the problems which result from living with chronic pain. The group format helped Mr. J. to realize that he was not alone and that other group members shared similar fears. By identifying with the fear responses of other members, patients are better able to accept and confront their own fears. Moreover, in a cohesive group setting, members often reinforce one another for mastering threatening situations (for example, riding in a car, shopping in a crowded mall). Group members are also instrumental as information providers, as patients are often able to give concrete suggestions that help the members to become more active.

In summary, inpatient treatment programs designed to reduce conditioned fear responses should utilize a comprehensive approach that encourages patients to confront and learn to control their reactions to situations that previously elicited a high degree of fear and anxiety.

Outpatient Program. Preparation for the transition from the hospital to the home environment is essential if progress on this protocol is to be maintained over time (refer to Figure 1). The gains acquired on the inpatient unit will be reversed if new skills are not generalized to the home environment. A home program is established using methods similar to those described for the operant protocol.

Involvement of family members is often critical during the initial transition period, as well as for maintenance of progress on this protocol. First, family members should be told that conditioned fear is a normal response and that there are ways that they can help the patient deal with this problem. When the family understands the treatment rationale, they can be instrumental in helping the patient to remain active. For example, Mr. J.'s spouse was told that activity would not exacerbate her husband's pain, and she was instructed to encourage her husband to socialize and participate in family activities. Spouse training is very important, as family members often give the patient a covert or overt message that activity might increase their pain. When the patient is able to master a task, such as shopping or visiting relatives, the spouse also recognizes that these activities need not be feared and avoided. Finally, spouses should be taught not to reinforce avoidance behaviors.

During the follow-up period, reinforcement is provided for further gains that have been made outside of the hospital. For example, Mr. J. was encouraged to return to work on a part-time basis, as this involved mastering a situation which had previously elicited fear. Ideally, the home environment should encourage increased activity while attempting to minimize fear, anxiety, and avoidance behaviors.

Indications and Contraindications. The conditioned fear response protocol is an effective intervention for a particular group of chronic pain patients. This approach should mainly be employed in cases where patients refuse to engage in activities that they are capable of doing because of fear and anxiety. In addition, those who display a high level of autonomic arousal such as increased heart rate, blood pressure, and sweating in feared situations are frequently good candidates. Those who respond to this protocol are also identified by the progressive restriction of their activity. Often there is a pattern of increasingly limited involvement in social, recreational, or vocational pursuits.

There are some pain patients who will not benefit greatly from this protocol. Individuals with pending litigation or pending disability are often reluctant to increase activity, as this may jeopardize the possibility of receiving financial compensation. As we have already stated, disability can be a powerful disincentive to overcome feared activities when there is the belief that mastery experiences might jeopardize the disability status.

A second contraindication for this protocol involves patients who are narcotic dependent. Unfortunately, the administration of pain medications are often made contingent on the presence of distress and the incapacitation resulting from pain. For example, there is frequently the fear that pain medications will not be delivered if there is improvement. Narcotic dependence can decrease motivation to confront the difficult task of mastering feared activities and situations.

In summary, a careful assessment of the pain patient should be undertaken prior to utilizing this protocol. If the candidate is suitable for the protocol, then a systematic intervention should be delivered that involves training in relaxation and graded exposure to a wide variety of feared activities.

MUSCLE REEDUCATION PROTOCOL

Conceptual Background

The major assumption underlying the muscle reeducation protocol is that pain is caused by musculoskeletal dysfunction such as muscle tension or muscle spasms. For many patients, this type of pain starts following an accidental injury such as a whiplash injury.

The muscle reeducation protocol begins with a comprehensive assessment of muscle function. Surface electromyography is used to objectively assess the functions of the involved musculature. In early neuromuscular research, this assessment was conducted from one muscle group while the subject was in one static position, such as reclining. However, there has been a growing trend in the literature to also include measures of EMG function of a variety of muscles during various movements (15). This approach developed because some individuals only display EMG abnormalities when required to perform certain movements. Thus, the muscle reeducation protocol often involves assessment of muscle function during static postures and patterns of muscle activity during movement.

Back pain frequently results from musculoskeletal problems. In this case, surface electrodes are placed on the left and right lumbar paraspinal muscles, and readings are obtained during static postures such as reclining, sitting, standing, and trunk movements such as extension, flexion, and rotation (15). Values obtained are compared to normative data (16). Research has shown that people without muscle pathology display low levels of muscle activity during static postures, symmetrical EMG patterns during trunk flexion and extension, and significantly greater muscle activity on the contralateral side during rotation (16). However, chronic low back pain patients with lumbar musculoskeletal problems display abnormal patterns of EMG activity such as elevated muscle tension at rest, asymmetrical activity at rest or during flexion and extension, or symmetrical activity during movements (15).

In the muscle reeducation protocol, treatment is designed to train patients to use the muscles affected by pain in a more normal fashion. For back pain, three major treatment approaches are evident in the literature. The earliest approaches utilized EMG feedback to assist patients in learning generalized muscle relaxation. Several studies have shown that generalized relaxation training using frontalis and trapezius EMG feedback, combined with relaxation practice during daily tasks, are effective techniques in reducing muscle tension and pain (17, 18). However, this method is an indirect means to achieve muscle relaxation and may not be useful for patients who need to learn specific muscle activation or certain patterns of muscle activity during movement. The second approach involves specifically training the lumbar paraspinal muscles during static postures (15). Nouwen and Solinger (19) demonstrated that feedback to the erector spinal muscles while patients are prone is helpful for patients with mechanical low back pain. Training in EMG biofeedback during movement in addition to static positions is the third and most recent approach. This approach follows logically from the findings of Wolfe and colleagues (15); that is, for some individuals abnormal patterns of activity only occur during movement. Research has shown that EMG feedback to the spinal muscles during trunk flexion, extension, and rotation is an effective means by which to train normal dynamic muscular patterns (15, 16).

In our laboratory, the treatment is selected to match the individual based on the assessment data. Typically for low back pain, EMG feedback to the spinal muscles is provided during reclining, sitting, standing, as well as trunk flexion, extension, and rotation. Training focuses initially on easy activities, and more difficult movements are added as training progresses. Activities and movements particularly problematic for the individual are targeted.

The neuromuscular protocol can also be applied to other rehabilitative problems where pain may not be the primary component. Basmajian (20) reviews the studies that have used EMG feedback to enhance neuromuscular control. In stroke patients, foot drop (21), shoulder subluxation (20), and reduced hand function have been treated with some degree of success. Also, some promising work has begun with spinal cord injury and cerebral palsy patients (20).

To illustrate this protocol, a patient recently seen in our laboratory with chronic neck pain will be presented.

Baseline Phase

The patient, Mrs. W., is a 38-year-old married woman who presents with a one-year history of neck pain. Mrs. W. experienced sudden onset of dull aching pain in her neck and shoulder after a motor vehicle accident in which she was hit from behind. She complained of radiating pain and numbness in her right arm and hand. Discogram and EMG conduction studies were positive and indicative of a C5-C6 radioculopathy. A C5-C6 fusion was performed. Following the operation, Mrs. W. wore a cervical brace for about six months. During this time, she experienced only minimal discomfort. However, only a few weeks after removal of the brace, she went on an extended vacation involving three weeks of driving. During the trip, she had recurrence of her symptoms.

At the time of admission to Duke University Medical Center, neurological evaluation including EEG and CT were within normal limits. Physical examination revealed normal muscle strength in the lower extremities and questionable decreased strength in the upper extremities. Tenderness and muscle spasms were noted at the base of her right neck and right shoulder.

During our interview, the patient rated her neck pain as a 6 on a 0- to 10-point pain rating scale. Her pain ranged from 0 to 10 on this scale and it was usually most severe in the late afternoon. Pain increased with activity and movement such as head rotation and, as a result, she limited her movement of her head and neck. Pain increased when driving and during stressful periods such as arguments with her teenagers. Although the patient was previously physically active, participating in sports such as tennis and swimming, she had drastically reduced her activity level to avoid pain episodes.

Recordings of muscle tension using surface electromyography (EMG) of the face, neck, and shoulder muscles were obtained. Significantly elevated muscle activity in the frontalis and trapezius muscles (20 uv to 30 uv) was found. In addition, comparison of left and right shoulder and neck muscles revealed relatively greater muscle tension on the right side corresponding with the patient's report of pain. During neck flexion and extension, asymmetrical muscle activity was noted with greater activity on the left (40 uv) versus the right side (10 uv). Every 5 minutes during the muscle evaluation, Mrs. W.'s pain rating was obtained using a 0 to 10 scale. A clear relationship was noted between the patient's self-reported pain level and EMG tension levels; that is, as tension increased, pain rating increased. When instructed to relax muscles, Mrs. W.'s EMG levels dropped somewhat, as did her subjective pain ratings.

Observation using our standard procedure yielded some interesting findings. When standing or walking, Mrs. W. held her shoulders rigidly and tilted her head forward. Whenever turning as to open a door, she turned with a stiff upper body posture rotating her entire upper body. Few other pain behaviors were observed except for occasional rubbing of the neck.

Mrs. W. described some variability of mood, minor sleep disturbance, and oversensitivity in stressful situations. In general, however, her psychological problems were not severe, and she appeared well adjusted emotionally.

From the evaluation it was concluded that Mrs. W.'s neck pain was primarily secondary to muscle tension and muscle spasms.

Treatment Phase

Patients are often unaware of their muscle problems, and thus it is important to prepare patients for treatment by giving them an explanation of the treatment protocol rationale. The pain–muscle tension/spasm cycle is explained in detail in a sharing conference format. Problems specific to the patient, identified in the baseline phase with regard to muscle tension and inappropriate muscle use, are pointed out. For example, Mrs. W. was told about her tendency to "favor" and protect her right side when at rest or moving. Showing her a videotape of this behavior helped make her aware of her tendency to use a stiff upper body posture when walking and opening doors. She was informed of her high EMG levels and abnormal muscle patterns during movement. In addition, Mrs. W. was informed about how her overall lack of exercise contributed to muscle weakness, atrophy, and pain. The development of these problems over a period of one year was highlighted.

Finally, Mrs. W. was familiarized with the goals of treatment. She was told she would learn to decrease tension and apply proper body mechanics to use muscles appropriately. The specifics of the treatment protocol were briefly explained. She was told how EMG feedback from her face, neck, and shoulder muscles would be used in combination with various relaxation strategies. Physical therapy techniques to improve muscle function also were explained briefly.

Biofeedback and Relaxation Strategies. During the first session, Mrs. W. was trained in the progressive muscle relaxation exercises described in the section on the psychophysiological protocol. The technician attached EMG electrodes to the patient's trapezius muscles, and tape-recorded relaxation instructions were played to the patient while EMG muscle activity was monitored. Following the relaxation practice, trapezius EMG biofeedback was given. As with the psychophysiological protocol example, a tone of increasing pitch signaled tension, whereas a decreasing tone pitch indicated relaxation. Criterion for shutting off the tone was initially set near Mrs. W.'s baseline level of tension, which was 30 uv, in order to ensure success during the first session. Mrs. W. was encouraged to pay close attention to what she did in order to achieve trapezius relaxation.

Mrs. W. was provided with a 20-minute tape of the relaxation exercises to practice with twice daily while she was in the hospital. Daily sessions were scheduled for her since she was an inpatient.

Once Mrs. W. was able to achieve relaxation while reclining, EMG feedback was given while sitting. Although her EMG levels were initially high, she quickly learned to reduce the tension. EMG feedback during movement was then introduced. Mrs. W. received extended practice with a portable EMG feedback unit while walking slowly, flexing and extending her head, and conducting activities of daily living such as opening doors. Initially, it took her a long time to return her muscles to a relaxed state after each task. Later, she could quickly bring EMG levels back to baseline.

Assignments to practice relaxing between sessions during activities on the unit were given. For instance, Mrs. W. was given daily assignments to practice relaxing while combing her hair, dressing, and carrying her meal tray.

By the sixth session, Mrs. W. was introduced to the mini-practice procedure, and she was instructed to do these 20 to 30 times daily. A knitting-tally counter was provided to record each mini-practice.

An evaluation of surface EMG activity was repeated at the final session. The results revealed near normal levels of trapezius muscle activity at rest and during movement. Mrs. W. was given a total of eight 50-minute sessions while she was in the hospital. Two outpatient sessions were scheduled after discharge to follow-up on her progress.

Record Keeping. Throughout her hospitalization, Mrs. W. kept a pain–tension diary form. Four times each day (breakfast, lunch, dinner, bedtime) she rated her pain on the 100-mm scale described in the section on psychophysiological protocol. A definite trend was observed for pain ratings to reduce as progress in EMG-assisted relaxation training was observed in the laboratory.

Pain Management Group. Another important feature of the muscle reeducation protocol is daily sessions in the pain management group. As previously described, this behavior therapy group emphasizes learning cognitive-behavioral strategies to help cope with pain. For Mrs. W., the group was especially useful in reinforcing the points reviewed in the rationale such as the relationship between pain, activity, and the body. She also learned more appropriate ways to deal cognitively with stressful situations.

Physical Therapy. Physical therapy is often used in conjunction with relaxation and biofeedback training as part of this protocol. Mrs. W. participated in daily individual physical therapy sessions and a group back school. In individual physical therapy, she was given a daily exercise program focusing on neck flexion and extension exercise. She started with a few repetitions of these exercises and gradually increased the number of repetitions to build strength, flexibility, and endurance. Mrs. W. was also given an individual aerobic program to increase her overall physical condition. In the back school, Mrs. W. was educated about the anatomy of the neck and back and taught proper body alignment and mechanics. She practiced appropriate ways to bend, reach, and lie down, as well as sweeping. She also learned a list of "don'ts" which apply to movements and activities.

Home Program. As with the other programs, home programs are a central component of this protocol. Home programs emphasize applying the relaxation techniques to reduce spasm and tension in activities of daily living. For Mrs. W., her *daily program* emphasized practice with muscle control during specific problem activities. Each day, she set aside 20 minutes when she was to select an activity from a list generated in the laboratory and practice muscle control and relaxation. Her list included unpacking groceries, sweeping, vacuuming, typing, and writing letters. Other aspects of her daily program were similar to those of patients on the psychophysiological protocol: a) practice with her relaxation tape twice daily; b) 20 mini-practices each day; c) daily physical therapy exercises; and d) 20 minutes daily of aerobic exercises such as walking or swimming. Mrs. W. kept records of her pain ratings as she did while in the hospital, in addition to recording compliance with her daily program, and listing any problem activities that she discovered. These problem areas then became part of her list of activities to practice.

Her *flare-up plan* was similar to that described for other patients in other protocols. She decreased her household activity by 50 percent, reduced her physical therapy repetitions, increased her relaxation practice, and eliminated her swimming. Over three days, she gradually was to build back up to her daily program.

As goals for the next two months, Mrs. W. wanted to increase her social activity with her husband and planned to have dinner out with him more often. She planned to resume three hours of volunteer work at the local hospital. On her *don't list,* Mrs. W. planned to avoid extended car trips without frequent rest periods. She also planned not to give in to her teenagers' requests for favors at the expense of her daily program.

Indications and Contraindications. Candidates for this protocol often have mechanical findings such as muscle spasm or limitation of movement on physical examination. Surface EMG evaluation often indicates muscle tension or spasm when engaging in activities such as extension, flexion, or rotational movements that involve the use of affected muscles. A clear relationship between increased pain and increased muscle tension levels is observed.

There are several contraindications for the muscle reeducation protocol. First, this protocol is usually inappropriate for patient who have undergone prior surgeries involving the pain affected musculature. Surgically cut muscles often result in artifacts that render feedback from the involved muscles invalid. For example, although a patient with prior back surgery may have elevated muscle tension and asymmetrical activity, he may not be a good candidate for surface EMG biofeedback because of muscle denervation. Denervation potentials produce highly variable surface EMG integrated readings. However, if diagnostic EMG with percutaneous electrodes fails to reveal denervation potentials, the patient may be an appropriate candidate for this protocol (15).

Second, this protocol emphasizes the use of self-control strategies on a daily basis. Thus, like the psychophysiological protocol, this protocol is contraindicated if the individual is not motivated due to operant or other factors, and/or lacks the intellectual skills and emotional stability necessary to profit from this learning experience.

REFERENCES

1. Fey SG, Williamson-Kirkland TE, Frangione RM: The return to work of injured workers following comprehensive pain management. Paper presented at the International Association for the Study of Pain Meeting, Seattle, WA, August 31–September 5, 1984
2. Rugh JD: Psychological factors in the etiology of masticatory pain and dysfunction. Invited address, American Dental Association, President's Conference on the Etiology, Diagnosis and Treatment of TMJ Disorders, Chicago, June 1–4, 1982
3. Thomas LJ, Tiber N, Schireson S: The effects of anxiety and frustration on muscular tension related to temporomandibular joint syndrome. Oral Surgery 36:763–768, 1973
4. Mercuri LG, Olson RE, Laskin DM: The specificity of response to experimental stress in patients with myofascial pain dysfunction syndrome. J Dent Res 58:1866–1871, 1979
5. Rao SM, Glaros AG: Electromyographic correlates of experimentally induced stress in diurnal bruxists and normals. J Dent Res 58:1872–1878, 1979
6. Christensen LV: Facial pain and internal pressure of masseter muscle in experimental bruxism in man. Arch Oral Biol 16:1031, 1971
7. Christensen LV: Some effects of experimental hyperactivity of the mandibular locomotor system in man. J Oral Rehabil 2:169–178, 1975
8. Scott DS, Lindeen TF: Myofascial pain involving the masticatory muscles: an experimental model. Pain 8:207–215, 1980

9. Clark GT, Rugh JD, Handelman SL, et al: Stress perception and nocturnal masseter muscle activity. J Dent Res 56 (Special Issue):161, 1977
10. Finch DP, Gale EN: Factors associated with nocturnal bruxism and its treatment. Behav Med 3:385–397, 1980
11. Evaskus DS, Laskin DM: A biochemical measure of stress in patients with myofascial pain–dysfunction syndrome. J Dent Res 51:1461, 1972
12. Lange AJ, Jakubowski P: Responsible Assertive Behavior. Cognitive/Behavior Procedures for Trainers. Champaign, IL, Research Press, 1976
13. Jacobson E: Progressive Relaxation. Chicago, University of Chicago Press, 1938
14. Wolpe J: Psychotherapy by Reciprocal Inhibition. Standford, CA, Standford University Press, 1958
15. Wolf SL, Nacht M, Kelly JL: EMG feedback training during dynamic movement for low back pain patients. Behav Ther 13:395–406, 1982
16. Wolf SL, Basmajian JV, Russel TC, et al: Normative data on low back mobility and activity levels: implications for neuromuscular reeducation. Am J of Phys Med 58:217–229, 1979
17. Keefe FJ, Block AR, Williams RB, et al: Behavioral treatment of chronic low back pain: clinical outcome and individual differences in pain relief. Pain 11:221–231, 1981
18. Keefe FJ, Schapria B, Williams RB, et al: EMG-assisted relaxation training in the management of chronic low back pain. American Journal of Clinical Biofeedback 4:93–103, 1981
19. Nouwen A, Solinger J: The effectiveness of EMG biofeedback in low back pain. Biofeedback & Self Regulation 4:103–112, 1979
20. Basmajian JV: Muscles Alive: Their Functions Revealed by Electromyography (fourth edition). Baltimore, William & Wilkins, 1979
21. Basmajian JV, Kukulka CG, Narayan MG, et al: Biofeedback treatment of foot drop technique after stroke compared with standard rehabilitation technique. Arch Phys Med Rehabil 56:231–236, 1975

Chapter 20

Analgesics in Chronic Pain

Randal D. France, M.D.
K. Ranga Rama Krishnan, M.D.
Ananth N. Manepalli, M.D.

Chronic pain patients frequently use a variety of analgesics. An understanding of the pharmacology, therapeutic rationale, and toxicology is essential for the appropriate use of these agents in chronic pain patients. A number of misconceptions and fears exist regarding the use of analgesic medication, especially opioid analgesics in chronic pain. When a patient has acute pain from an organic basis, physicians frequently use the medications without hesitation. Even under these conditions they tend to underestimate the severity of the pain complaint and often threat the pain with both an inadequate dose and inappropriate frequency. The primary fear in the physician's mind is that the patient will abuse the analgesic and become addicted. This fear is most prominent in treating chronic pain patients, which produces a limited evaluation of the pain complaint. This restricted assessment of the patient and the pain complaint can lead to unwarranted use of analgesics. For a more detailed discussion on substance abuse in chronic pain patients, see Chapter 12.

It must be kept in mind that opioids and other analgesics may be beneficial for some patients in chronic pain and help them lead productive lives. In assessing a given patient, one must bear in mind the individual's characteristics, including personality, drug-seeking behavior, presence of affective disorders and other psychiatric illnesses, plus the etiology of the chronic pain, before deciding on a particular type and regimen of analgesic use. This chapter provides a review of the clinical pharmacology of analgesics so that physicians can make intelligent and medically rational use of these drugs.

We will first discuss the nonsteroidal anti-inflammatory analgesic drugs, to be followed by a review of opioid analgesics.

Nonsteroidal Anti-Inflammatory Analgesics in Chronic Pain

Nonsteroidal anti-inflammatory analgesic (NSAIA) drugs are commonly used in the management of chronic pain, sometimes appropriately and at other times inappropriately. Many of these drugs, while useful in modulating peripheral pain in the acute states, are less useful in modulating chronic pain. In general, the efficacy of these drugs in most types of chronic pain can best be described as unproven and equivocal. Many of the nonsteroidal anti-inflammatory analgesic drugs have both anti-inflammatory and analgesic action, while others have primarily an analgesic effect. Drugs belonging to the former class are more useful than those belonging to the latter class in treating chronic pain secondary to inflammatory processes such as rheumatoid arthritis. As many of these NSAIAs are available as over-the-counter preparations, they are commonly used (abused) by patients with chronic pain syndromes.

In this section we will briefly review some of the commonly used NSAIAs.

415

Classification

Nonsteroidal anti-inflammatory analgesics can be classified in several different ways. A simple and practical classification is given in Table 1.

Salicylates

The three common salicylates used as analgesics are acetylsalicylic acid (aspirin), salicylic acid, and methyl salicylate. Of these, acetylsalicylic acid is the most commonly used.

Acetylsalicylic acid (aspirin).   Although some pharmacologists have contended that the analgesic effect of salicylates might be centrally mediated (1), at the present time it is generally held that the site of action

Table 1.   Classification of Nonsteroidal Anti-inflammatory Analgesic Drugs Based on Therapeutic Use

---

Salicylates—Anti-inflammatory Antipyretic Analgesics
  Acetylsalicylic acid (aspirin)
  Salts of salicylic acid
  Sodium and magnesium salicylate
  Choline magnesium trisalicylate
  Methyl salicylate diflumisal

Propionic Acid Derivatives—Anti-inflammatory
  Ibuprofen
  Naproxen
  Fenoprofen

Pyrazolone Derivatives—Anti-inflammatory
  Phenylbutazone
  Oxyphenbutazone

Indole Derivatives—Anti-inflammatory
  Indomethacin
  Sulindac

Tolmetin Sodium

Para-aminophenol Derivatives—Antipyretic Analgesics
  Acetaminophen
  Phenacetin

Anthranilic Acid Derivatives—Antipyretic Analgesics
  Mefenamic acid
  Fenfenamic acid

---

is probably both central and peripheral. Lim and colleagues (2) have reported that salicylates interfere with pain reception and/or transmission at the peripheral receptors. In addition, salicylates inhibit the synthesis of prostaglandin by acetylating cyclooxygenase. This reduces inflammation and reduces pain secondary to inflammatory processes. Acetylsalicylic acid is the most potent of the salicylates in anti-inflammatory action.

The primary indication for aspirin is acute pain of mild to moderate severity. Its utility in chronic pain is unclear. In general, in our opinion, the drug is not effective in the management of chronic pain that is not associated with inflammatory processes. It is effective for rheumatoid arthritis and osteoarthritis. The dose for rheumatoid arthritis is 2.6 to 5.2 grams per day in divided doses. The contraindications are: 1) hypersensitivity to salicylates; 2) bleeding ulcers; and 3) hemophilia. A complete list of side effects is beyond the scope of this book; however, of the many side effects of chronic salicylate use, salicylism is an important one to note. Mild, chronic salicylate intoxication is termed salicylism. The condition can occasionally be seen in chronic pain patients taking large doses of salicylates. The syndrome is characterized by headache, ringing in the ears, impaired hearing, lassitude, fatigue, thirst, hyperventilation, nausea, vomiting, epigastric pain, diarrhea, restlessness, cognitive impairment, and dimness of vision. When the intoxication is severe, delirium, hallucinations, and convulsions may occur.

Diflunisal. This is a derivative of salicylic acid. It is a peripherally acting nonopioid steroidal analgesic. The primary indications are: 1) acute pain of mild to moderate severity; 2) chronic pain secondary to osteoarthritis and rheumatoid arthritis; and 3) other chronic pain syndromes (efficacy uncertain). The dose commonly used is 500 mg to 1.5 grams per day in divided doses.

The side effects include: 1) gastrointestinal—nausea, vomiting, abdominal pain, and peptic ulcer; 2) central nervous system—headache, dizziness, vertigo, and, in rare cases, depression; 3) skin—rash, pruritus, and stomatitis; and 4) miscellaneous—tinnitus, fatigue, edema, and transient visual disturbances. The side effects appear to be related to length of treatment.

Propionic Acid Derivatives

These drugs are primarily anti-inflammatory analgesics. They are useful for the relief of mild to moderate pain. Ibuprofen, naproxen, and fenoprofen are the three propionic acid anti-inflammatory analgesics. The mechanism of action of these drugs is still unknown.

Ibuprofen. The indications are for rheumatoid arthritis, osteoarthritis, and relief of mild to moderate pain. Ibuprofen is also useful for primary dysmenorrhea. The efficacy for other chronic pain syndromes is uncertain. The dose used is 300 to 600 mg three to four times a day. The side effects are: 1) gastrointestinal—bleeding, peptic ulcer, nausea, and vomiting; 2) central nervous system—depression, headache, and somnolence; 3) cardiovascular system—peripheral edema and water retention; 4) hematological—anemia, leukopenia, and thrombocytopenia; 5) ophthalmological—blurred vision and corneal deposits; and 6) hepatic—transient elevation of serum glutamic-oxaloacetic transaminase (SGOT), serum glutamic-pyruvic transaminase (SGPT), lactic acid dehydrogenase (LDH), and alkaline phosphatase activity. Skin rash can occur quite commonly.

Fenoprofen. The indications for fenoprofen are the same as those for ibuprofen. The dose is 300 to 600 mg three to four times a day. The maximal dose is 3200 mg a day. The contraindications are the same as for ibuprofen. In addition, it should not be used in patients with impaired renal function or in patients with impaired hearing. The side effects are similar to those of ibuprofen. In addition, nephrotic syndrome, dysuria, hematuria, and allergic nephritis have been reported in patients on fenoprofen. Headache has been reported to occur in about 15 percent of patients.

Naproxen. The indications are similar to those for ibuprofen. Naproxen's efficacy in chronic pain syndromes is uncertain. The dosage is 250 to 375 mg twice daily. The maximum dose is 1250 mg per day. The contraindications and side effects are similar to those of ibuprofen. Drowsiness is quite common among patients on naproxen. Tinnitus and pruritus are also common side effects.

Pyrazolone Derivatives

The two main drugs belonging to this class are phenylbutazone and oxyphenbutazone. Neither drug is indicated for chronic pain of a noninflammatory nature. Even when the pain is secondary to inflammatory processes, the drug should be used with caution.

Both drugs are contraindicated in children. Hypersensitivity to the drugs is another contraindication. A number of medical conditions also preclude the use of the drug. These include incipient cardiac failure, blood dyscrasias, temporal arteritis, senile dementia, pepitc ulcer, and severe renal, cardiac, or hepatic disease. In elderly patients, drug treatment should be discontinued as quickly as possible due to the high risk of severe, often fatal, side effects. The side effects are: 1) gastrointestinal—vomiting, constipation, epigastric pain, parotitis, and peptic ulcer; 2) hematological—anemia, thrombocytopenia, leukopenia, agranulocytosis, aplastic anemia, and hemolytic anemia; 3) skin—rash, erythema multiforme, and purpura; 4) cardiovascular—salt and fluid retention, hypertension, pericarditis, and interstitial myocarditis; 5) renal—glomerulonephritis, nephrotic syndrome, and hematuria; and 6) endocrine—thyroid hyperplasia, hyper- and hypothyroidism. In addition, numerous other severe side effects and hypersensitivity reactions have been reported. Thus, if the drug is used, several precautions to assess occurrence of their side effects is essential. In addition, numerous interactions with other drugs have been reported. This necessitates caution when using these drugs concomitantly with other drugs.

Indole Derivatives

Sulindac. The indications for sulindac are similar to those for ibuprofen. Its efficacy in chronic pain syndromes, not secondary to clear peripheral nociceptive processes, is uncertain. The dose is 150 to 200 mg twice daily. The contraindications and side effects are similar to those of ibuprofen. Diarrhea has been reported to occur among patients taking sulindac.

Indomethacin. The drug is used to treat moderate to severe rheumatoid arthritis. It should not be used in the treatment of other chronic pain syndromes, as the efficacy is uncertain and potential toxicity is high. The dose is 50 to 200 mg in divided doses. The contraindications for indomethacin are similar to those for ibuprofen. It should not be used in patients with peptic ulcer disease. The side effects are similar to those of ibuprofen. Indomethacin can invalidate the dexamethasone suppression test by producing false negatives. It has been reported to cause depression and should be avoided if possible in chronic pain patients, especially those vulnerable to depression. Headache has been reported to occur in about 10 percent of patients. Indomethacin can mask the development of infection. Indomethacin can elevate plasma lithium levels secondary to reduction in renal lithium clearance. Indomethacin can reduce the antihypertensive effect of beta-blockers and thiazide diuretics, and it is also reported to aggravate parkinsonism and epilepsy.

Tolmetin Sodium. The indications are for rheumatoid arthritis and osteoarthritis. Efficacy in other chronic pain syndromes has not been proven. The dose is 400 mg three times a day. The contraindications and side effects are similar to those of ibuprofen. Unlike other nonsteroidal anti-inflammatory analgesics, tolmetin does not alter prothrombin time. Headache is reported to occur in about 10 percent of patients on tolmetin.

Para-aminophenol Derivatives

The two main derivatives clinically used are phenacetin and acetaminophen. Of the two, acetaminophen is more popular. Phenacetin has a higher potential for renal toxicity. Irreversible renal damage following long-term use has been reported with phenacetin. It is usually available as part of various combination drugs. Phenacetin is reported to increase pain threshold.

The mechanism of analgesic action of these drugs is unclear, but is believed to be primarily peripheral. These drugs do not have the same anti-inflammatory potency as aspirin; thus, they are not as effective as aspirin for chronic arthritic pain. Among the various nonsteroidal anti-inflammatory analgesics, these drugs are probably the one most commonly used by chronic pain patients. Their efficacy in the treatment of headache, musculoskeletal pain, and other acute pain is clear. However, their utility in the long-term management of chronic pain syndromes is uncertain. In chronic pain syndromes secondary to rheumatoid arthritis and osteoarthritis, salicylates are probably more effective.

The dose is 325 to 650 mg every four to six hours for both phenacetin and acetaminophen. The drugs are contraindicated in patients with glucose-6-phosphate dehydrogenase deficiency. Although safe when used in therapeutic doses, the drugs can cause acute hepatic necrosis in excess, and severe liver damage can occur (3). Repeated administration can cause a headache and a hangover. These drugs can impair concentration, attention, and retention. Anxiety is said to be diminished with use of these drugs. They may, on occasion, cause drowsiness and sedation. Hematologic, gastrointestinal, and cardiovascular effects are rare. Para-aminophenol derivatives at one time were considered to be a major cause of analgesic nephropathy, characterized by interstitial nephritis, tubular and papillary necrosis, and chronic pyelonephritis. At the current time, it is not certain whether acetaminophen should be singled out as the main cause of these side effects. It is noted that most of these cases occurred following chronic long-term use of analgesic drug mixtures.

Anthranilic Acid Derivatives

Mefenamic acid is one of the anthranilic acid derivatives. The drug is primarily used as an analgesic rather than as an anti-inflammatory. It is used for short-term treatment of moderate pain. Its utility in chronic pain syndromes has not been demonstrated. The dose is 250 mg four times a day given after meals. It is contraindicated in patients with hypersensitivity to nonsteroidal anti-inflammatory analgesics and impaired renal function. The side effects are similar to those of ibuprofen. Mefenamic acid may cause diarrhea, rash, and hematological abnormalities. It can give false positive test results for proteinuria when the sulfosalicylic acid test is used.

In summary, nonsteroidal anti-inflammatory analgesics, which have anti-inflammatory properties, are useful in the management of rheumatoid arthritis/osteoarthritis when there is an inflammatory process. Nonsteroidal anti-inflammatory analgesics may be useful in short-term management of musculoskeletal pain and headache. Their use in the management of chronic pain syndromes of central or peripheral origin has not been proven. They are not useful in the management of pain seen in psychiatric disorders. It must be kept clearly in mind that although these drugs are widely used, their usage is not necessarily indicated for their efficacy. Another issue is the trade-off between therapeutic effects and risk.

OPIOID ANALGESICS IN CHRONIC PAIN

This section presents the pharmacological properties the physician should be familiar with when prescribing opioid analgesics for use in chronic pain states. The use of opioid analgesics in the management of chronic pain, especially cancer pain, is indicated when less potent analgesics fail to relieve the pain. In nonmalignant chronic pain states, the continuous use of opioid analgesics remains controversial (4). Some physicians and patients are reluctant to use opioid analgesics for fear of habituation and drug dependency (5–7). In many instances, exaggerated concerns about physical dependency cause the physician to prescribe low and infrequent doses of opioid analgesics (5, 7–16). Concomitantly, many physicians believe that opioids prescribed on an as-needed basis minimize the overall dose of opioid analgesics and tolerance, and yet provide effective pain control. This is an erroneous concept that usually leads to poor utilization of pain medications and control of pain (13, 17, 18). Opioid abuse in general medical practice is uncommon despite the frequent use of these drugs (5, 6, 11, 17, 19, 20). In addition, opioid drugs are not positively reinforcing to normal subjects as they are to narcotic addicts (21).

If opioid analgesics are indicated in the management of chronic pain states, the physician and patient need to be aware that habituation and possible physical dependency will occur. For a more detailed discussion of opiate abuse, see Chapter 12. When the guidelines noted in Table 2 are followed, opioid analgesics can be used effectively and safely for the management of pain. Opioid analgesics, when used as part of a comprehensive treatment approach for the management of chronic pain, minimize the potential for abuse and dependency. In using opioid analgesics, a good understanding of the clinical pharmacology of these drugs is required.

Pharmacology

The use of opium dates to antiquity. The word *opium* is derived from the Greek word *opion,* meaning the juice of the poppy. Opium is obtained

Table 2.   Guidelines for Opioid Analgesic Use in Chronic Pain

---

1. Identifiable cause of chronic pain
2. Failure of nonopioid analgesic to relieve pain
3. Negative history of alcohol or substance addiction
4. No concomitant use of minor tranquilizers or sedative hypnotics
5. Informed consent of parent
6. Treatment initiated with weak opioid analgesic
7. Avoidance of parenterally administered medications
8. Progress to potent opioid analgesic after failure of weaker agents
9. Regular follow-up visits
10. Stabilized maintenance dose low
11. Records of type, frequency, and prescription of opioid analgesics
12. Use of nonmedical therapeutics for chronic pain

---

from the milk-like exudate of the incised unripe seed capsule of the poppy plant (Papaver somniferum). The milky juice is air-dried, forming a brownish gummy mass. Further drying produces a powder containing the alkaloids morphine and codeine (Table 3). In 1803, Serturner isolated morphine and in 1832, Robiguet discovered codeine. The term *opiate* refers to the naturally occurring alkaloids, morphine and codeine, plus the semisynthetic congeners of morphine (oxycodone, diacetylmorphine, and hydromorphine). Synthetic morphine-like drugs are designated as opioid drugs. The term *narcotic* is derived from the Greek word for stupor, referring to the group of strong morphine-like analgesics. Since the development of synthetic opioid analgesics and mixed agonist, and antagonist analgesic drugs, the term has little meaning. The word *opioid* is the term now applied to exogenous substances binding specifically to the opiate receptor and producing agonist action (22).

Mechanism of Action

Opioid agonists bind to opiate receptors in the central nervous system (CNS). Opiate receptors are unevenly distributed throughout the CNS, with the highest concentration of receptors in the limbic system (temporal cortex, amygdala, hippocampus), thalamus, hypothalamus, midbrain, and spinal cord (23–25). The affinity of the opioid analgesics for the opiate binding sites correlates with their pharmacological activity (11, 22). Opioid analgesics that have a high affinity for the opioid receptor have significant analgesic properties. The binding sites appear to be the normal sites for the endogenous opioid substances, met-enkephalin, leu-enkephalin, and beta-endorphin.

Pert and Snyder, in 1973, demonstrated the presence and activity of the opioid binding sites in brain membrane (26). Opioid antagonists compete with the opioid agonist for positions at the opioid binding site. Snyder has suggested that the relative ability of an opioid to have antagonistic versus agonist properties is predicted by the effects of sodium on the drugs binding to the receptor (27). Sodium markedly increases the binding of opiate antagonists while decreasing the binding of pure agonists. This interaction may be of value in the development of opioid antagonists that have effective analgesic properties without the risk of dependency.

There are five known opioid receptors: mu, delta, sigma, kappa, and epsilon (see Chapter 5) (28, 29). Morphine and its derivatives bind mainly with the mu receptors. Other opioid agents have been shown to bind with the delta, sigma, and kappa receptors. It is known that sodium selectively inhibits opioids that bind to high affinity sites and has little or no effect on low affinity binding sites (30). It has been suggested that those receptors with high affinity sites are responsible for analgesia and low affinity sites are responsible for many of the undesirable effects of opioids (sedation and respiratory depression) (31). With these new findings, new opioids may be developed that have effective analgesic properties without the unwanted side effects such as respiratory depression and sedation.

Table 3.   Classification of Opioid Analgesics

Natural opium alkaloids
  morphine
  codeine

Semisynthetic analogues of natural opium alkaloids
  oxycodone
  hydromorphine
  hydrocodone
  oxymorphine
  diacetylmorphine

Synthetic compounds
  methadone
  meperidine
  levorphanol
  fentanyl
  propoxyphene

Mixed agonist–antagonist compounds
  pentazocine
  butorphanol
  nalbuphine
  buprenorphine

Central Nervous System

Exogenous opiates induce mood alterations, analgesia, drowsiness, and mental clouding (Table 4). The euphoric effects produced by these drugs is variable, and often in pain-free patients dysphoria may be produced. Patients in pain will report a decrease in the intensity and discomfort of the pain or disappearance of the pain. As the dose of the opiate is increased, the analgesic effects of the drug, as well as the sedating, mental clouding, and mood changes, will be magnified. Opiate analgesics have been shown to increase the level of pain threshold in experimentally induced pain (32), but these effects have not been seen in other studies (33). Clinically, a moderate dose of morphine is quite effective in relieving pain. Dull continuous pain is relieved more effectively than sharp, intermittent pain, but with an increase in the dose, severe colic can be relieved (22). Not only is the painful sensation altered by opiates, but the affective response is also modified (22). With a lessening of the fear, anxiety, and suffering associated with pain, the patient's tolerance to pain will increase. Slurred speech and incoordina-

Table 4.   Pharmacological Effects of Opioids

Central Nervous System
   Analgesia
   Mental clouding
   Mood changes
   Drowsiness
   Nausea/vomiting
   EEG changes
   Miosis
   Respiratory depression
   Suppression of cough

Cardiovascular
   Orthostatic hypotension

Gastrointestinal Tract
   Decrease in biliary and pancreatic secretion
   Decrease in pulsitive peristalsis in small and large intestines
   Increase sphincter tone
   Increase tone of biliary tract smooth muscle

Other Effects
   Increase tone urinary tract smooth muscle
   Increase vesicular sphincter tone
   Release of histamine
   Dilation of cutaneous blood vessels

tion is unusual with opioid analgesics. The absence of slurred speech distinguishes the sedating effects of opioids from those of sedative hypnotic drugs (33).

Another CNS effect of opioids involves stimulation of the chemoreceptor trigger zone producing nausea and vomiting. The opioids also act on the respiratory center in the brain stem, inducing respiratory depression. This effect increases as the dose is advanced. Irregular breathing may occur when opioids are used in therapeutic levels (22). However, respiratory depression of clinical significance is rarely reported in patients with severe pain, even with large doses of morphine (34). Opioids suppress the cough reflex. An opioid's ability to suppress coughing may vary in its potency to suppress respiration (17). Miosis occurs with opioid administration, and tolerance to the miotic effects is limited (22). Heroin addicts continue to have constricted pupils. Opioids produce altered temperature regulation (21). Opioids increase voltage and lower frequencies on the EEG (35).

Opioids stimulate the release of antidiuretic hormone and urinary output falls (Table 5). Opioids inhibit the adrenocorticotropin hormone (ACTH), decrease secretion of corticotropin-releasing factor (CRF), and decrease adrenal cortical activity (36–38). The stress-induced release of ACTH is also blocked by opioids (22). The opioid antagonist (naloxone) increases the level of ACTH and cortisol (39). Chronic morphine administration results in a decrease in the level of urinary 17-ketosteroids and 17-hydroxycorticosteroids, with the development of some tolerance to this effect (40). During chronic administration of opioids, plasma concentrations of cortisol may be within normal ranges (22). During the withdrawal syndrome, there is a marked increase in plasma in urinary 17-hydroxycorticosteroid and in urinary 17-ketosteroids (37, 38). Morphine inhibits the release of thyroid-stimulating hormone (TSH) (40).

Table 5. Opioid Effects on the Endocrine System

Secretion Of:	Opioid Agonist	Opioid Antagonist
Corticotropin-releasing factor (CRF)	↓	
Adrenocorticotropin hormone (ACTH)	↓	↑
Plasma cortisol	↓	↑
Thyroid-stimulating hormone (TSH)	↓	
Luteinizing hormone (LH)	↓	↑
Follicle-stimulating hormone (FSH)	↓	↑
Growth hormone	?	
Antidiuretic hormone (ADH)	↓	

↓ = decrease   ? = unknown
↑ = increase

Opioids suppress the release of luteinizing hormone (LH) and follicle-stimulating hormone (FSH), and enhance the release of prolactin (41). Naloxone increases the plasma concentrations of LH and FSH (41).

Cardiovascular System

Opioids have little effect on the heart. They do lessen peripheral vessel resistance leading to vasodilatation. Orthostatic hypotension may occur. Cerebral circulation is not affected (22).

Gastrointestinal Tract

Opioids diminish biliary and pancreatic secretions. The propulsive peristaltic waves of the small intestine and colon are diminished. This promotes increased water absorption from the bowel content. These factors account for constipation and there is little or no tolerance to this effect. The tone of the atrium of the stomach, sphincter of Odi, ileocecal valve, and anal sphincter is increased. The pressure in the biliary tract is greatly increased. Patients may develop epigastric pain after administration of opiates by the induction of biliary colic. This pain is relieved by naloxone or nitroglycerine.

Other Effects

Opioids increase the spasm of urinary tract smooth muscle and the vesicular sphincter tone. Clinically, urinary retention may develop, especially in patients with prostatic disease. Histamine release is caused by opioids and may be responsible for the pruritus and sweating seen after a dose of opioids. Opioids dilate cutaneous blood vessels and induce warmth and flushing in patients taking opioids. Ciliary activity is diminished and bronchial motor tone is increased with opioid use. These effects, plus suppression of the cough reflex, can lead to pulmonary congestion, especially in patients with chronic obstructive pulmonary disease.

Tolerance and Physical Dependency

With the repeated administration of opiate drugs, tolerance and physical dependency will develop. Tolerance occurs when the opiate drug is given repeatedly and there is an increase in the dose of the drug to produce the same desired effects, or the same dose of the drug produces a decrease in effect after repeated administration (42). The tolerance to the CNS effects (analgesia, sedation, respiratory depression, and mood alteration) of opiates does not occur at similar rates and does not necessarily occur in a uniform pattern (19). Tolerance to the opiate effects of miosis and constipation develops slowly or not at all (22, 43). Tolerance is initially exhibited clinically by a shortening of the duration of action (6). Cross-tolerance among the opiates does occur and changing agents appear to have little effect on the lessening of tolerance (42). Although cross-tolerance does occur with the opiates, this appears not to be complete in chronic cancer pain patients (6). If a cancer pain patient develops tolerance to an agent, it may be useful to change to another opiate to increase the analgesic effect. The development of tolerance is quite variable from patient to patient (42). The rate in which tolerance develops is dependent upon the dose, frequency of dose, and duration of treatment (11, 22, 42). Physical dependency refers to the physiological state that develops with continuous use of the opiate, and repeated administration of the drug is necessary to prevent the appearance of the withdrawal syndrome. The withdrawal syndrome (rebound hyperexcitability) of opiates is characterized by: request for the drug; lacrimation; rhinorrhea; yawning; sweating; restlessness; dilated pupils; anorexia; gooseflesh; tremor; nausea and vomiting; periods of chills and fever; muscle spasms; and cramps) (Table 6). The request for the drug during the withdrawal period is highly dependent upon the setting and patient. Hospitalized or medically ill patients express little demand for opiate drugs during the withdrawal period (19). Physical dependency develops simultaneously with tolerance. Tolerance to opioid drugs is an indication that the patient has some degree of physical dependence.

For morphine and its derivatives, withdrawal symptoms develop 8–12 hours after the last dose of opioid and reach their peak in 48–72 hours. Minor symptoms may be present for seven days. The time course of withdrawal symptoms varies from one opioid to another (19). Generally, the longer the duration of action of the opioid, the more slowly withdrawal symptoms develop, and intensity of symptoms is less (19). Methadone withdrawal symptoms may occur 24–48 hours after the last dose and continue with minor symptoms for about three weeks (43). Meperidine, which has a relatively short duration of action, has the appearance of withdrawal symptoms three hours after the last dose, and peak intensity is 8–12 hours. Minor symptoms may be present for four to five days. Muscle spasm and fewer gastrointestinal symptoms occur more frequently with meperidine withdrawal than with morphine (44).

The severity and type of withdrawal symptoms when the opioids are discontinued are dependent upon the type of opioid drug, total daily dose, frequency of dose, duration of use, and health and personality of the patient. Mild withdrawal symptoms include anxiety, lacrimation, rhinorrhea, sneezing, sweating, and yawning. Moderate withdrawal symptoms include all of the mild withdrawal symptoms plus anxiety, nausea, tremor, gooseflesh, and dilated pupils. Severe withdrawal symp-

Table 6. Clinical Characteristics of Opioid Withdrawal

Early	
Anxiety	Rhinorrhea
Lacrimation	Sweating
Restless sleep	Yawning
Prior to Peak	
Anorexia	Gooseflesh
Dilated pupils	Restlessness
Irritability	Tremor
Peak	
Insomnia	Increased irritability
Anorexia	Nausea and vomiting
Diarrhea	Abdominal cramps
Sneezing	Weakness
Violent yawning	Lacrimation
Fever	Periods of chills and flushing
Gooseflesh	Increased heart rate
Muscle cramps	Increased blood pressure
Musculoskeletal pain	
Late	
Depression	Diminished self-confidence
Irritability	Somatization
Weakness	

toms include all of the previously mentioned withdrawal symptoms, plus vomiting, diarrhea, abdominal pain, muscle spasms and pain, elevated blood pressure, fever, and chills (see Table 6). The withdrawal symptoms appear with the discontinuation of the opiate or administration of an opioid antagonist (naloxone). The higher the degree of physical dependency, the lower the dose of opioid antagonist needed to precipitate withdrawal symptoms. After the withdrawal of opioids is complete, the tolerance to these drugs disappears. Cross-dependency between the opioids allows for the substitution of one opioid for another, and a dose-equivalent basis without the emergence of the withdrawal syndrome.

The time required to produce physical dependency on an opioid is variable. Medically ill patients receiving full therapeutic doses of morphine (20–40 mg daily) for one to two weeks usually have subclinical to mild withdrawal symptoms on discontinuation of the drug. These mild withdrawal symptoms are insomnia and slight irritability. The symptoms are fewer if the drug is slowly tapered or if an opioid is used that is slowly eliminated (methadone). For discussion on the treatment of withdrawal syndrome and detoxification from opiate drugs, refer to Chapter 21.

Abuse Liability

All opiate agonists have abuse potential. The abuse potential varies considerably among the opioid analgesics. Morphine and its derivatives have a higher index for abuse compared to codeine and propoxyphene, and agonist–antagonist drugs (pentazocine, butophanol, nalbuphine, and buprenorphine) (45–47). The abuse potential for an opioid drug is not based on one property but on a combination of several factors. These factors include: 1) ability of the drug to produce physical dependency and its absence to induce drug-seeking behavior; 2) ability of the agent to suppress the withdrawal of other opiates; 3) degree to which it produces euphoria; 4) type of toxicity produced by the drug; and 5) physical characteristics of a particular opioid (that is, water solubility would determine whether the drug could be used by the parenteral route (29). For a more detailed discussion on the abuse and addiction to opioid drugs, see Chapter 12.

Absorption, Distribution, Metabolism, and Excretion

All opiates are absorbed from the gastrointestinal tract (48, 49). In addition, they are readily absorbed from the nasal mucosa, lung, and after subcutaneous and intramuscular injection. However, opioids differ widely in the extent of biotransformation to inactive metabolites as they are absorbed from the gastrointestinal tract (48, 49). The metabolism of opiates occurs in the liver, and it is this first pass-through phenomenon that accounts for the difference in potency of the oral (PO) versus intramuscular (IM) route of administration. The oral to intramuscular (PO/IM) potency ratio for morphine, hydromorphine, and oxymorphine is 1:5 to 1:6. The PO/IM potency ratio for methadone, oxycodone, buprenorphine, and levorphanol is 1:2. For meperidine, pentazocine, and codeine the PO/IM potency ratio is 1:3. It is important to keep these potency ratios in mind when changing from one opioid to another and when changing routes of administration. Failure to do so will result in incorrect dose and poor pain control. The duration of action is also modified by first-pass effect, and when the drug is given parenterally it is prolonged as compared to when the drug is given by oral route (50).

Opioids are bound to plasma proteins in an unbound state (48, 49). Free opioids accumulate quickly in the kidney, lung, liver, spleen, and muscle tissue. The short-acting opioids (such as morphine) do not persist in the tissue, and tissue accumulation after the last dose is low within 24 hours. The plasma half-life of the opioids varies considerably (51). Morphine, pentazocine, meperidine, hydromorphine, codeine, and butorphanol have a plasma half-life in a range of two to four hours, whereas methadone, levorphanol, and propoxyphene have a range of 15 to 30 hours. Opioids are detoxified to inactive metabolites in the liver. Certain opioids are metabolized to active metabolites such as codeine, heroin, oxycodone, meperidine, and propoxyphene (52). Metabolism of opioids in the liver can be altered by certain drugs. Diphenylhydantoin increases the metabolism of meperidine (53), methadone metabolism is increased by rifampin (54), and opioid metabolism is decreased by certain anti-depressants (55, 56). The clearance of opioids is delayed in patients over the age of 50 (57, 58). In patients with impaired liver function (cirrhosis), there is an increase in the plasma half-life and a decrease in the systemic clearance of the opioid drugs (48, 59, 60). However, Patwarda and colleagues (60) did not observe toxic accumulation of morphine when used in cirrhotic patients. This possibly suggests, and is yet to be proven, an extrahepatic metabolism of opioids.

The major route of elimination for the active and inactive metabolites of opioids is by renal excretion (48, 49). Less than 10 percent is found in the feces (22). Patients with impaired renal function have a resulting accumulation of opioids (17). In summary, patients with cirrhosis (61, 62), renal failure (63), and the aged (64, 65) have increased sensitivity to opioid agonists and the dose and frequency of administration should be adjusted accordingly.

OPIOID ANALGESICS IN CLINICAL USE

Morphine

Morphine is the protype of the strong opioid analgesics and is commonly used to treat acute pain by the parenteral route (Table 7). Due to the reduced potency by the oral route, oral morphine has limited use in chronic pain states. However, oral morphine for the control of chronic cancer pain can provide effective pain relief if the dose is increased by a factor of five to six times the effective parenteral dose of morphine. The duration of effective analgesia is three to five hours. Sustained release preparations of morphine sulfate are now available for use. If a patient is on a stable morphine dose and in a stable clinical state, the sustained preparation has the advantage of a less frequent administration schedule.

Meperidine

Meperidine is similar in its pharmacological properties and clinical use to morphine (Table 7). Meperidine is one-eighth as potent as morphine and one-third as potent orally as parenterally. The duration of action is shorter than that of morphine. Unlike morphine, meperidine is associated with CNS hyperactivity including seizure, tremor, and muscle

Table 7. Opioid Analgesics: Comparison of Dosage, Duration of Action, Time of Peak Effects, and Equianalgesic Dose to Morphine

Generic Name	Trade Name	Route	Dose (mg)	Duration of Action (hr)	Peak Effects (hr)
morphine		I.M.	10	4–5	0.5–1
		P.O.	60	4–5	1.5–2
meperidine	Demerol	I.M.	75–100	2–4	0.5–1
		P.O.	225–300	2–4	1.0–2
codeine		I.M.	120	4–6	0.5–1
		P.O.	200–240	4–6	1.5–2
methadone	Dolophine	I.M.	7.5–10	4–6	0.5–1
		P.O.	20	4–6	1.5–2
oxycodone		I.M.	10–15	4–5	1
		P.O.	30	4–5	1
levorphanol	Levo-dromoran	I.M.	2	4–5	0.5–1
		P.O.	4	4–5	0.5–1
hydromorphine	Dilaudid	I.M.	1.5	4–5	0.5–1
		P.O.	7.5	4–5	1.5–2
diacetylmorphine (heroin)		I.M.	3–5	3–4	0.5–1
		P.O.	60	3–4	1.5–2

Route:
  P.O. = oral
  I.M. = intramuscular

twitching. It also has an atropine-like effect. Meperidine produces less constipation and urinary retention than does morphine. In addition, meperidine has less of an effect on the spasm of the biliary tract, and a diminished rise of pressure in the common bile duct. Meperidine has little antitussive activity. Older patients have an increased sensitivity to meperidine (64). Normeperidine, the metabolite of meperidine, has greater CNS excitation than does meperidine. The accumulation of meperidine and normeperidine can lead to toxicity in patients with renal failure. This can lead to a clinical state characterized by stuper and seizures (66). Meperidine should be the preferred opiate analgesic in patients with biliary or ureteral colic and prostatic hypertrophy, and where constipation is to be minimized. However, its use should be limited in patients with renal failure, liver disease, and in the elderly. Meperidine should be avoided in patients receiving MAO inhibitors.

Codeine

Codeine is effective for mild to moderate pain. It is one-twelfth as potent an analgesic as morphine (Table 7). Ten percent of codeine is metabolized to morphine by the liver. Codeine has a low affinity for the opioid receptor, and the conversion to morphine may account for the analgesic effect of codeine (67). The oral parenteral ratio for codeine is 2:3, and duration of action is four to six hours (22). Codeine is an effective analgesic for mild pain, and intensity of the withdrawal symptoms is milder than with morphine. Codeine has significant constipating and antitussive effects.

Methadone

Methadone, a synthetic opioid analgesic, is similar in potency to morphine by the parenteral route (68) (Table 7), and possesses similar pharmacological properties to morphine. The oral to parenteral ratio is 1:2, making it an effective analgesic by the oral route. The side effects caused by methadone are similar to those caused by morphine. Tolerance appears to develop more slowly to methadone than to morphine (22). The overall abuse potential of methadone is similar to that of morphine (43). The duration of action to a single dose is four to six hours, and plasma half-life is 15 to 20 hours (69). Regular doses of methadone increase the plasma half-life to two to three days (70). Repeated doses of methadone may result in marked sedation (44). When methadone is given in repeated doses, it is more potent than morphine because of the cumulative effect of methadone. This effect increases the duration of action to six to eight hours (14). While the cumulative effects of methadone are desirable in providing effective analgesia orally, methadone should be limited in the elderly and demented patients, and patients with respiratory, hepatic, and renal failure. Cimetidine (14) and diazepam (71) inhibit the metabolism of methadone, and rifampicin increases the metabolism of methadone (54). Methadone is an excellent oral analgesic producing steady blood levels over six to eight hours. Little or no impairment of cognitive function (memory, visual, and motor perceptual skills) were seen in the study by Lambordo and colleagues with methadone at doses seen in clinical practice (72).

Oxycodone

Oxycodone is a semisynthetic morphine-like opioid that is an effective oral analgesic, with an oral to parenteral ratio of 1:2 (Table 7). The duration of action is four to six hours. Oxycodone is commonly mixed with either aspirin or acetaminophen in oral preparations. Oxycodone is slightly less potent than morphine and 10 to 12 times more potent than codeine.

Levorphanol

Levorphanol is four to eight times as potent as morphine via parenteral administration (Table 7). It has similar pharmacological properties to morphine (73). Oral potency is one-half the parenteral dose; duration of action is six hours. These two characteristics make it a useful agent in the management of chronic pain. Levorphanol may produce less nausea and vomiting than morphine.

Hydromorphine

Hydromorphine is eight times as potent as morphine and has a shorter duration of action (four hours) than morphine. The drug is one-fifth as potent orally as parenterally.

Propoxyphene

Propoxyphene, a derivative of methadone, is a commonly used oral analgesic, especially in combination with aspirin, acetaminophen, and caffeine (Table 7). Propoxyphene is available in the hydrochloride or napsylate form. Propoxyphene hydrochloride is more readily absorbed than napsylate but the peak concentration of the true drugs are similar (22). Propoxyphene is absorbed after oral and parenteral administration. The duration of action is 4 to 5 hours and the mean half-life after oral administration is 12 hours (22). Parenterally, 240 mg of propoxyphene is equipotent to 10 mg of morphine. After oral administration, 30 to 70 percent of the drug is eliminated by the first pass effect. Propoxyphene is one-half to two-thirds as potent as codeine, and 65 mg of propoxyphene hydrochloride is approximately as effective as 650 mg of aspirin (17). Propoxyphene is recommended for mild to moderate pain. Dependency liability of propoxyphene is less than that for codeine (17).

Agonist–Antagonist Opioids

Agonist–antagonist opioids are agents that have agonist effect (morphine-like) and, when given with a pure agonist opioid (morphine), they have antagonistic properties. There are currently four agonist–antagonist opioids approved for use as analgesics: pentazocine, butorphanol, nalbuphine, and buprenorphine (Table 8). The agonist–antagonist drugs can be divided into two types based upon their subjective and objective actions: morphine and nalorphine-types. Buprenorphine is the

Table 8.   Agonist-Antagonist Opioid Analgesics: Comparison of Dosage, Duration of Action, Time of Peak Effects, and Equianalgesic Dose to Morphine

Generic Name	Trade Name	Route	Dose* (mg)	Duration of Action (hr)	Peak Effects (hr)
pentazocine	Talwin	I.M.	60	4–5	0.5–1
		P.O.	180–300	4–5	1.5–2
nalbuphine	Nubain	I.M.	10	4–5	0.5–1
butorphanol	Stadol	I.M.	2	4–5	0.5–1
buprenorphine	Buprenex	I.M.	0.4	6–8	0.5–1
		S.L.	0.8	6–8	2.0–3

Route:
  P.O. = oral
  I.M. = intramuscular
  S.L. = sublingual

* Dose is equivalent to 10 mg of morphine I.M.

morphine-type and pentazocine, butorphanol, and nalbuphine are the nalorphine-types. The morphine-type has no antagonist activity at low dose and the nalorphine-type has antagonist properties at any dose. It is important to be aware of the opioid analgesic being used and to avoid using an agonist–antagonist in a patient chronically receiving a pure agonist drug. This combination may precipitate a withdrawal syndrome.

   Buprenorphine.   This morphine-type agonist–antagonist analgesic has similar effects to morphine. Buprenorphine has a high affinity for the opioid receptor. Parenterally it is 25 to 50 times more potent than morphine and has a relatively low sealing effect as compared to morphine (74). The abuse potential of the agent is less than that of morphine-like agonists. The duration of action is six to eight hours, and the sublingual dose is 50 percent as potent as the dose given by the parenteral route. Currently, buprenorphine is an investigational drug but in clinical studies it has been proven to be an effective analgesic in acute and chronic pain syndromes (47). Although respiratory depression has not been a major problem in clinical studies, the respiratory depression is not readily reversed even with high doses of naloxone (4–16 mg) (75). Psychotomimetic effects are rare with buprenorphine (47). A major advantage to this drug, when available, will be the sublingual form in chronic pain patients. The ease of administration and long duration of action provide major benefits for these patients. However, more clinical studies in chronic pain patients need to be performed to establish its clinical usefulness.

Pentazocine. Pentazocine was the first agonist–antagonist analgesic to be available in the U.S. It is a nalorphine-type agonist–antagonist drug. The drug is effective at relieving moderate pain. Pentazocine is absorbed well by all routes of administration, but first pass metabolism reduces the bioavailability of the drug by 80 percent when given orally. Approximately 10 percent of hospitalized patients receiving pentazocine for analgesia develop psychotomimetic effects (76, 77). This reaction includes dysphoria, vivid dreams, nightmares, hallucinations, delusions, and panic. Naloxone 10–15 mg can reverse these effects (22). High doses of pentazocine cause increase in blood pressure and heart rate unlike the morphine analgesics. The abuse potential for pentazocine is lower than that for morphine, but drug dependency can occur.

Other Agonist–Antagonist Analgesics. Butorphanol and nalbuphine are nalorphine-type agonist–antagonist analgesics. They are effective parenterally in moderate to severe pain, and present studies indicate usefulness in acute pain states but not in chronic pain. They have similar psychotomimetic effects to pentazocine. On chronic administration they produce physical dependency.

Opioid Analgesics in Combination with Other Drugs

The addition of an opioid analgesic in combination with certain adjunctive drugs enhances analgesia. Aspirin or phenacetin increase the analgesic effects of opioids (78). These drugs are frequently combined with oxycodone, codeine, and propoxyphene. Hydroxyzine produces additive analgesic effects to morphine (79, 80). Hydroxyzine has analgesic properties of its own (80). In postoperative patients, 100 mg of IM hydroxyzine has analgesic activity similar to 8 mg of morphine (81). Parenteral morphine 5 mg and hydroxyzine 100 mg provide analgesia similar to morphine 10 mg in postoperative patients (82).

Dextroamphetamine (10 mg IM) combined with morphine enhances its analgesic effects in postoperative pain (83). This enhancing effect occurs also when small amounts of morphine are used. In chronic pain patients where the dose of opioid is high, or when sedation and lack of concentration are present, the addition of 2.5–5 mg of dextroamphetamine in the morning and midday can be of benefit. It is wise to avoid late afternoon and bedtime doses of dextroamphetamine due to its alerting effect. Tolerance to this effect can develop, and in the cancer pain patient the dose may need to be increased. Benzodiazepines do not produce additive analgesic effects with morphine, but the sedating effects are additive (84). As stated in Chapter 18, phenothiazines do not enhance the analgesic activities of morphine. However, the antiemetic properties of neuroleptics are effective in controlling the nausea associated with opioid use. Twycross demonstrated that cocaine, when combined with a narcotic, does not provide additive analgesia effects (81).

Opioid analgesia has been shown to be potentiated by antidepressants in numerous studies (85–101). In vitro and animal studies suggest that there may be at least two mechanisms responsible for this effect:

1. inhibition of opioid biotransformation: antidepressants inhibit the hepatic metabolism of opioid drugs, prolonging the bioavailability of the drug and thereby potentiating its effect (91).
2. alteration of monoamines, especially serotonin, in the central nervous system.

Opioid analgesia is affected by changes in serotonin and norepinephrine in the central nervous system. Antidepressants block serotonin and norepinephrine reuptake, thus increasing synaptic concentrations of norepinephrine and serotonin. This has been postulated as the reason for potentiation of opioid analgesia. It has been suggested that alterations in serotonin may be more important for analgesia than changes in norepinephrine (see Chapter 4). This appears to be the case even for the potentiation of opioid analgesia. Antidepressants that primarily block norepinephrine reuptake do not potentiate as consistently or effectively as opioid analgesia, as antidepressants are more specific serotonin reuptake blocks (85–89, 91–93, 95–97, 100–103). Kellstein and colleagues (97) studied the effects of acute and chronic administration of clomipramine and desipramine on the potentiation of opioid analgesias in rats. Acute administration of both antidepressants shared enhancement of opioid analgesia, but with continued administration of antidepressants, the potentiation decreased. After a washout period, the enhancement returned. This study suggested that the increase in monoamines in the CNS with antidepressants may not be the sole reason for potentiation of opioid analgesia. Opioid analgesics, when combined with antidepressants, neuroleptics, benzodiazepines, sedative hypnotics, and alcohol enhance the opioid depressant effects (Table 9). When opioid analgesics are combined with antidepressants or neuroleptics, there is a potentiation of hypotensive effects.

Administration of Opioid Analgesics in Chronic Pain

More effective pain control can be achieved in chronic pain provided the analgesic is administered on a time-contingent basis rather than on an as-needed basis. The dose and frequency of dose is individualized according to the duration of action, efficacy of the analgesic, and physical health and response of the patient. Opioid analgesics with a long dura-

Table 9. Interaction of Opioid Analgesics with Other Drugs

Drug	Effect
Heterocyclic antidepressant	Potentiate orthostatic hypotension Enhance opioid depressant effects Potentiate opioid analgesia
Neuroleptic	Enhance opioid depressant effects Potentiate hypotension
MAO inhibitors	Enhance opioid depressant effects Toxic syndrome (meperidine)
Benzodiazepines	Enhance opioid depressant effects Reduce opioid analgesia (?)
Sedative-hypnotics	Enhance opioid depressant effects
Alcohol	Enhance opioid depressant effects
Amphetamines	Potentiate opioid analgesia

tion of action and effective orally (methadone, oxycodone, codeine, and levorphanol) are preferred. Careful titration of the dose and selection of the drug can minimize the development of tolerance and other undesirable side effects. The "pain cocktail" is an effective method to administer opioid analgesics to chronic pain patients. The pain cocktail is a mixture of aqueous opioid analgesics diluted in a liquid vehicle (cola or cherry syrup) given at regular intervals. Adjuvant medications (acetaminophen, hydroxyzine, neuroleptics) can be added to the pain cocktail to treat side effects (nausea) and potentiate the effects of the opioid analgesics (Table 10). The pain cocktail with a progressive decrease in the opioid analgesic is an effective method to detoxify and discontinue the use of opioid analgesics in patients with chronic pain. In patients who have been on opioid analgesics for a long period of time and have physical dependency to them, a decrease in the total daily dose of the opioid analgesic by 10 percent every two to three days provides smooth effective taper of the drug. For additional discussion and methods for opioid withdrawal, see Chapter 21. This approach, combined with behavioral strategies, is an effective means of treating the chronic pain patient (104). No tolerance to the constipating effects of opioid analgesics develops. Constipation can be controlled by fiber diet, stool softeners, or occasional use of laxatives. Patients on continuous opioid analgesics, especially when combined with nonsteroidal anti-inflammatory drugs, often develop peripheral edema. Low sodium diet or reduction in the dose of either drug

Table 10.   Example of "Pain Cocktail" in the Treatment of Chronic Pain

Medication:	methadone (1 mg/cc) hydroxyzine (25 mg/5cc)
Vehicle:	cola
Frequency of Dose:	q. 6 hours
Schedule:	methadone 5 mg (5 cc) plus hydroxyzine (5 cc) in 20 cc of cola given every 6 hours P.O.

can control this effect. Although tolerance may develop with the continuous use of opioid analgesics, opioid abuse and addiction is seldom a problem in chronic pain patients with organic symptomatology (1, 105).

In patients with chronic benign states who have anxiety, depression, and/or severe character pathology, the potential for abuse is high and opioid analgesics are not effective drugs for the management of pain. Similarly, caution should be exercised in prescribing opioid analgesics to patients who have a history of substance abuse. Informed consent from the patient should be obtained before using opiates for the management of chronic pain. The patient needs to have a clear understanding of the possible side effects, habituation, and physical dependency that may occur with opioid drugs. More potent opioid analgesics (methadone, morphine, oxycodone) should be used only when weaker opioid analgesics do not provide effective pain control. Regular follow-up visits are essential to monitor dose, to prevent or minimize tolerance, and to monitor side effects. The goal is to establish the lowest effective maintenance dose with a minimum of side effects.

Guidelines from the Federal Bureau of Narcotics state that physicians may use narcotics to relieve acute pain. Physicians directly in charge of patients suffering from a chronic disease can use opioid analgesics for the relief of pain over an extended period if the doses are kept within limits accepted by other physicians, and if proper care and reasonable precautions are taken to prevent illicit diversion of the drugs (106). It is advisable that physicians document the indication for continuous use, maintain records of the drugs used, and obtain consultation for the use of opioid analgesics in chronic pain patients (107).

CONCLUSIONS

In this chapter we presented an overview of the pharmacology, rationale for analgesic use, and the practical aspects of analgesic management in chronic pain. It is important to keep in perspective the distinction between analgesic use and abuse in chronic pain patients. For effective management of these patients, it is important not to confuse use with abuse, so that patients needing analgesics receive them in an appropriate manner, and so that patients whose analgesic use is likely to complicate their management do not receive analgesics inappropriately. Chapter 12 addresses the issue of analgesic abuse in chronic pain patients. Chapter 21 discusses and presents strategies for the management of opioid dependency as it pertains to chronic pain patients.

REFERENCES

1. Dubas TS, Parker JM: A central component in the analgesic action of sodium salicylate. Arch Int Pharmacodyn Ther 194:117–122, 1971
2. Lims RKS, Gruzman QW, Rogers T, et al: Site of action of narcotic and non-narcotic analgesics determined by blocking bradykinin evoked visceral pain. Arch Int Pharmacodyn Ther 152:25–58, 1964
3. Prescott LF: Poisoning with salicylates, paracetamol and other analgesics. Prescribers Journal 19:169–178, 1979
4. France RD, Urban BJ, Keefe FJ: Long term use of narcotic analgesics in chronic pain. Soc Sci Med 19:1379–1382, 1984
5. Perry SW: The undermedication for pain. Psychiatric Annals 14:808–811, 1984
6. Houde RW: The use and misuse of narcotics in the treatment of chronic pain. Advances in Neurology, vol 4. Edited by Bonica JJ. New York, Raven Press, 1974
7. Dewi-Rees W: The distress of dying. Br Med J 3:105–107, 1972
8. Beaver WT: Management of cancer pain with parenteral medication. JAMA 244:2653–2657, 1980
9. Twycross RG: Relief of terminal pain. Br Med J 4:212–214, 1975
10. Reuler JB, Girard DE, Nardone DA: The chronic pain syndrome: misconceptions and management. Ann Intern Med 93:588–596, 1980
11. Stimmel B: Pain Analgesics and Addiction. New York, Raven Press, 1983
12. Marks RM, Sachar EJ: Undertreatment of medical inpatients with narcotic analgesics. Ann Intern Med 78:173–181, 1973
13. Shimm DS, Logue GL, Maltbie AA, et al: Medical management of chronic cancer pain. JAMA 241:2408–2412, 1979
14. Twycross RG: Narcotics, in Textbook of Pain. Edited by Wall PD, Melzack R. London, Churchill Livingstone, 1984
15. Cohen FL: Postsurgical pain relief: patient's status and nurses's medication choices. Pain 9:265–274, 1980
16. Arivatonakul K, Weis OF, Alloga JL, et al: Analgesia or analgesic use in the treatment of postoperative pain. JAMA 250:926–929, 1983
17. AMA Division of Drugs: General analgesics, in AMA Drug Evaluation. Chicago, American Medical Association, 1983
18. Charap AD: The knowledge, attitudes, and experience of medical personnel treating pain in the terminally ill. Mt. Sinai J Med 45:561–580, 1978

19. Jaffe JH: Drug addiction and drug abuse, in The Pharmacological Basis of Therapeutics. Edited by Gilman AG, Goodman LS, Gilman A. New York, 1980

20. Porter J, Jicks H: Addiction rare in patients treated with narcotics. N Engl J Med 302:123, 1980

21. Smith GM, Beecher HK: Subjective effects of heroin and morphine in normal subjects. J Pharmacol Exp Ther 136:47–52, 1962

22. Jaffe JH, Martin W: Opioid analgesics and antagonists, in The Pharmacological Basis of Therapeutics. Edited by Gilman AG, Goodman LS, Gilman A. New York, 1980

23. Beaumont A, Hughes J: Biology of opioid peptides. Annu Rev Pharmacol Toxicol 19:245–267, 1979

24. Snyder SA: The opiate receptor and morphine-like peptides in the brain. Am J Psychiatry 135:645–652, 1978

25. Terenius L: Endogenous peptides and analgesia. Annu Rev Pharmacol Toxicol 18:189–204, 1978

26. Pert CB, Snyder SH: Opiate receptor: demonstration in nervous tissue. Science 179:1011–1014, 1973

27. Synder SH: Opiate receptors and internal opiates. Scientific American 236:44–56, 1977

28. Chang K-J, Cooper BR, Hazum E, et al: Multiple opiate receptors: different regional distribution in the brain and differential binding of opiates and opioid peptides. Mol Pharmacol 16:91–104, 1979

29. Chang K-J, Cuatrecasas P: Multiple opiate receptors. J Biol Chem 254:2610–2618, 1979

30. Pert CB, Pasternak GW, Snyder SH: Opiate agonists and antagonists discriminated by receptor binding in brain. Science 182:1359–1361, 1973

31. Pasternak GW: Endogenous opioid system in brain. Am J Med 68:157–159, 1980

32. Gracely RH, McGrath D, Dubner R: Narcotic analgesia: fentanyl reduces the intensity but not the unpleasantness of painful tooth pull sensations. Science 203:126–1263, 1978

33. Beecher HK: The Measurement of Subjective Responses: Quantitative Effects of Drugs. New York, Oxford University Press, 1959

34. Walsh TD, Baster R, Bowman K, et al: High-dose morphine and respiratory function in chronic cancer pain. Pain Suppl 1:39, ;1981

35. Fink M, Zaks A, Volavka J, et al: Electrophysiological studies in man: opiates and antagonists, in Narcotic Drugs, Biochemical Pharmacology. Edited by Clouet D. New York, Plenum Press, 1971

36. Zis AP, Haskett RF, Albala AA, et al: Escape from dexamethasone: possible role of an impaired inhibitory opioid mechanism. Prog Neuropsychopharmacol Biol Psychiatry 7:563–568, 1983

37. Eisenman A, Fraser HF, Brooks JW: Urinary excretion and plasma levels of 17-hydroxycorticoids during a cycle of addiction to morphine. J Pharmacol Exp Ther 132:226–231, 1961

38. Wexler BC: Effects of bacterial polysaccharide (Piromen) on the pituitary adrenal axis: modification of ACTH release by morphine and salicylates. Metabolism 12:49–56, 1963

39. Volavka J, Cho D, Mallya A, et al: Naloxone increases ACTH and cortisol levels in man. N Engl J Med 300:1056–1057, 1979

40. George R: Hypothalamus: anterior pituitary gland, in Narcotic Drugs, Biochemical Pharmacology. Edited by Clouet D. New York, Plenum Press, 1971

41. Bruni JF, Von Vugt D, Marshall S, et al: Effects of naloxone, morphine, methionine enkephalin on serum prolactin, luteinizing hormone, follicle stimulating hormone, thyroid stimulating hormone, and growth hormone. Life Sci 21:461–466, 1977

42. Jaffe JH: Narcotics in the treatment of pain. Med Clin North Am 52:33–45, 1968

43. Martin WR, Jasinski DR, Haertzen CA, et al: Methadone—a reevaluation. Arch Gen Psychiatry 28:286–295, 1973

44. Isbell H, White WM: Clinical characteristics of addiction. Am J Med 14:558–565, 1953

45. Deem J, Blasig J, Herz A: Buprenorphine: demonstration of physical dependence liability. Eur J Pharmacol 70:293–300, 1981

46. Graham JDP, Lewis JW: The assessment of abuse potential drugs of the opiate type, in Pain: New Perspectives in Measurement and Management. Edited by Harcus AW, Smith R, Whittle B. Edinburgh, Churchill Livingstone, 1977

47. Zola EM, McLeod DC: Comparative effects and analgesic efficacy of the agonist–antagonist opioids. Drug Intell Clin Pharm 17:411–417, 1983

48. Misra AL: Metabolism of opiates, in Factors Affecting the Action of Narcotics. Edited by Adler ML, Manara L, Samanin R. New York, Raven Press, 1978

49. Way EL, Alder TK: The pharmacologic implications of the fate of morphine and its surrogates. Pharmacol Rev 12:383–446, 1960

50. Houde RW, Wallenstein SL, Beaver WT: Clinical measurement of pain, in Analgetics. Edited by de Stevens G. New York, Academic Press, 1965

51. Inturrisi CE: Narcotic drugs. Med Clin North Am 66:1061–1071, 1982

52. Inturrisi CE, Foley KM: Narcotic analgesics in the management of pain, in Analgesics: Neurochemical, Behavioral and Clinical Perspectives. Edited by Kuhar M, Pasternak G. New York, Raven Press, 1984

53. Pond SM, Kretschzmor KM: Effects of phenytoin on meperidine clearance and normeperidine formation. J Clin Pharmacol Ther 30:680–686, 1981

54. Kreek MJ, Garfield JW, Guljahr CL, et al: Rifampin-induced methadone withdrawal. N Engl J Med 294:1104–1196, 1976

55. Goldstein FJ, Mojaverian P, Ossipav MH, et al: Elevation in analgetic effect and plasma level of morphine by desipramine in rats. Pain 14:279–282, 1982

56. Leu SJ, Wang RIH: Increased analgesia and alterations in distribution and metabolism of methadone and desipramine in the rat. J Pharmacol Exp Ther 195:94–104, 1975

57. Brunks SF, Delle M: Morphine metabolism in man. Clin Pharmacol Ther 16:51–57, 1974

58. Kaiko RF, Wallenstein SL, Rogers AG, et al: Narcotics in the elderly. Med Clin North Am 66:1079–1089, 1983

59. Neal EA, Meffin PHJ, Gregory PB, et al: Enhanced bioavailability and decreased clearance of analgesics in patients with cirrhosis. Gastroenterology 77:96–102, 1979

60. Pond SM, Tang T, Benowitz NL, et al: Presystemic metabolism of meperidine to normeperidine in normal and cirrhotic subjects. Clin Pharmacol Ther 30:183–188, 1981

61. Patwardan RV, Johnson RF, Hayumpa A, et al: Normal metabolism of morphine in cirrhosis. Gastroenterology 81:1006–1011, 1981

62. Laidlow J, Read AE, Sherlock S: Morphine tolerance in hepatic cirrhosis. Gastroenterology 40:389–396, 1961

63. Fabre J, Balont L: Renal failure, drug pharmacokinetics and drug action. Clin Pharmacokinet 1:99–120, 1976

64. Mather LE, Tucker GT, Pfug AE, et al: Meperidine kinetics in man. Clin Pharmacol Ther 17:21–30, 1975

65. Kaiko RF: Age and morphine analgesia in cancer patients with postoperative pain. Clin Pharmacol Ther 28:823–826, 1980

66. Szeto HH, Inturrisi CE, Houde RW, et al: Accumulation of normeperidine, an active metabolite of meperidine in patients with renal failure or cancer. Ann Intern Med 86:738–741, 1977

67. Findlay JWA, Jones EC, Butz RF, et al: Plasma codeine and morphine concentrations after therapeutic oral doses of codeine-containing analgesics. Clin Pharmacol Ther 24:60–68, 1978

68. Nathon PW: Newer synthetic analgesic drugs. Br Med J 2:903–908, 1952

69. Inturrisi CE, Verebely K: Disposition of methadone in man after a single oral dose. Clin Pharmacol Ther 13:923–930, 1972

70. Inturrisi CE, Verebely K: The levels of methadone in the plasma in methadone maintenance. Clin Pharmacol Ther 13:633–637, 1972

71. Spaulding TC, Minium L, Kotake AW, et al: The effects of diazepam on the metabolism of methadone by the liver of methadone dependent rats. Drug Metab Dispos 2:458–463, 1974

72. Lombardo WK, Lombardo B, Goldstein A: Cognitive functioning under moderate and low dosage methadone maintenance. Int J Addict 2:389–401, 1976

73. Eddy VD, Halback H, Braenden OJ: Synthetic substance with morphine-like effect—Clinical experience: potency, side-effects, addiction liability. Bull WHO 17:569–863, 1957

74. Jasinski DR, Pevnick JS, Griffith JD: Human pharmacology and abuse potential of the analgesic buprenorphine. Arch Gen Psychiatry 35:501–516, 1978

75. Lewis JW, Rance MJ, Sanger DJ: The pharmacology and abuse potential of buprenophine: a new antagonist analgesic. Advances in Substance Abuse 3:103–154, 1983

76. Woods AJJ, Moir DC, Campell C, et al: Medicine evaluation and monitoring group: central nervous system effects of pentazocine. Br Med J 1:305–307, 1974

77. Taylor M. Galloway DB, Petric JC, et al: Psychotomimetic effects of pentazocine and dihydrocodeine titrate. Br Med J 2:1198, 1978

78. Beaver WT: Mild analgesics: a review of their clinical pharmacology. Am J Med Sci 251:576–599, 1965

79. Beaver WT, Feise G: Comparison of the analgesic effects of morphine, hydroxyzine, and their combination in patients with postoperative pain, in Advances in Pain Research and Therapy, vol. 1. Edited by Bonica JJ, Albe-Fessard D. New York, Raven Press, 1976

80. Kanton TG, Steinberg FP: Studies of tranquilizing agents and meperidine in clinical pain: hydroxyzine and meprobamate, in Advances in Pain Research and Therapy, vol. 1. Edited by Bonica JJ, Albe-Fessard D. New York, Raven Press, 1976

81. Twycross RG, Lack SA: Symptom Control in Far Advanced Cancer: Pain Relief. London, Pitman, 1983

82. Hupert C, Yocoub M, Turgean LR: Effects of hydroxyzine and morphine analgesia for the treatment of postoperative pain. Anesth Analg 59:690–696, 1980

83. Forrest WH, Brown BW, Brown CR, et al: Dextroamphetamine with morphine for the treatment of postoperative pain. N Engl J Med 296:712–715, 1977

84. Singh PN, Sharma P, Geysta S, et al: Clinical evaluation of diazepam for relief of postoperative pain. Br J Anaesth 53:831–835, 1981

85. Spencer PSJ: Some aspects of the pharmacology of analgesia. J Int Med Res 4:1–14, 1976

86. Lee RL, Spencer PSJ: Effects of tricyclic antidepressants on analgesic activity in laboratory animals. Postgrad Med J 56:19–24, 1980

87. Lee RL, Spencer PSJ: Antidepressants and pain: a review of the pharmacological data supporting the use of certain tricyclics in chronic pain. J Int Med Res 5:146–156, 1977

88. Messing RB, Lytle LD: Serotonin containing neurons: their possible role in pain and analgesia. Pain 4:1–21, 1977

89. Ogren SO, Holm AC: Test specific effects of the 5-HT reuptake inhibitors alaproclate and zimelidine on pain sensitivity and morphine analgesics. J Neurol Transm 47:253–271, 1980

90. Malseed RT, Goldstein FJ: Enhancement of morphine analgesics by tricyclic antidepressants. Neuropharmacology 18:827–829, 1979

91. Leu SJ, Wang RH: Increased analgesia and alterations in distribution and metabolism of methadone and desipramine in the rat. J Pharmacol Exp Ther 195:94–104, 1975

92. Sparkes CG, Spencer PSJ: Antinociceptive activity of morphine after injection of biofenic amines in the cerebral ventricles of the conscious rat. Br J Pharmacol 42:230–241, 1971

93. Tofanetti O, Albiero L, Galatulas I, et al: Enhancement of propoxyphene-induced analgesia by doxepin. Psychopharmacology 51:213–215, 1977

94. Bensemana D, Gasion AL: Relationship between analgesics and turnover of brain biogenic amines. Can J Physiol Pharmacol 56:722–730, 1978

95. Tenen SS: Antagonism of the analgesic effect of morphine and other drugs by p-chlorophenylalanine, a serotonin depletor. Psychopharmacologia 12:278–285, 1968

96. Vogt M: The effect of lowering the 5-hydroxytryptamine content of the rat spinal cord on analgesia produced by morphine. J Physiol 236:483–498, 1974

97. Kellstein DE, Malseed RT, Goldstein FJ: Contrasting effects of acute or chronic tricyclic antidepressant treatment on central morphine and analgesia. Pain 20:323–334, 1984

98. Tauvo YO, Fabian A, Pazoles CJ, et al: Potentiation of morphine antinociception by monoamine reuptake inhibitors in the rat spinal cord. Pain 21-329–337, 1985

99. Hatangdi VS, Boas RA, Richard ED: Postherpetic neuralgia: management with antiepileptic and tricyclic drugs, in Advances in Pain Research. Edited by Bonica JJ, Albe-Fessard D. New York, Raven Press, 1976

100. Mayer DJ, Price DD: Central nervous system mechanisms of analgesia. Pain 2:379–404, 1976

101. Larsson AA, Takemori AE: Effects of fluoxetine hydrochloride, a specific inhibitor of serotonin uptake, or morphine analgesia and the development of tolerance. Life Sci 21:1807–1812, 1977

102. Rochat C, Cervo L, Romandini S, et al: Differences in the effects of d-fenfluramine and morphine on various responses of rats to painful stimuli. Psychopharmacology 76:188–192, 1982

103. Spiegel K, Kalb R, Pasternak GW: Analgesic activity of tricyclic antidepressants. Ann Neurol 13:462–465, 1983

104. Fordyce WE: Behavioral methods for chronic pain and illness. St. Louis, C. V. Mosby, 1976

105. Portenoy RK, Foley KM: Chronic use of opioid analgesics in non-malignant pain: report of 38 cases. Pain 25:171–186, 1986

106. Treasury Department, Bureau of Narcotics: Prescribing and Dispensing of Narcotics Under Harrison Narcotic Law: Pamphlet No. 56. Washington, DC, Bureau of Narcotics, 1966

107. Tennant FS, Uelmen GF: Narcotic maintenance for chronic pain: medical and legal guidelines. Postgrad Med J 73:81–94, 1983

Chapter **21**

Management of Opioid Dependence

Randal D. France, M.D.
K. Ranga Rama Krishnan, M.D.

In assessing opioid dependence in chronic pain patients, it is important to keep in mind some of the concepts and definitions discussed in Chapter 12. Once a diagnosis of opioid dependence is established and a treatment decision is made to detoxify the patient, the detoxification can proceed using one of several methods.

Prior to describing various detoxification methods, however, it is advisable for the reader to review some of the common symptoms of opiate withdrawal. A brief listing of the signs and symptoms is given in Table 1. In opioid withdrawal it must be noted that mental functions are almost always intact. Hallucinations, tremors, and delusions are uncommon during opioid withdrawal. The most frequent symptoms seen during opioid withdrawal resemble an influenza-like syndrome lasting a few days. The duration of withdrawal symptoms is related to the pharmacokinetics of each opioid. The intensity of the withdrawal syndrome is dependent on the following: duration of treatment, amount of drug administered, type of opioid, concomitant illnesses, and psychological state of the patient. It is also worth noting that unlike withdrawal from sedatives or alcohol, withdrawal from opioids, although intensely dysphoric, usually occurs without any associated mortality (except in medically ill patients or in patients undergoing withdrawal from multiple drugs where tolerance is present).

METHODS OF DETOXIFICATION

Detoxification Using Methadone

This is the common method used for treating opioid dependence in patients who may or may not have other chronic diseases including pain. Methadone is substituted for whatever opioid is responsible for the withdrawal syndrome, such as codeine, morphine, and the like. Meth-

Table 1. Clinical Features of Opiate Withdrawal Syndrome

Autonomic Symptoms	Psychological	Vital Signs	Other
Piloerection	Severe anxiety	Increased temperature	Yawning
Dilated pupils	Restlessness	Increased pulse	Insomnia
Sweating	Depression	Increased blood	Rhinorrhea
Flushing		pressure	Lacrimation
Diarrhea		Acid base imbalance	Aches and
Abdominal			pains
cramps			Anorexia
			Muscle spasm

adone is then withdrawn gradually over a period of days, weeks, and occasionally months. This withdrawal depends upon the dose and the clinical condition of the patient. To establish a regimen, a small dose of methadone, usually about 5 mg, is given and the effects are noted. The regimen is then constructed on the basis of the clinical observations made. As the dose of opioids involved in dependence increases, the length of the withdrawal regimen is also increased. Another method of recognizing the equivalent dose of methadone to whatever drug was being used can be assessed by using potency ratios. An approximation of the equivalent dosages needed are given in Table 2. The most common initial dose is 5 mg four times a day. Higher doses are rarely necessary. In patients who are using very high doses of opioids, extended withdrawal tends to be better than attempting to withdraw over a short period of time. The relationship between dose level, dose increment, and opioid withdrawal symptoms is not a linear one. It is highly individual and can vary from subject to subject and within subjects at different points in time. Another factor that has to be kept in mind is that as the dose gets lower, one should take time in producing further decreases in dose. In other words, as the amount of methadone is being lowered, and once it reaches very low levels, withdrawal needs to be slowed down even further.

Detoxification Using Pain Cocktail

The use of a pain cocktail is probably the most popular method used for detoxifying chronic pain patients from opioids. The patient is first started on a dose of methadone equivalent to the dose of the opioid he or she has been using. The dose is then gradually tapered over a period of time. The taper is very similar to what we have described under detoxification using methadone. The usual dose of methadone used is 5 mg four times a day. Rarely are higher doses used. An approximation of the equivalent dosages needed are given in Table 2.

Table 2. Relative Potency of Commonly Used Narcotic Drugs

Drug	Half-Life (hrs)	Relative Potency Compared to 100 gm of Methadone
Morphine	1.5 to 2	100
Hydromorphine	2.6	15
Codeine	3	100 times greater
Pentazocine	2–3	600
Meperidine	3–4	800
Propoxyphene	12	2000

The methadone is usually mixed in a sweet and colored base, usually cola or cherry syrup. Sometimes an acetaminophen syrup or elixir is used along with the sweet base. The volume of the sweet base is gradually increased as the dosage of methadone is decreased, so that the volume of medication the patient receives remains the same although the dose has been decreased. Our experience is that this method is probably the most effective one for use with chronic pain patients. For any patient sensitive to methadone, other opioids can be substituted for detoxification. The other opioid that is commonly used (other than methadone) is codeine. Methadone, however, is usually preferred to other opioids in the pain cocktail. Methadone is the logical narcotic for substitution because it is effective orally, it suppresses abstinence symptoms for up to 24 to 32 hours, and it has fewer euphoric effects compared to other narcotics. Methadyl acetate or alpha acetylmethadol (LAAM, a methadone congener) is also effective orally and suppresses opioid withdrawal symptoms for even longer durations up to 72 hours. This drug is, however, not yet commonly used for detoxification in pain patients. When side effects such as sedation or altered mentation occur, this may indicate that the substituted dose is too high. On the other hand, if the substituted dose is not sufficient, sweating is the most common symptom seen. In patients who may be feigning withdrawal symptoms to obtain more opioid or resist detoxification, the clinician should observe for the appearance of gooseflesh and borborygmus. These two withdrawal symptoms are difficult for the patient to reproduce and sustain. As we have noted in earlier chapters, it is best to reduce the dose of the methadone to the minimum required, and once dependence is no longer a problem or when the drug is definitely needed, it should not be kept from the patient. For further details, see Chapter 20.

Opioid Withdrawal Using Alpha Adrenergic Agonist

Gold and colleagues reported that clonidine hydrochloride can ameliorate opiate withdrawal signs and symptoms (1). Clonidine at a dose of 17 μg/kg per day was given in three divided doses by Gold and his colleagues to safely withdraw patients from opioids (2). The protocol that they used requires a 14-day inpatient stay. This method may be a useful alternative to the methods described above. As currently practiced, it begins with a complete cessation of opioid intake with concurrent administration of .1 to .5 mg of clonidine which is given on day one. Over the next 9 to 10 days, the clonidine dose may need to be increased to a maximum of 1 to 1.5 mg per day. After that dose is reached, the clonidine is tapered over a four- to five-day period. Side effects of sedation and postural hypotension can occur in some individuals. This can be managed with a reduction of the dose of clonidine. Gradual reduction of a narcotic with concurrent use of clonidine does not appear to be feasible. This is probably because clonidine and the narcotic potentiate the sedative properties of each other. Another drug that appears useful is lofexidine. This drug is currently being evaluated. It is an alpha-adrenergic agonist that blocks narcotic withdrawal symptoms, but unlike clonidine has less sedation. In chronic pain patients, opioid withdrawal using clonidine is not used commonly. This is because many patients with chronic pain often have other medical problems. These medical problems may preclude the use of clonidine to withdraw from opiates.

Opioid Withdrawal Using Haloperidol

Maltbie and colleagues (3) reported that haloperidol may be used as an adjunctive to safely detoxify patients who are dependent on opioids. In an earlier study, Karkalas and Lal (4) reported that haloperidol 1–2 mg three times a day was as effective as methadone taper in opioid withdrawal. Again, this method may be a useful alternative to using a methadone taper. This method may be more applicable to chronic pain patients.

Opioid withdrawal using propoxyphene napsylate has also been attempted. Propoxyphene napsylate can suppress the narcotic withdrawal symptom. It is a weak opioid agonist; therefore, if it needs to be used to withdraw patients from high doses of other opioids, one would require quite large amounts of propoxyphene, as much as 1 to 1.5 grams a day. At these doses, side effects such as sedation can occur. However, for withdrawal from lower doses, this may be quite an effective drug to use. Since propoxyphene is occasionally used for the management of chronic pain patients, propoxyphene substitution for other opiates prior to withdrawal may be one way of reducing opioid dependence in chronic pain patients.

Long-Term Management of Opioid Dependence

As we noted earlier, opioid dependence per se is very rare in chronic pain patients. When opioid dependence is seen, it is important to investigate what the other antecedents could be in relation to the opioid dependence, such as prior history of drug abuse, drug dependence, and so on. In managing the chronic pain patient with opioid dependence, it is important to evaluate all of these possibilities before trying to manage the patient on a long-term basis. Emphasizing that the drug is primarily effective for treating pain when it is kept within the medium dose range (less than 20 mg of methadone equivalent per day), it is important in these patients to try to keep the methadone equivalent to around 20 mg for the long-term management of chronic pain. In those few patients who use pain as a method of obtaining narcotics, it will be extremely hard to manage these patients unless they are willing to seek treatment for their addiction. However, it would be well worthwhile not to fall in the trap of prescribing the narcotic medications when such circumstances are suspected, especially in individuals who attempt to go doctor shopping in order to obtain narcotics. Long-term management of narcotic dependence is beyond the scope of this book. For further details regarding this, several textbooks are available on the subject.

REFERENCES

1. Gold MS, Pottash AC, Sweeney DR, et al: Opiate withdrawal using clonidine: a safe, effective and rapid nonopiate treatment. JAMA 243:343–346, 1980
2. Gold MS, Redmond DE Jr, Kleber HD: Clonidine in opiate withdrawal. Lancet 1:929–930, 1978
3. Maltbie AA, Sullivan JL, Cavenar JO, et al: Haloperidol treatment of a sixty-year narcotic addiction. Milit Med 144:251-252, 1979
4. Karkala J, Lal H: A comparison of haloperidol with methadone in blocking heroin withdrawal symptoms. International Pharmacopsychiatry 8:248-251, 1973

Chapter **22**

Physiotherapy in Chronic Pain

Linda M. Lawrence, L.P.T.

This chapter delineates the physiotherapy assessment and treatment of chronic pain patients. As noted in Chapter 14, a variety of physical changes occur in chronic pain syndromes. In chronic pain patients one sees physical sequelae not only from the initiating illness or trauma, but dysfunctional syndromes resulting from inactivity and disease. Progression and extension of the physical sequelae seen in dysfunction syndromes often occur with an associated psychiatric disorder (depression) or learned pain behavior (inactivity). Given the interaction of physical and psychological/behavioral impairments in chronic pain patients, an integrated treatment approach is essential to restore or maintain function. Lack of appreciation by the psychiatrist of the physical impairments and treatment methods in physiotherapy, or by the physiotherapist of the psychological/behavioral disorders and psychological treatments of chronic pain patients, can result in incomplete rehabilitation of the patient.

The first section of this chapter addresses the assessment of the chronic pain patient and is followed by a discussion of the appropriate physiotherapy treatments for chronic pain, including exercise, modalities, and back school. Description of the assessment and treatments is brief and, for the interested reader, more detailed explanations may be found in the references listed at the end of the chapter.

The assessment of the chronic pain patient by a physiotherapist will be described. In Chapter 14, the physical sequelae from chronic pain is discussed. A variety of dysfunctional and derangement syndromes can develop in the chronic pain patient. These diverse physical changes require a complete musculoskeletal evaluation for each chronic pain patient. The findings from this assessment are essential to devise a physiotherapy treatment program for the individual requirements of the patient. The assessment includes: 1) history of pain complaints and physical function; 2) observation of gait, posture, and activities; and 3) test of the musculoskeletal system. Each test places stress on selected tissues to determine the involvement in the pain syndrome and their functional ability. This method of testing was initially described by James Cyriax (1). Following the discussion of the assessment, an evaluation of a chronic low back pain patient will be presented.

ASSESSMENT

History

The evaluation begins with a review of the patient's record (Table 1). Interview of the patient is directed to obtain the following information: onset and history of the pain, previous and present treatments, activity limitations, pain description, and history and response to previous phys-

453

Table 1.   Components of the Evaluation

History:	chart review
	subjective complaints
Observations:	general body size, appearance, condition
	posture
	gait
	activities of living
	inspection of body part
	palpation
Functions:	active range of motion
	passive range of motion
	determine end feel
	capsular pattern
	noncapsular pattern
	joint mobility testing
	isometric muscle contractions
Neurological Examination:	traditional manual muscle test
	sensory
	reflexes
	coordination
	balance
Special Tests:	ligamentous stress testing
	compression of joints
	distraction of joints
	muscle length testing
	cardiovascular tests
	pulses
	foraminal closure
	leg length
	circumference testing
	sacroiliac provocation
	dural stretch

iotherapy treatments. Activities of daily living, occupation, participation in physical activities, and positions and activities that affect the pain are discussed in detail. Careful assessment of these data will often identify problems with the musculoskeletal system and help organize proper treatment.

Observation

Observation of the patient's posture, gait, movements, deformities, functional range of motion, appearance, body type, color, and muscle bulk is initially considered. A more detailed evaluation is then started.

Posture. A patient is observed from the front, back, and side to check bony alignment symmetry, curvatures, soft tissue bulk, and presence of deformities. A plumb line helps to visualize alignment problems. A more detailed discussion can be found in a reference book (2).

Gait. Visual observation or video recording of gait patterns is done from three views—front, back, and side. Heel to toe pattern, joint flexion and extension, trunk rotation, step length, center of gravity, and arm swing and cadence are noted. Gait abnormalities imply dysfunction in several of these components. Normal gait requires coordination, a certain amount of muscle strength, joint range of motion, balance, and trunk rotation. The gait evaluation identifies abnormalities and poss ble causes that are more thoroughly assessed during the muscle and joint examination. Devices measuring weight bearing, inked foot prints, force plates, and treadmills may be used to document gait dysfunction.

Activities. Functional movements (squatting, walking up stairs, dressing, lifting, writing, and so on) identify problems in activities of daily living and screen for joint motion strength, body mechanics, and coordination. It may illustrate a discrepancy between the patient's abilities in a natural movement versus their tested functions. This inconsistency may be seen in patients with secondary gain issues, somatoform disorder, malingering, depression, or dementia.

Palpation

Palpation and observation of the painful area are performed for changes in color, temperature, skin texture, circulation and presence of scars, neuromas, infection, abrasions, edema, and deformity. If observations suggest a problem, more specific tests are done. Palpation of bony landmarks, joint lines, and soft tissues determine the presence of deformity, effusion, tenderness, and scar formation with adherence to pain sensitive tissues.

Active Motion

The patient moves the body or part by contracting and relaxing opposite muscles. This places stress on all tissues, both inert (bone) and contractible (muscle). The information gained is the patient's willingness to move, quality of the movement, available active range of motion, and ability of the muscle to perform locomotion. Range of motion may be limited by willingness of the patient, strength of the muscle, pain, or tissue tightness. Individual strength of each muscle group is tested later. Repeated active movements may be needed to evaluate minor injury or symptoms of overuse syndromes.

Passive Range of Motion

The physiotherapist moves the part of the body through the available range of motion while noting the quality and amount of motion. At the limitation in the movement end feel, overpressure is given to determine a comparison to the unaffected side. Examples of end feel include: 1) bone contacting bone; 2) muscular spasm; 3) length or capsular restriction; 4) soft tissue bulk; and 5) empty end feel (subjective complaint that pain limits motion). The pattern of lost motion is examined for capsular and noncapsular patterns. The former involves a proportional limitation of motion in a joint (arthritis or inflamed joint). Noncapsular pattern involves any limitation that does not fit into these proportional limitations (muscle tightness, adhesions, tumor, and so on). Passive range of motion tests eliminate the muscular unit to focus the examination more on the joint and surrounding inert structures.

Muscle Integrity

Resisted motions are done with the joint in a position of rest without joint movement in an attempt to determine whether pain originates from the contractible unit (muscle, tendon, area of bone around the muscle insertion). If the joint moves during this test, it is impossible to determine whether the source of the pain lies in the contractile elements or noncontractile components (joints). Resisting muscle contraction will produce joint compression and possibly cause joint pain resulting in a false positive test.

Possible results include: 1) strong and painless—normal muscle; 2) strong and painful—minor lesion of contractile structure; 3) weak and painless—nerve lesion or old complete tear of muscle or tendon; 4) weak and painful—gross lesion of bone or muscle or chronic pain state; 5) pain with repetition—chronic tendonitis, overuse syndrome, vascular lesion, or minor trauma; and 6) all painful—gross lesion, psychogenic pain, or chronic pain syndrome.

Joint Mobility Testing

Joint mobility testing is a passive examination of the available joint play (3). Each joint has a certain amount of movement not under voluntary control, allowing for motion in the joint. It is tested by passively gliding or distracting joint surfaces. They are classified as follows:

1. fused—no motion
2. hypomobile—a loss in joint motion
3. normal movement

4. hypermobile—some excessive motion in the joint
5. unstable—excessive motion leading to a dysfunctional joint

Neurological Examination

Traditional manual muscle testing is performed and graded as follows:

Grade 0—no palpable contraction
Grade 1—palpable contraction
Grade 2—able to complete range with gravity eliminated
Grade 3—able to complete range against gravity
Grade 4—able to complete range against resistance
Grade 5—able to hold against maximal resistance

These grades must only be given if the proper test position or acceptable variation is used. Retesting under the same conditions becomes more reliable.

Reflexes are tested and comparison to the uninvolved side is made. Reflexes can be scaled as follows:

0—absent
1—diminished
2—normal
3—increased
4—clonus

Light touch, pinprick, temperature discrimination, proprioception, and vibration are components of the sensory examination to be performed. Coordination and balance of limbs, trunk, and head are done.

Special Tests

There are a variety of specific tests for each joint, testing structures that are essential to normal function of the joint. These examinations may involve stress testing of ligament stability, compression/distraction of joint structures, and provocation test of certain joints (sacroiliac joint). Other procedures must be objectively evaluated if a problem is noted. These tests may include: leg length measurements, circumferential measurements, and pulses. A review of radiographic and vascular studies may be of assistance. Before initiating a vigorous exercise program or abrupt changes in a patient's level of activity, the physiotherapist may need the evaluation of the physician on general health status of the patient and stability of the musculoskeletal system. Communication among the treating team members can assure the most comprehensive evaluation of the patient and establish an appropriate physiotherapy program for each patient.

EVALUATION OF A CHRONIC LOW BACK PAIN PATIENT

The physiotherapy evaluation begins with a chart review of the patient's pertinent medical history. Interview with the patient is initiated with a description of the present pain complaints and previous treatments. An assessment of the pain complaints is similar to that outlined in Chapter 16, but a more detailed account of pain modifying positions and activities is obtained. These activities may be associated with work, hobbies, chores, or sports. The patient is asked to estimate the duration of walking, sitting, and standing tolerance without intensifying the pain. The patient can give many clues to the underlying pathology and effective treatment through a discussion of what makes him or her feel better and worse. For example, a patient with an acute posterior lateral disc bulge has more pain while sitting but less with walking short distances, whereas a patient with degenerative disc disease has less pain while sitting and more pain while standing.

Description of previous and present treatments is obtained. Previous physiotherapies are documented as to type (modalities, traction, exercise), duration of treatment, and outcome. It is important to assess the patient's attitude toward physiotherapies. A description and understanding of the family structure is helpful to facilitate a home physical therapy program and utilize the family members to support the patient in the treatment. A history of previous operations to treat the pain is taken. Physical changes prior to and preceding the operations are recorded. Effects of medications or other medical illnesses on the back pain are noted.

The objective evaluation begins with an evaluation of the patient's standing posture by comparing bony landmarks to the plump line. Asymmetries in the postural alignment are noted. Symmetry of shoulder levels, pelvic crest, anterior and posterior superior iliac spines, popliteal creases, and gluteal folds are examined. Asymmetry may indicate leg length discrepancies, scoliosis, muscle tightness, and areas of stretch and compression. From the side position, the patient is viewed for head position, rotation of the shoulders or pelvis, deformities, and cervical, thoracic, and lumbar curvatures. The patient is asked to slowly bend forward to evaluate spinal motion, reversal of curves, muscle length, nerve stretch, and deviations to one side. Side bending is evaluated to see if it is equal in both directions, and if it produces or increases pain symptoms. If pain is elicited on the bending side, then a structure could be pinched; or if the pain is on the opposite side, a structure could be causing pain from stretch. The ability to extend the spine, the amount of motion, and the effect on peripheral pain is assessed. Repeated movements of the trunk help distinguish a bulging disc in a younger person from a dysfunction or postural syndrome. A posterior lateral disc bulge (with an intact annulus) with repeated forward bending should increase the peripheral signs, whereas with a dysfunction (adaptive shortening), pain should be at end range and it will not necessarily increase with these movements (4). With a pure postural syndrome, pain should not be elicited with forward bending unless the position was held for a long period of time.

Gait is evaluated for changes in swing or stance phase, decreased cadence, decreased step length, and an antalgic pattern. Frequently back pain patients will show a decrease in hip and knee flexion during swing, causing excessive circumduction of the leg, abnormal heel to gait patterns, decreased arm swing, decreased trunk rotation or excessive trunk motion, and abnormal alignment, especially with a forward head position. If a patient has a foot drop or weakness in the quadriceps, hip abductors, gastrocnemius, or hip extensors, they can frequently be discovered during observation of gait. The problems are documented for further use in devising a treatment plan. Occasionally, balancing difficulties need to be evaluated in greater detail, especially if the history or the evaluation suggests more neurological problems such as loss of position sense.

In the sitting position, trunk rotation is evaluated and unsupported and supported sitting postures are observed. Muscle strength can be tested for the psoas, quadriceps, hip rotators, tibialis anterior, toe extensors, toe flexors, extensor hallicus, and peroneals. Lower extremity reflexes (quadriceps and ankle jerk) can be tested in this position as well as a plantar response. Sensation to pinprick, light touch, temperature, vibration, and position sense of the lower extremities is tested. In the chronic pain patient, scapulothoracic rhythm is evaluated during arm elevation looking for secondary loss of motion and abnormal patterns of motion. Cervical range of motion is recorded. Cervical and upper extremity strength can be tested, with the exception of the posterior deltoid and scapular muscles, which are tested in the prone position. Sitting straight leg raising is compared to the results in the supine position.

Straight leg raising is again tested and compared with sitting with the patient in the supine position. Dorsiflexion of the foot and head raising are combined with this movement to give more clues to nerve root involvement and dural irritation. Hip range of motion is assessed for secondary loss, tightness on the posterior aspect, and other problems associated with this joint. These may include: degenerative joint disease, bursitis, decreased flexibility, tendonitis, and piriformis syndromes. Upper and lower abdominal muscle strength is recorded. If presenting with possible sacroiliac lesions, compression of the anterior and posterior aspects of the joints should be screened. Pectoralis length, anterior cervical muscle strength, Faber's test, and leg length can also be tested is pertinent to the patient.

In the side lying position, hip abduction and adduction are tested for strength. Tensor fascia latae length is examined. Passive lumbar mobility is done in flexion, extension, rotation, and side bending. This is passively done by the therapist in an effort to determine movement at each segment of the spine and to grade the movement. If a patient has limited spinal motion for a long period, one would expect to see tightening of the facet capsules. This would cause increased joint compression, decreased joint lubrication, pain, and excessive mobility at other spinal levels above or below the injury. This frequently occurs in patients who limit their spinal motion following a lumbar laminectomy. The limited lumbar motion can lead to hyper- or hypomobility and pain in the thoracic region. Muscular and ligamentous tightening is evaluated with both active and passive range of motion tests. If the sacroiliac joint is thought to be a problem, provocation tests can be done by pressing downward on the ilium.

The long sitting position is used to examine the back extensor length, hamstring length, and reversal of the lumbar curve in the forward bent position. The hamstrings are put on slack and the patient bends forward at the lumbar area to assess low back flexibility.

In the prone position, the strength of the gluteus maximus, hamstring, and back extensors are assessed. Prone knee flexion with hip extension is tested for femoral nerve stretch as well as the amount of knee flexion. Passive trunk extension is done with the patient pushing the upper body up with the arms and allowing the stomach to sag toward the plinth. This will determine range of motion and assess for radicular pain. Strength of the scapular muscles and posterior deltoids is examined in this position. The passive lumbar mobility testing can also be done in this position instead of side lying to determine joint play. Pressure on the sacrum and flipping of the iliac crests can be tested to help rule out sacroiliac pathology. Some practitioners prefer to test the ankle jerk in this position. Gastrocnemius and soleus muscle length are checked. Observation and palpation of the back may help give information on muscle tone, histamine reaction, temperature, scar mobility, skin and fascia mobility, and vertebral positional defects.

In addition, the patient's hip flexor length is tested in the Thomas test position with one knee drawn to the chest to the point of flattening the lumbar spine, and the other knee and foot over the end of the bed. One assesses the hip flexion with the knee extended and with it flexed. Compression and distraction of the joints can be done as well as positioning the patient in maximal foraminal closure to see whether peripheral pain increases, which could indicate something in the space pressing the nerve root.

Sleep positions are evaluated for spinal alignment. Transfers out of bed and out of a chair are observed for proper body mechanics. Other activities such as sitting at a desk, reaching to the floor, squatting, climbing stairs, and lifting can be observed.

Cardiovascular endurance should be assessed prior to any vigorous exercise or increase in activity. In many patients this may be a simple assessment of pulse during activity, and in patients with a predisposition for cardiovascular disease, a stress test and electrocardiogram may be suggested.

After the evaluation is completed, abnormalities are identified. Positions and pain are correlated with the findings. Problem areas in posture and activities of daily living are noted. Cardiovascular endurance and other medical problems are assessed. Pain behavior, cooperation of the patient, and the patient's awareness of the problems are noted.

Treatment is prioritized and put into a sequence. For example, if you want to correct an excessive lumbar lordosis but the lumbar extensors are tight and the abdominals are weak, the patient will not be able to correct his or her posture until the lumbar extensors are lengthened and the abdominal muscles are strengthened. The treatment for the problem needs to be addressed in the proper order. The following section describes the treatment for the above-mentioned problems.

Physiotherapy Treatment in Chronic Pain

Physical therapy treatment must begin after a complete evaluation of the patient as described above. The stresses from improper body mechanics and pathological structures are identified and an individualized treatment program initiated. Programs need to be supervised until techniques are well understood by the patient. The physiotherapist designs treatment consisting of a prescribed exercise program, modalities, and back school. The following section will briefly describe exercise selection and type, commonly used modalities, and back school.

Exercise Selection

General exercise programs are minimally beneficial for the chronic pain patient, as they may not address the problem areas. Specific exercises are selected for each patient to meet individual needs. The classification of exercise as seen in Tables 2 and 3 indicates various exercises a physical therapist may select for the most appropriate treatment. Each type of exercise is designed to accomplish the desired goals. For example, if one wants to increase the strength of the quadriceps throughout the knee

Table 2. Types of Exercise (Active)

Free	Cardiovascular
Assisted	Posture
Resisted	Relaxation
isometric	Breathing
isotonic	Gait
isokinetic	Coordination and balance

range of motion, there must be active participation from the patient. To increase muscle strength, resistance must be great enough; otherwise, endurance may be the only gain. For some patients this resistance is the friction of the leg on a powder board; for others, the weight of the leg itself; and for stronger individuals, resistance from an outside source. Isometrics (maximal contraction of the muscle without joint motion) increase strength in one position but there is no carry-over throughout the range. No amount of passive motion will increase the strength of the muscle.

Two major categories of exercise are active and passive movements (Tables 2 and 3). Each category has a wide selection which will briefly be described in order to give the reader some indications on how exercise selection is made. This chapter outlines the various exercises important in the physical therapy program for the chronic pain patient.

Active

Active exercises are done with the patient moving the part of the body by voluntarily contracting and relaxing the muscles (Table 2).

Free.   No external help or resistance is given to the patient. Examples could be movements done with gravity to assist the part or antigravity which would give resistance to the part. Calisthenics are a type of active free exercise.

Assisted.   External assistance is given to help move the part or to control motion. The assistance may be the patient's or another person's uninvolved extremity. Mechanical devices such as pulleys, slings, and springs are another form of assistance.

Resisted.   Movement is performed voluntarily against some form of resistance. Such types of movement include isometric, isotonic, and isokinetic.

Isometric: Isometric is stable resistance without change in muscle length or motion of the joint. This may be done by tightening the muscle without joint motion or by pushing against an immovable object. The strengthening caused by this type of exercise is specific to the position in which it is performed (5). There is no carry-over throughout the range. To increase the strength throughout the range, the exercise must be done at different joint positions.

Isotonic: Isotonic is stable resistance given throughout the range, with the muscle changing lengths. The joints are moved through the range of motion and this will increase the circulation and endurance. This is done with free weights, weighted pulleys, bar bells, and other similar gym equipment. To strengthen the muscles, the resistance must achieve near maximum performance from the muscles. These exercises should always be done with a warm-up set of repetitions (at one-half resistance and then two-thirds prior to maximum resistance) in order to avoid straining the muscles. A cool-down period in the reverse order should be done to help remove metabolic build-up. This will decrease muscle soreness. During the exercise the weight is the same throughout the range and for both concentric and eccentric contractions. There is no accommodation, for varying strength throughout the range of muscles becomes more or less efficient. This means the muscles cannot work at maximum potential throughout the range. The maximum level of strength gained will be that which the part can move at the least efficient angle. Frequently this type of exercise will cause muscle soreness and joint stresses. Advantages include ready availability and low cost. Patients can make or obtain the equipment for home use.

Nautilis equipment is slightly different, since variability in resistance with the use of pullup occurs throughout the range. This piece of equipment is frequently found in health clubs and spas. It has been found to give less muscle soreness. This is not an isokinetic piece of equipment.

Isokinetic: Isokinetic gives accommodating resistance throughout the range while maintaining the speed for the agonist and antagonist muscle groups. It takes into account fatigue, joint angle, inertia, and pain. It allows for exercising at various speeds that are similar to normal functional movements. Patients also do not experience as much muscle sore-

Table 3. Types of Exercise (Passive)

Passive range of motion	Nonthrust articulation
Mobilization	Oscillation
Distraction	Stretch
Traction	Functional
positional	Muscle energy
adjustive	Thrust articulation
inhibitory	
manual	
mechanical	

ness after this exercise. Isokinetic equipment is very effective in rehabilitating sports injuries and patients with chronic pain. The availability of the equipment is limited by its cost. If this equipment is used by the patient while in the hospital, other methods of exercise must be taught for the home program.

Cardiovascular. Cardiovascular exercise is training before the patient's maximum target heart rate is maintained for more than 20 minutes. This is to improve circulation, strengthen the heart so it pumps a greater stroke volume at a reduced heart rate, and improve oxygenation and vital capacity. This type of exercise is also linked to relieving depression, improving absorption and utilization of medication, decreasing body weight, and stimulating the production of endorphins to control pain. All chronic pain patients are started on a program including walking, exercycling, bicycling, or swimming. The choices of walking and bicycling are the least expensive and most readily available. The disadvantages include stress of weather and uneven terrain or hills. If the patient has leg pain, this may aggravate the condition. In addition, the exercycle or bicycle can cause compression by sitting and bicycle handle bars may not be adjustable allowing improper sitting posture. Swimming is a good exercise but frequently is unavailable.

Posture. Posture exercises are listed separately in this classification due to their significance in the chronic pain patient's treatment program. In order to correct poor postural habits, practice is necessary. Frequently supervision by a physical therapist or nurse is needed until the patient is aware of his or her body alignment. Exercises may be in the form of breaking activities into parts and exercising in the functional position, increasing the patient's body image by utilizing mirrors, viewing video tapes, or using plumb lines. Patients are given a new component to practice daily. By breaking the activities into components, it allows the patient to concentrate on one area. The activities are consolidated only after the patient has mastered each of the separate exercises.

Relaxation. Relaxation exercises are emphasized in a pain program. Pain increased tension even in areas remote from the injury or painful part. Patients are frequently unaware of facial tension, shoulder tension, and jaw clenching. This leads to increased muscle tone, increased pain, increased energy requirements, and fatigue. Biofeedback plays an important role in giving patients visual or auditory cues to their tension level. Like all other exercises, the patient must practice for it to be effective.

Breathing. These exercises are components of all exercise. Patients should be encouraged to utilize proper breathing patterns during exercise routines. Pain patients frequently guard, increase their muscle tension, and decrease the depth of each breath. Many pain patients hold their breath during exercise, breathe shallowly, or hyperventilate when in pain. Education, awareness, and practice can help control these patterns. Increasing the depth and slowing the pace may actually increase the oxygen to the tissues and increase relaxation. In patients with thoracic or rib pain, breathing exercise is incorporated to increase rib mobility, increase movement of the costovertebral joints, and increase separation between the ribs.

Activities of daily living, gait, transfers, stairs, squatting, and dressing are broken into parts and practiced as exercise. These may be included in an exercise program. The coordination of movements and improved strength enable the patient to satisfactorily perform the motion. For example, a patient may have the strength in the quadriceps and sufficient range of motion in the foot, ankle, knee and hip, but still be unable to squat. The exercise to practice is one in a functional position, such as a partial squat while getting up and down from a chair, until the patient can perform an isolated squat. Eventually the whole maneuver is done.

Gait Training. Gait is another area where components are isolated to improve the functional movement. Antalgic gait patterns do more harm than good. Patients get into this habit because they think it is easier on the back or leg. Education and retraining in the components of gait can effectively eliminate many of these deviations. This reduces stress on the lumbar complex, decreases energy requirements, and improves walking.

Coordination and Balance. These exercises help improve joint receptors' response to proprioception, speed of righting and protective reactions, weight bearing, and eye-hand coordination. The outcome is improved with controlled functional activities. If a person has not used an extremity for an extended period of time, the receptors are slow in their ability to respond. Exercise includes one-leg balancing, toe walking, reciprocal motions, balance board or beam activities, and ball catching or kicking.

Passive

External forces are applied to a patient's joint or body part to create motion without the assistance or resistance of the individual. Two major categories are passive range of motion and mobilization (Table 3).

Passive Range of Motion. An external force is applied causing a movement of the extremity or body part through all or part of the available range. Frequently it is termed physiological motion. This movement of the joint will change the length of tendons and muscles. The goal is to maintain joint movement and to increase flexibility of muscles. A chronic pain patient usually has dysfunctional joint biomechanics in the affected areas. If passive range of motion is performed by an unskilled therapist, the joint can be subjected to further injury, decrease joint play, and increase pain. Passive range of motion does not increase muscle strength since there is no active contraction of the muscle.

Mobilization. External forces are applied to a joint improving joint mobility and decreasing pain originating in joint structures. Joint play is motion occurring in the joint but not under voluntary control. It is generally limited when loss of motion is due to the joint capsule or ligamentous structures. For example, normally when the arm is actively elevated, the muscle activity causes the humeral head to glide downward on the joint to avoid impingement at the acromion. This downward motion cannot be voluntarily done without the active joint motion. When a person develops a frozen shoulder, the inferior capsule adheres to itself, preventing this downward motion. Whenever the arm is actively or passively elevated, the subacromial tissues are pinched between the humeral head and the acromion causing pain. The only method to restore this joint play is by mobilization. This will cause less pain and a return to normal joint mechanics. There are four types of mobilization: 1) distraction; 2) traction; 3) nonthrust articulation; and 4) thrust articulation.

Distraction: External force perpendicular to the joint line is applied in the direction of the separating joint surface. The external force is graded (1–3) to produce a variable amount of joint motion. A weak force is used for articulation and pain relief. Greater force is used to increase joint motion and decrease compression.

Traction: External forces are applied to separate the joint surfaces. A few types of traction are briefly discussed.

Positional: The joint surfaces are opened by placing the patient in a static position that anatomically opens the joint surfaces. This is used in the cervical and lumbar spine where flexion, rotation, and side bending open the foramin to relieve compression or to stretch structures.

Adjustive: Manual traction is used in conjunction with articulation (thrust or nonthrust). Thrust is designed to relieve structural impingement, float a loose body, or break an adhesion.

Inhibitory: Joint traction is applied with pressure on the muscle tendon to inhibit the stretch reflex and gain muscle relaxation. It is used in tension headaches and cervical pain by placing pressure just below the occipital line.

Manual: Traction is done by a therapist applying an external force in a static (constant) or intermittent (interval) method. Static traction is frequently used for disc lesions or nerve root impingement to create a suction force relieving pressure or stretch structures. Intermittent traction is used for relieving pain by joint stimulation, relaxing muscle tension, or increasing motion.

Mechanical: The traction is done by a mechanical device applying the external force. Methods are similar to manual traction but there is less joint specificity and less control of pain. The advantage is the availability of heavier poundage for longer periods of time. The angle of pull can be in the direction of the long axis of the body or in a three-dimension position to maximize the biomechanics of the joint efficacy of the traction. Poundage for both the manual and mechanical types of traction must be sufficient enough to cause the desired effect. Bed traction with minimal weight is ineffective to cause joint separation.

Nonthrust Articulation. This involves small external forces directed to increase joint play. There are four types: 1) oscillations, 2) stretch, 3) functional, and 4) muscle energy.

Oscillations: In this method, small rhythmic movement is applied by an external force to a joint. The force is graded from one to five. Grades one and two are used for relaxation, pain relief, and stimulation of circulation. Grades three to five are used to increase range of motion, increase joint motion, and break adhesions.

Stretch: This involves large oscillations that occur throughout the range of motion in a joint.

Functional: Articulations are used in normal motion to help increase joint play.

Muscle energy: Muscle contractions are used to move a joint by fixation of the muscle insertion or origin while the free end moves an attached bony structure.

Thrust Articulation: In this method, high velocity external forces are applied to the joint at end range. Thrusting forces are isolated to one joint. These techniques are used to create a suction force, break adhesions, and move a loose body or compressed structure.

Exercise has multiple components. It is essential to recognize the structure one wishes to change and the desired response. Passive joint play can affect an increase in mobility within the joint but not increase the muscle flexibility or strength. Joint range of motion can increase the muscle flexibility but if loss of motion results from a tight joint capsule, it will not be an efficient exercise. After increasing the motion of a joint, one needs to increase the strength in that newly acquired range so that the patient can functionally use the new movement. This will take an active contraction of the muscle. Specificity of the results of each exercise type needs to be remembered and used in the proper place.

EXERCISE PROGRAM

Once problems are identified and treatment sequenced, the exercise mode must be selected which will affect the problem. Duration of the hold, selection of speed, number of repetitions, and frequency need to be established. The patient's activity level is evaluated for a decision on where treatment should occur. If the patient is on an activity/rest cycle of

5 minutes up and 55 down, it is frequently more beneficial to see the patient in his or her room. If the patient is up to 10 minutes or more, that usually allows enough time for the patient to be seen in the physical therapy department.

The advantages of utilizing the physical therapy treatment are the availability of firm exercise mats and other equipment, the stimulation of exercising with other people, and the observation of progress and/or compliance. Equipment may include mirrors, parallel bars, and stairs or ramps for gait training. Weights, milk crates, and shelves at varying levels are used for lifting practice. Weights, pulleys, exercycle, and isokinetic equipment may be used for exercise. A variety of chair styles, foot stools, and lumbar supports are tried for sitting posture. A sink, refrigerator, stove, and cupboards are useful for practice in body mechanics in the kitchen. Also, modalities are available for preparing tissue for exercise. The therapist's time is also used more efficiently when observing several patients at a time. This is cost-effective and encourages a patient's independence with the program.

Patients are taught the rationale behind the exercise and the techniques. A program begins on a level where the patient can succeed, utilizing a small number of exercises and limited repetitions. Written directions are given that patients are expected to bring to physical therapy so they can follow the same directions they will have at home. Decisions as to frequency per day and number of repetitions are discussed with the patient. The extent and duration of the exercise program must not exceed the capabilities of the chronic pain patient. If the exercises are too difficult and the program confusing, the patient's compliance will likely be compromised. A deliberate approach may delay progress in some patients, but promotes compliance in most chronic pain patients. Patients are reminded that their physical problem did not develop overnight and correction of these problems by the exercise program will take time. Progression with the program occurs over a period of several months. After the initial treatment phase, pain patients are seen at three- to six-month intervals for two to three years.

Patients with severe chronic pain limited in function by musculoskeletal problems can achieve a higher level of activity with the application of the proper exercise program extending over two to three years. Even though these patients continue to have some pain and exacerbations of intense pain, improvement in their functioning level occurs. Follow-up visits, monitoring of the exercise program, support from family members, and a goal based on realistic expectations are essential components of a successful program. As the patient progresses in the exercises, functional activities, hobbies, or sports are substituted for specific exercises. If no change has occurred, the types of exercises are modified to make the program more effective. Often changes in frequency and duration of exercise can transform an unsuccessful program to a successful one.

Exercise programs are an important component of the treatment of the chronic pain patient. Generally, these programs are incorporated into pain management programs with both inpatients and outpatients. An inpatient pain program is designed to treat patients with severe pain and physical limitations. These patients usually need a comprehensive physical therapy program to achieve a higher level of physical function. The exercise program is combined with a back school. After the initial evaluation, the pain patient is seen daily in the physical therapy department, and other exercise sessions occur independently on the pain unit. This also allows the patient to assume responsibility for their program.

The physiotherapist supervises and monitors the program of the patient. One or two repetitions of each exercise are reviewed by the physiotherapist to assure proper technique. Patients are given new exercises and these increase in repetition as progress develops. A component of body mechanics is reviewed daily with the patient. This material is also incorporated in the back school. The patients are given assignments that concentrate on one aspect of proper posture so they can practice during the day.

Frequently patients are asked to chart the progress in their program. This can be done by graphing the number of repetitions completed per day. This identifies progress or inconsistencies in the exercise program. The goal should be a line that may have plateaus, but overall, there should be a slow progression. If a patient exercises too vigorously, the graph will show an irregular pattern indicating poor progress. This pattern may also indicate poor technique, poor compliance, or too difficult a program. Graphs give feedback to the patient and other pain team members to encourage the patient's progress. Patients will likely have pain flare-ups requiring a modification in the exercise program. Patients are taught how to manage the flare-ups. During these periods, many pain patients become discouraged. Support from other patients and team members plus skill in management of the pain flare-ups counteract this discouragement.

It is the expectation that the exercise program will continue and not be interrupted by weekend home passes from the hospital or visitors. Emphasis is placed on compliance, and responsibility for the outcome is placed on the patient.

BACK SCHOOL

The back schools vary in content, length, and style, but the concept is to teach a group of individuals body mechanics and ways to care for their backs. Some programs are very complete and done by qualified health professionals, while others are presented during one- or two-hour sessions by laymen in health clubs. Some programs are geared toward the prevention of injury, especially in industry. Other programs are designed for the patient experiencing a first episode of back pain. A majority of the programs are written for the patient who is able to return to the work force or maintain a somewhat normal life-style. In today's economic environment in health care, this is an efficient use of the therapist's time and provides the patient with the most information at a reduced cost.

In studies comparing no treatment, physical therapy alone, back school alone, and physical therapy with back school, the latter, combined treatment, gives greater pain relief and a higher percentage of persons returning to the work force. Those industries starting back school programs show a decrease in back injuries (6–10).

The Physical Therapy Department at Duke University Medical Center runs two separate back school programs. The first is designed for the outpatient with back pain referred by a physician for back care treatment. Frequently the referral is initiated by a Workmen's Compensation carrier, rehabilitation nurse, or family physician. A referral from a physician is necessary for the patient's participation in the program. The other back school is an inpatient program started for patients with chronic pain. Patients are accepted from the orthopedic, neurosurgery, neurology, rheumatology, and psychiatry services.

Outpatient Program

After physician referral to physical therapy for back school evaluation, the physical therapist does a complete musculoskeletal evaluation of the patient. The patient is started on an exercise program tailored to his or her needs and instructed in basic body mechanics. The patient is assessed for back school. The principles are discussed with the patient to gain his or her acceptance to the idea. The program occurs on two consecutive days, from 9:00 A.M. to 5:00 P.M. and is held approximately every two months. Twenty patients are accepted for each class. The back school is held in a room with plinths, a variety of chairs, foot stools, and pillows. Few back pain patients can sit or maintain one position for two days.

After completion of the back school, patients are encouraged to make an individual appointment in one month and again in three months to assess their exercise ability and answer questions. Individual problems are addressed. This method leads to an efficient use of the therapist's time and makes the patients responsible for treatment and care of their backs.

Inpatient Program

The inpatient program is designed for chronic pain patients. The program meets one hour per day for a total of six treatment sessions. Each day a separate unit of the program is presented. The patients can enter at any point, although it is better if the patient starts during one of the first three sessions. The room has recliners, chairs, wall space, black-board, screen, counter with cupboards, and bathroom. Patients are en-couraged to change positions during the class and informality is encouraged as long as it does not interfere with the class. Instructional aids include a series of nine slide tapes, a model of the spine, types of pillows, lumbar roll, and seats. Before entering the class, patients have completed their skeletal evaluation and appropriateness for back school has been determined. The following outline is the basis of the back school program.

Outline of Back School Program

DAY 1: Instruction in the anatomy and pathology of the spine (disc bulge, prolapse, degenerative disc, sciatica, osteoarthritis, laminectomy, fusion, scar tissue, myelogram) is initially discussed. Emphasis is placed on how the muscles of the back, abdomen, and legs control the pelvis. The relationship between muscle length and strength is explained. Normal and abnormal curves of the spine are shown. The spinal motion during flexion and extension is demonstrated. Intradiscal pressures affected by posture and exercise are illustrated (11).

DAY 2: The force of gravity affecting body mechanics in the overweight patient, during pregnancy, and while lifting and carrying objects is demonstrated. The importance of a support base and center of gravity through the center of the support base during activities is emphasized. Application of these principles to everyday activities such as counter work, brushing one's teeth, getting dishes out of the cupboard, carrying laundry, or doing yard work is demonstrated. Principles of leverage, friction, and inertia, and how they apply to various activities, are explained. Special attention is directed toward understanding how the forces generated for or produced by pushing and pulling, lifting, or carrying objects affect the supportive structure of the body. Improper techniques in these activities will likely increase pain in the chronic pain patient. The members of the class are asked to identify problem areas for themselves and devise a solution to make their tasks easier following the principles just discussed.

DAY 3: Anterior and posterior pelvic tilt of the pelvis are described as well as how this relates to posture and exercise. Standing posture is reviewed. Sleep positions are demonstrated and reviewed as well as methods of getting into and out of bed while maintaining proper body alignment. Selecting a bed for good spine support is discussed.

DAY 4: The pain cycle and how it relates to the patient's total treatment with activity, rest, exercise, biofeedback, medications, modalities, and pleasurable activities are reviewed. The effects of each type of treatment on the pain cycle are illustrated. The effects of rest and activities on intradiscal pressure are explained. Proper sitting posture, selecting a chair, driving position, getting up and down from a sitting position, and getting in and out of a car are demonstrated. Ways to modify chairs to fit are reviewed.

DAY 5:   The correct standing posture is reviewed. Gait is observed for antalgic patterns and the stresses it puts on the lumbar complex are reviewed. The rationale for strong legs is emphasized. Stooping, squatting, and kneeling positions are demonstrated for proper technique and their use in various activities explained. The beneficial effects of proper foot wear are described.

DAY 6:   Lifting techniques for objects of different sizes, shapes, and weights are explained and demonstrated. Emphasis is on keeping the back straight and on normal lordosis. Physiological response to modalities (heat and cold) is reviewed. Differences between moist and dry heat and how to utilize these at home are discussed. Treatment times are set during their individual sessions. Patients should experience moist heat, cold pack, and ice massage by the time of their discharge. This again allows the patient to use the modality throughout the day and at home. There is greater benefit if these modalities are used frequently, as they increase the blood flow, decrease the waste products, and decrease muscle tension. If patients have access to health clubs, whirlpool, sauna, and steam rooms, these are also reviewed with the patient.

Exercise principles and types are discussed. Inclusion of a cardiovascular program of swimming, walking, or exercycling into a patient's exercise program is encouraged. Pain flare-up plans are reviewed in detail (Table 4). It is important for patients to develop a plan under the supervision of the pain team and while in the hospital. As flare-ups occur at home, patients are less frightened by these periods if they have a specific treatment approach to deal with them. Flare-up plans are individualized for each patient and reviewed in back school. Patients are instructed to reduce or stop certain exercises and re-introduce the easier exercises, increase the use of modalities, decrease certain activities, correct poor posture, increase rest time, and use relaxation techniques. A review of the patient's activities prior to the flare-up is emphasized to enhance the patient's ability for self-monitoring.

A patient's exercise should not cause more than a 30-minute increase in pain. If so, he or she is over-stretching, rocking the back too much, or attempting too difficult an exercise program. The patient is taught to recognize the difference between a stretch pain, muscle fatigue, and their baseline pain.

The proper exercise program for each chronic pain patient is an essential part of treatment if the goal is to activate the patient to a higher level of function. The appropriate exercises can only be selected after the patient has had a complete musculoskeletal evaluation. The desired

Table 4. Pain Flare-up Plans

Exercise:
  Reduce or stop exercise for 8–16 hours
  Reintroduce easiest exercise (3 or 4 preselected)
  Do exercise less vigorously
  Cut repetitions in half
  Slowly over the next 24–48 hours reinstate all exercise with reduced repetitions (not all during one session)
  Try to get back to pre-flare-up levels within 3 days
  Try to do some exercise every day
  If you miss a session, do not double the repetitions the next time
  If you need to break exercise sessions up, do them more frequently with fewer repetitions

Modalities:
  Use every 2–3 hours
  Try packs
  Use before and after the exercise session
  Do not wait for excruciating pain before beginning
  Do not double the time used, but use more frequently

Activity:
  Decrease sitting time
  Correct posture
  Decrease activity and increase rest accordingly
  Use relaxation tapes and pleasurable activities
  Utilize a graph or chart to note progress on exercise or activity
  Recognize the frustration with flare-ups
  Assess noncompliance or activity to identify the cause

effects of such a program on activity and pain level are not readily apparent. Compliance with an exercise program and adherence to the principles demonstrated in the back school are necessary if these goals are to be met. Support and participation by family members are beneficial in the attainment of the patient's goals.

MODALITIES

Just as exercise is specific to the goal and structure, modalities need to be selected in the same manner. In order to choose the most appropriate modality, the type, depth of the tissue or structure, and desired response is determined. Other considerations include type of nerve fibers being affected, circulation to the part, contraindications to the modality, availability of equipment, frequency of treatment, and status of the patient. For example, if one wants to increase the capillary blood flow frequently during the day, a method of increasing tissue temperature will have to be directed to home treatment. If the therapist considered using electrical stimulation for relaxation but finds the patient afraid of any electrical equipment, the desired response will be negated by the attitude of the patient. Another type of modality needs to be selected. If one desires the decrease of acute edema of the foot or hand, a whirlpool may not be the best choice because of the dependent position of the part during the treatment. There may be greater benefit from elevating and using an intermittent compression pump.

In the acute injury, modalities can speed the healing process and assist with acute pain relief. This may reverse the problem with minimal efforts on the part of the patient. In chronic pain the time involved in the acute healing process has lapsed and secondary problems (disease, scarring, loss of motion, and postural defects) have developed. The pain cycle is well in effect. Total obliteration of pain is not a realistic goal. Modalities are used to lessen the pain cycle or the secondary problems. Modalities are used in conjunction with exercise, postural correction, improved body mechanics, and relaxation. One of the major goals is to prepare tissues for stretching and mobilization techniques, or to decrease the pain so the patient can successfully carry out their exercise program.

The use of modalities at home will offer the chronic pain patient optimal benefit. To go to a health practitioner for heat, ultrasound, and massage may feel good, but it is impossible to accomplish the needed change in the anatomical structures with these alone. By the time the patient dresses, drives to the clinic, waits for the therapist, undresses for treatment, and then reverses this procedure to get home after treatment, the benefit from treatment has probably been lost. The additional

Table 5. Modalities in Chronic Pain: Heat and Cold

Types of Heat	Deep
Superficial	Shortwave diathermy
Dry	Microwave diathermy
Electric heating pad or blanket	Ultrasound
Hot water bottle	
Sauna	*Types of Cold*
Paraffin	Cold pack
	Ice towels
Moist	Ice bag
Hot packs	Ice massage
Moist heating pad	Ice whirlpool
Wet towels	
Shower/bath	
Whirlpool/hot tub	
Steam room	
Infrared	

stresses will overshadow improvement. The use of modalities has a greater chance of benefitting the patient when combined with home treatments, exercise, and body mechanics. Modalities can be used at home many times per day. In the long run, it is less expensive, more beneficial, and gives the patient the responsibility for his or her own care. They can be used before and after the exercise program, which is an essential part of home treatment. The modalities at home can include heat (dry or moist), cold packs, ice massage, massage, and transcutaneous nerve stimulation (TENS).

Various modalities used in clinics for chronic pain are listed in Tables 5 and 6. A brief discussion of each appears below. It is not the purpose of this section to give a detailed physiological basis for the mechanics, indications, contraindications, or methods of application. Those can be found in basic textbooks on therapeutic modalities (12). The goal is to familiarize one with the name of various modalities and the type of response that may be beneficial to the chronic pain patient.

Superficial Heat

Superficial heating methods include electrical heating pads and blankets, hot water bottles, moist warm towels, hydrocollator packs, whirlpools, saunas, ultraviolet sources, and paraffin (Table 5). All increase the superficial temperature of the body part. For use with chronic pain patients, moist heat is usually more comfortable and a better conductor of heat. None of these methods can directly increase the temperature in a joint covered by muscle or subcutaneous tissues. Therefore, the structures affected are limited by the depth of penetration.

During the acute stage of injury, superficial or deep heat may increase the extravasation of plasma from capillary beds causing an increase in

Table 6. Modalities in Chronic Pain: Electrical Stimulation, Massage, and Other Types

Electrical stimulation	Massage
Transcutaneous nerve stimulators (TENS)	Traditional
	Connective tissue
High voltage galvanic stimulators	Myofascial
	Friction
Inferential stimulators	Transverse friction
Low voltage stimulators	Acupuncture
Neuroprobes	
	Other types
	Jobst pump (intermittent compression)
	Laser

edema, and is therefore not recommended. In patients with chronic pain, the goal is to increase relaxation, increase circulation, decrease accumulation of waste products in muscle, and increase nutrition to the area. Different types of superficial heat have certain advantages. In treating a hand injury, whirlpool or paraffin can surround all the fingers. Whirlpool leaves the extremity in a dependent position but, utilizing paraffin by dipping and wrapping, the body part can be elevated. Patients can do this at home using a mixture of paraffin and mineral oil, and using a crock pot or double-boiler for heating purposes.

Ultraviolet radiation allows immediate inspection of the body part and no heavy packs are placed on the body part. Hydrocollator packs work well in the clinic due to ease in positioning, relatively low cost, and versatility. At home, hot packs have to be heated on the stove in large pots and are relatively heavy for some patients. Electrical moist heating pads are extremely effective for the lumbar and thoracic area, but difficult to wrap around the cervical spine. Saunas, steam rooms, and whirlpools in clubs require the expense of membership, whereas showers and baths at home are more readily available.

All heat treatments are used for a limited period of time, usually 15–30 minutes. They are then removed and as the body part returns to its resting temperature, then they may be used again. Patients should not sleep on heat; if the area receives too much heat, the surrounding area will protect itself by decreasing in circulation. This increases the risk of a burn because the heat is not dissipated. Caution should be exercised over bony areas, areas with poor circulation, and areas without sensation, as burns can occur without the patient's awareness.

Deep Heat

Deep heat can only be done in a clinical setting as it requires special equipment. These methods include shortwave diathermy, microwave diathermy, and ultrasound.

Shortwave diathermy applies a high frequency oscillating electrical current to deep tissues in the body (12). This provides a source of heat, the depth of penetration of which will depend on the technique of application and the body part being treated. When applied to joints surrounded by soft tissue, the heating will probably be limited to subcutaneous tissue and superficial muscles. If applied to joints with little muscle, there will be a good heating effect around the joint.

During treatment patients should only feel a very mild warmth with correct dosage. If the part feels hot to the patient, the dosage is too high and a burn will develop under the skin. The major effect is achieved by increasing the tissue temperature and reflexively increasing the circulation. Shortwave is used frequently with musculoskeletal pain and spasm, pelvic inflammatory conditions, and sinus congestion. Applicators include air space plates, drum electrodes, induction coils, pads, and internal pelvic applicators.

Microwave diathermy is a form of electromagnetic radiation. Therapeutic frequencies of microwave are higher and wave lengths shorter than radio waves. This type of treatment is similar to shortwave diathermy in that the major effects are due to the heating. Depth of heating of tissues depends on the frequency used. This type is not used in clinics as frequently as shortwave diathermy. It has the advantage of easier observation of the part being treated.

There are many contraindications in the use of this device. Some of these include sensory and circulation impaired areas, metal implants, contact lenses, cardiac pacemakers, malignancies, hemorrhagic diseases, thrombophlebitis, intrauterine devices, pregnancy, heavy menstrual flow, or acute infections. All treatments need to be done on wooden beds or with metal parts adequately padded. Jewelry and watches must be removed. Knowledge of the equipment, careful screening of patients, and appropriate treatment areas are of prime concern.

Ultrasound has a crystal that turns electrical energy into acoustic vibrations occurring at inaudible frequency. The compression waves cause movement of particles, creating an increase in the tissue temperature. Other studies have indicated some effects not related to the heating mechanism. These include changes in ion transfers across cell membranes, reactions to gaseous cavitation, changes in tissue extensibility, and changes in nerve conduction.

Frequently used as a source of deep heating, ultrasound will penetrate to the joint capsules and periosteum. This makes it a valuable tool in preparing joints for stretching or to effect change in joint adhesions. In addition to its heating effect, ultrasound produces extensibility of connective tissues. Other uses have included pain relief, resolution of hematomas, and resolution of calcium deposits. The latter has been refuted by some. Clinical studies have found ultrasound to be a valuable tool but the mechanisms are not fully understood.

Contraindications include ischemia on sensory deprived areas, tumors, pregnancy, epiphyseal areas in children, areas of high fluid content, and reproductive organs.

In patients with chronic pain, ultrasound is used to prepare tissues for stretching, decreasing joint irritations, and decreasing pain. Ultrasound needs to be combined with exercise to achieve changes in the anatomical structures. Alone, it is ineffective for this purpose. Frequently, this modality is overutilized in clinics where patients receive multiple treatments with no long-term improvement. If a patient's pain is not improved and maintained after 3–10 treatments of a modality, one can judge treatment to be ineffective. If pain reductions occur only for hours, no long-term benefit is gained. Research findings are inconclusive as to the long-term effects of overutilization of ultrasound. As with all treatments and modalities, a reevaluation needs to be frequent, and treatment adjusted appropriately.

Ultrasound is also utilized for phonophoresis, which drives topical medications into underlying tissues. Specially prepared ointments such as hydrocortisone cream or xylocaine are used to help reduce inflammation and to decrease pain of tendonitis, bursitis, or strain. Ultrasound can also be used in conjunction with electrical stimulation. This modality can be beneficial in treating muscle spasms, trigger points, and mobilization of fluid collection. Another common term for this is medcosonalator.

Therapeutic Cold

Theories on the therapeutic effect of cold have been proposed for years. Initially it causes vasoconstriction but reflex vasodilatation occurs to bring blood into the area to protect the tissues from ischemia. If the cold treatment continues at a significant level to keep the temperatures abnormally cold, the body protects itself by causing vasoconstriction in the area. Therefore, irreversible damage to the tissues will occur.

Therapeutic cold is an effective treatment if used properly to avoid the irreversible damage. In acute injuries it can reduce the extravasation of plasma from capillary beds, making it a vital modality in the control of edema. It also has an analgesic effect in the treatment of pain. In inflammatory conditions such as arthritis, it has been shown to be beneficial.

Techniques of application are simple and readily available for home treatments. These include ice bags, ice packs, slush buckets, ice towels, and ice massage. There are also electrical machines that create cold pads. As with heat, therapeutic effects occur with a specific duration of application so that overexposure does not damage the tissues. Usually treatment is 10–20 minutes in length, but can be repeated frequently during the day.

Patients with chronic pain may alternate heat and cold during the day. Some patients find cold to be of greater benefit during flare-ups. Cold is effective for the patient with local edema or nerve root irritation. Caution and contraindications are observed in patients with sensory and circulatory impairments.

Electrical Stimulation

Electrical stimulation devices apply alternating or direct currents to the muscle or peripheral nerve, with the intent of causing continuous or intermittent muscle contractions and relaxations, and increasing large nerve fiber input into the cutaneous sensory nervous system (Table 6).

This stimulation causes a reduction in pain. Direct current was widely used for decades in patients having peripheral nerve damage to stimulate the muscle directly, thereby keeping the contractile elements functional while nerve regeneration occurred. In patients who had nerve function, alternating currents were used to stimulate axons to cause a muscle contraction for muscle re-eduction, increasing circulation, and decreasing pain. Alternating currents are more comfortable for these patients.

In the 1970s, the development of a high voltage (galvanic) current made it more comfortable without the skin irritation under the electrodes (13). Today high voltage is used in many areas of muscle reeducation, improvement in circulation to the muscles, relaxation, and pain relief. This modality is used in musculoskeletal treatment, wound healing, pain, and tension headaches.

Muscle stimulating currents have also been used in combination with strengthening exercises to improve the strength of muscle contractions. These machines have an adjustable pulse parameter, which can evoke very strong muscle contractions at lower levels of energy and yet be comfortable for the patient. The results show improvement in the strengthening abilities of muscles.

Interferential stimulators deliver alternating currents from two sets of electrodes at medium but different frequencies to the same muscle mass. At these frequencies the skin resistance is much lower. The effect to the area is a composite of the difference in frequencies. Therefore, painless low frequency alternating current is delivered. This is used for the relief of pain from a variety of musculoskeletal problems.

Transcutaneous electrical nerve stimulation is used to treat pain caused by a large variety of problems. Physical therapists are frequently responsible for applying these devices and educating the patient in their use. Patients must be thoroughly instructed in skin care, care of the device, as well as the use of the equipment for optimal benefits.

Electrical stimulation has also been used to drive ions into underlying tissue (iontophoresis). Preparations are used to decrease inflammation, decrease adhesions and scar tissue, decrease pain, and improve some skin disorders.

Massage

Massage, utilizing the traditional strokes, is one of the oldest therapeutic techniques to increase blood flow, mobilize fluid, relax muscle spasms, and manipulate soft tissue. Specialized methods have developed over the years with modification of strokes and techniques.

Friction massage is a stroke utilizing a strong circular motion. This is done over areas of scarring, adhesions, and around joints and fascia to increase mobility and over trigger points to decrease pain.

Transverse friction massage is a technique in which the force is given by way of a very small area (fingertip) perpendicular to the tendon or muscle belly. This method is used to maintain or increase mobility of a tendon, tendon sheath, or muscle fibers without putting undue strain on the entire length of the structure. It is frequently used in tendonitis, small tears of muscle fibers on tendons, tendosynovitis, sprains, and strains. The technique will cause a localized hyperemia from increased blood flow to the area.

Connective tissue massage is a series of strokes which originate in the lumbar area and move to the extremities. It is associated with reflex responses in the tissues, which include increased blood flow and sympathetic response. This procedure is not always comfortable while being done. Myofascial massage is another technique advocated for mobilization of fascial structures.

Acupressure is the stimulation of certain acupuncture points along the meridians and trigger point areas outside the meridians using finger pressure or electrical stimulation (14). These points will frequently be along nerve trunks or at motor points of the muscles. The points can be detected by electrical devices that detect areas of low electrical resistance. Studies show that stimulation along these points can decrease pain, although the mechanism is not known. Theories include the gate control theory and the release of endorphins. Used with exercise programs, instruction in body mechanics, transcutaneous nerve stimulation, and other pain management techniques, acupressure can be helpful in certain patients with chronic pain. Painful trigger points, pain from excessive scarring, areas of point tenderness, painful ligamentous insertions on bony areas, and painful neuromas are indications for its use. It can be used with visceral organ pain with selection of a referred pain point, or used with musculoskeletal problems.

Acupressure is done with finger pressure held over the acupuncture point for a period of minutes. Acustimulation is produced with an electrical stimulation machine, ultrasound, TENS, or neuroprobe. Neuroprobe stimulation of the point should be strong but tolerable for 15 to 60 seconds.

Other Types

High power lasers have been used to retard or arrest physiological activity for medical purposes. These procedures produce incisions during surgical procedures and destroy tumors. The effect is destruction of tissue by high level heat and dehydration. Using ultra low output laser light below the level of thermal vibration, heat production and tissue dehydration create a cellular micro-response. These low level lasers have the effect of increasing the metabolic process of healing and increasing phagocytosis. Increases in tissue granulation rate, faster epithelization, activation of collagen in ulcers, increases in vascularization and post-traumatic regeneration, and decreases in pain have occurred with its use. This device has had widespread use in Europe and Russia for the past 15–17 years. Clinical studies are being conducted in this country but the Food and Drug Administration classifies low power lasers as investigational. Documented studies with low power lasers in the treatment of chronic pain patients have been encouraging but limited in scope. In the future, we may see more of this device in clinics for wound healing, acute injuries, treatment of scar tissue, and treatment of chronic pain.

The advantage of this treatment is that the patient feels nothing, treatment is relatively quick (seconds per area), and the placebo effect of "hands on" may be reduced. Used in conjunction with exercise programs, instruction in body mechanics, and other pain management techniques, it may be a valuable tool.

Intermittent compression pumps are machines that intermittently inflate a sleeve applied to an extremity to reduce edema. They are used in acute injuries with secondary edema, postoperative amputations, and lymphedema.

In summary, physiotherapy for the chronic pain patient provides effective management for the pain complaints and a means to activate the patient to a higher level of function. In acute injury and pain, the treatment promotes healing and pain relief, whereas in the chronic pain state, treatment is directed toward management of the condition. A physical therapy program including an exercise program, modalities, and back school are individualized after a complete musculoskeletal evaluation to insure maximum benefit from treatment.

REFERENCES

1. Cyriax J: Textbook of Orthopaedic Medicine: Diagnosis of soft tissue, volume 1, 8th edition. London, Bailliere, Tindall, 1982
2. Kendall F, McCreary E: Muscles Testing and Function. Baltimore, Williams & Wilkins, 1983
3. Saunders HD: Evaluation, Treatment and Prevention of Musculoskeletal Disorders. Minneapolis, Viking, 1985
4. McKenzie R: The Lumbar Spine. Waikanae, New Zealand, Spinal Publications, 1981
5. Gould J, Davies G: Orthopaedic and Sports Medicine. Saint Louis, C.V. Mosby, 1985
6. Hall HMD: The Canadian back education unit. Physiotherapy 66:115–116, 1980
7. Forssell-Zachresson M: The Swedish back school: Physiotherapy 66: 112–114, 1980
8. Kennedy B: An Australian programme for management of back problem. Physiotherapy 66:108-111, 1980

9. Mattmiller AW: The California back school. Physiotherapy 66:118-122, 1980
10. White A: Back School and Other Conservative Approaches to Low Back Pain. Saint Louis, C.V. Mosby, 1983
11. Nachemson A: The lumbar spine: an orthopaedic challenge. Spine 1:50-71, 1976
12. Krusen F, Koltke F, Ellwood P: Handbook of Physical Medical and Rehabilitation. Philadelphia, W.B. Saunders, 1971
13. Griffen J, Karselis T: Physical Agents for Physical Therapist. Springfield, IL, Charles C Thomas, 1982
14. Brickey R: Acupuncture and Transcutaneous Electrical Stimulation Techniques. Acutherapy, Waukegan, IL, Post Graduate Seminars, 1978

Chapter **23**

Nursing in Chronic Pain

Mary Trainor, R.N.

Nursing practice mandates responsible pain management. In spite of this mandate, a significant void exists in nursing education regarding pain assessment and treatment. This is especially true in the area of chronic pain. Lacking an adequate knowledge base, nurses have fallen short of the goal of responsible pain management. Attempting to function in this void often results in patient management that is counterproductive. Examples occur all too often in inpatient settings. For instance, when deciding whether or not to administer pain relief measures, a nurse often makes a judgment about whether the pain is "real." This judgment, coinciding with a misconception about the addictive qualities of medications, and especially of narcotics, often means that treatment is withheld from the patient.

This deficiency in knowledge and lack of an organized approach to treatment is most apparent when we look at how chronic pain is handled. In response to the need for increased education and training in this area, nurses are actively pursuing opportunities for dialogue with other nurses and health professionals in such organizations as the International Association for the Study of Pain and the American Pain Society. Comprehensive pain clinics, with nursing actively involved in the ongoing clinical design, are becoming more common. "Pain consult nurses" in the general hospital are helping other professionals manage the patient in pain who presents with the typical complex of treatment needs. Nursing research is attempting to answer the many questions being asked by nurses who are struggling to care responsibly for the patient in pain.

This chapter will focus on the nursing management of the patient with chronic pain and will primarily address the inpatient treatment phase, as this is where nurses are primarily utilized. Though the nursing care to be described is that found on a comprehensive inpatient chronic pain management unit within a university medical center's department of psychiatry, many aspects of the total nursing program could easily be transferred to another setting with minimal adaptation.

SYSTEM OF CARE DELIVERY

Basic to the nursing care provided on any unit is the system that defines the manner in which it is organized. We believe that nursing care on an inpatient chronic pain unit is most effectively organized with a primary nursing focus. Patients admitted to such a unit often have been treated in a number of settings previously, usually unsuccessfully. Their dependency needs are intense and they function with minimal or no trust in the health care system. It is important that the patient feel cared for and that the system be organized tightly enough to prevent the all-too-common splitting and manipulating that may occur with this patient population. A primary nurse who consistently and totally cares for the patient can provide assurance that his or her needs will be met. This is an important first step in reestablishing the trust that will be important for compliance with the program and a positive treatment outcome.

STAFFING

The nursing care on a pain unit differs significantly from that provided on a medical/surgical unit or on a psychiatric unit. While such nursing closely resembles that found on a combined medical/psychiatric unit, it actually combines *surgical* and psychiatric nursing. Thus, the concept of a surgical/psychiatric nurse or a "pain nurse" emerges. This is a nurse who is skilled in both medical/surgical and psychiatric skills. Nurses who are experienced in pain management or who have had experience in both surgery and psychiatry are few in number. Thus, a head nurse responsible for hiring a nursing staff must decide between staffing the unit with surgical nurses who possess strong interpersonal skills, and psychiatric nurses who are technically skilled.

In describing the nursing care on combined medical/psychiatric units, several authors have stated their opinion regarding the type of nurse to recruit and hire. Hoffman (1) prefers nurses with medical/surgical experience. Fogel (2) describes the conversion of a psychiatric unit to a psychiatric/medical unit using the psychiatric nurses who staffed the unit at the time of the conversion. In describing staffing for a pain unit, Pinsky and colleagues (3) discuss what behaviors and personal qualities are necessary in staff members, and assert the importance of an ability to work as a team member. In order to function effectively as part of a team, a nurse must be comfortable with a higher level of involvement and sharing of clinical experiences than is the norm in a medical/surgical area. The nurse must also feel free to question other staff members and be questioned in return. Communication among the nurses and other health care professionals must remain open. These are personal behaviors and qualities that are more often found among nurses with psychiatric experience. For these reasons, my preference is to hire psychiatric nurses who are motivated to further develop their medical/surgical skills.

A further rationale for this preference is the importance of the milieu as a treatment modality. Establishing and maintaining a unit's milieu is almost solely a nursing function and psychiatric nurses are skilled in this. Psychiatric nurses can, as well, generally effectively deal with patients' psychological distress and maladaptive coping behaviors. As stated, however, motivation to acquire expanded medical/surgical skills is essential.

The psychological needs of chronic pain patients vary widely. Some patients require minimal psychological interventions since they have a psychologically intact premorbid personality and their adaptation to their pain and disability is adequate. However, other patients require sophisticated psychological and behavioral interventions, as their chronic pain and disability have precipitated intense psychological symptoms and regressed behavior. The nurse working on a psychiatric unit expects that patients admitted have significant psychopathology that requires intense psychological and behavioral care. On a chronic pain unit, however, the level of psychological dysfunction varies greatly. The nurse on a chronic pain unit must be able to assess patients' level of psychopathology, pre-morbid personality, psychological reactivity to the pain, and maladaptive behavior. After this assessment is made, the nurse is required to implement an individualized psychological and behavioral nursing care plan. Job performance expectations require that a skilled nurse be able to apply a variety of therapeutic interventions in response to the varied intensity of need. Hence, psychiatric nurses who have interest only in dynamic, insight-oriented nursing care may not be able to respond to the variety of needs exhibited by chronic pain patients. If the nurse is unable to respond to these varied needs, she often becomes obstructive to the individual patient's treatment and to the overall functioning of the milieu.

Two types of nurses seem to be the most effective on a chronic pain unit. The first is the experienced and highly skilled psychiatric nurse who is also highly motivated to expand his or her medical/surgical skills. While experienced and skilled enough psychiatrically to respect the importance of psychological defenses, this nurse's professional identity is not dependent on the patient achieving a higher level of intrapsychic awareness. If the pain unit has in place an experienced and skilled nursing group, then the second type, a relatively new nurse who has had minimal experience in either a medical/surgical or psychiatric area, can be incorporated into available positions. It is essential that he or she possess the maturity to function as a member of a complex team and desire to acquire new skills. Given this, the nurse can be educated effectively in the specifics of chronic pain management.

DELIVERY OF CARE

Assessment

Responsible nursing care begins with a thorough nursing assessment. The American Nursing Association's First Standard of Nursing Practice and its rationale state, "Comprehensive care requires complete and on-going collection of data about the client/patient to determine the nursing care needs of the client/patient. All health status data about the client/patient must be available for all members of the health care team." The standard states: "The collection of data about the health status of the client/patient is systematic and continuous. The data are accessible, communicated, and recorded." (4)

Accurate assessment of pain is a difficult process. Initially, the most readily available source of data comes from the admission interview with the patient. By focusing this interview on the collection of objective data related to the pain that is being experienced, the patient is reassured that the nurse views his pain as "real." This point is especially important when the patient is being admitted to a unit that is associated with psychiatry. The Nursing Pain Assessment form used by the admitting nurse on the Clinical Specialty Unit at Duke University Medical Center (see the Appendix) emphasizes the patient's individual perception of his or her pain. Gathering these data enables the nurse to structure a more complete nursing care plan. It is also especially useful in gauging the effectiveness of treatment interventions as the patient proceeds with hospitalization.

Along with a thorough interview, an important aspect of the initial assessment is the nurse's observation of the patient. Gait, posture, and range of motion should be observed and recorded. It is important to observe for any skin color or temperature differences or edema. An assessment of any displayed pain behaviors is also an important aspect of the pain assessment. Specific behaviors, such as guarding, bracing, rubbing, grimacing, and sighing, have been shown to provide valuable data to clinicians in evaluating a patient's progress during the course of treatment (5).

Of special importance in any assessment is an emphasis on what significance the pain has for the patient. What the pain *means* for patients may increase or decrease their suffering. Many patients assume that if their pain is severe, then the disorder is getting worse. This, of course, may or may not be true. A person's cultural, educational, and religious background all influence the perception of pain and its significance. We always assess the patient's level of depression, since many of our chronic pain patients are also significantly depressed. Certain symptoms in depression are almost always part of the chronic pain picture and include sleep disorders and a decrease in general daily activities (6).

In assessing the chronic pain patient, the nurse cannot rely only on demonstrated pathophysiology. A patient admitted with a chronic low back pain diagnosis may also be experiencing muscle spasms, including weakness and atrophy, a significant sleep disturbance, social isolation, decreased interest, irritability, feelings of helplessness and worthlessness, personality changes, and even suicidal ideation. This patient may be unemployed and experiencing significant financial problems, which have stressed the marital and family relationships as well as relationships in general. To determine which of these issues is the cause and which the effect of the pain problem is a difficult task. What is clear is that the demonstrated pathophysiology is only a small part of the complex problem. To organize the variety of clinical data and formulate a comprehensive nursing care plan, the nurse may utilize the model for assessment that was presented in Chapter 16. The advantages of a thorough nursing assessment are obvious.

Milieu Therapy

The creation and support of a carefully designed milieu is one of the primary functions of nursing on a chronic pain unit (7). Several authors have described the importance of the milieu in the effective treatment of chronic pain patients. Wilson and Aronoff (8) describe the therapeutic community as the basic formulation upon which all the treatment modes of an inpatient pain unit are built. In this environment, communication is open and direct between staff and patients, and patients are expected and encouraged to participate in their treatment. Emphasis on the medical model of physician authority is reduced. Individual psychotherapy is only occasionally used as a supplement to group therapy. The milieu emphasis is on exploring the ways in which pain has affected the person's life and family and on how well the patient has adjusted to these changes. Morse (9) explains that careful structuring of milieu results in the pain patient replacing pain-related behavior with normal activity. The milieu is a source of information, authority, and support.

Many pain patients have the impression that they are alone with their mysterious illness. To discover that others have the same problem is an important and salutary experience. Progress made by one patient is very encouraging to others and is more convincing than any promise made by a professional. Thus, patients become teachers and models for each other.

The difference between a traditional psychiatric milieu and that of a pain unit is subtle but important. The nurses on a pain unit take a more direct role in manipulating the milieu than they do on a traditional psychiatric unit. There is also more somatic treatment offered in response to the fact that our patients' goals for hospitalization are organized less around insight and personality reconstruction and more around support, grief resolution, and pain relief.

On a psychiatric unit, a somatizing depressed patient would be allowed to be active in the milieu, attend community meetings, participate in group activities, and carry on social interactions. The goal of the hospitalization would likely involve helping the patient gain some level of insight into the cause of his or her symptoms. During the process, discussions centered around childhood experiences that may have contributed to the adoption of somatic symptoms as a way of expressing feelings, would be encouraged. These discussions would be rewarded, while the symptoms would be allowed to persist. This would, in effect, lead to the patient's temporary regression and would be displayed by increased somatic symptomatology and psychological distress. Fellow patients would be encouraged to interact with this patient. All patients on the unit would to some degree participate in the patient's therapy. With increased insight, the symptoms would gradually diminish and the patient would be functioning at a more sophisticated level.

The somatizing patient on a pain unit, however, would be managed differently. Displays of somatic symptoms would be viewed as destructive to other patients. Since the primary goals of hospitalization center around adaptation and not insight, the somatizing patient is isolated from his fellow patients, which prevents him or her from negatively affecting the optimistic, coping-oriented "feeling" of the milieu. Attempts to interpret repressed conflicts are not usually made, and when they are, further regression in the patient is quickly evident. These patients have too often been told that there is no somatic explanation for their pain. Continuous reinforcement for nonsomatizing behavior is given and the isolation continues until the symptoms diminish. When this occurs and adaptive pain coping skills are firmly in place, the intrapsychic and interpersonal conflicts contributing to the chronic pain state are then addressed utilizing more traditional psychotherapies.

In this and many other examples, the nursing staff relies less on the natural group process as a tool in resolving conflicts and more on direct interventions to channel interactions into more constructive behavior. Patients are not expected to independently plan activities, resolve group living difficulties, or confront inappropriate behavior in fellow patients. Though these behaviors are expected to a greater degree than they would be on a medical/surgical unit, they are not expected to the same degree that they are on a psychiatric unit. A highly structured milieu involving group meetings, educational classes, and scheduled leisure activities is essential.

Understanding the dynamics of a traditional psychiatric milieu, however, is very important to the nursing staff responsible for the pain unit milieu. Nurses need to understand that patients interpret the meaning of unit events in terms of their own needs. The nurse must assess a patient's interpretations and attempt to reinterpret or reshape the meaning of the event if the meaning is disruptive. A properly structured milieu provides a social support system, a network of relationships, a source of information, and an arena for working out issues of trust, conflict, and cooperation. This milieu is a valuable therapeutic tool providing an environment in which the rest of the pain management program operates. Locating and implementing the various treatment modalities (physical therapy, nerve blocks, biofeedback, back school, and group therapy) on the pain unit itself greatly enhances patient comfort and compliance.

Supportive Psychotherapy

In formulating the psychotherapy portion of the nursing care plan for the chronic pain patient, it is important to assess the etiologies and emotional and behavioral sequelae of the chronic pain state. To illustrate the importance of this approach, two examples of patients from either end of the continuum—from an organically based pain syndrome to a psychologically based pain syndrome—will be described (see Table 1). It should be noted that these examples are artificial and do not necessarily represent a majority of chronic pain patients. Most patients' chronic pain has various etiologies, both organic and psychological in nature. The patient who has a significant medical illness over an extended period of time will often develop psychological distress and symptoms. On the other hand, a patient who has a psychopathological psychiatric disorder can develop a chronic pain complaint. This condition can, in turn, lead to physical changes such as poor exercise tolerance, muscle weakness, posture changes, changes in weight, or discoordination. These patients tend to exaggerate their physical changes or other bodily symptoms. The pain complaint is used defensively to cope with underlying intrapsychic and interpersonal emotional conflicts.

It is, therefore, important that the nurse be able to identify whether the psychological and behavioral symptoms are a cause of or a reaction to the chronic pain. The nursing care plan will be different for each of these patients. For instance, for the patient with organic pain who displays reactive psychological and behavioral symptoms, supportive psychotherapy is aimed at the various losses that most of these patients have experienced. Helping these patients deal with changes in themselves, in

Table 1. Nursing Interventions Based on Etiological Classification

Organically Based Pain with Reactive Psychological Symptoms	Psychologically Based Pain
1. Recognize that much of psychopathology is result of pain	1. Recognize that much of psychopathology existed prior to pain
2. Encourage ventilation of feelings	2. Minimize patient's expressions of feelings
3. Confront maladaptive defenses	3. Support defenses
4. Approach interactions allowing patient to determine topic, flow of conversation	4. Approach with present goals defining topic of conversation, length of interaction
5. Concern regarding number of staff not an issue	5. Limit number of staff interacting with patient
6. Support paperwork if helpful to patient, deemphasize if not	6. Encourage paperwork such as graphing, record keeping, pain rating
7. Encourage involvement in group discussions about the physical aspects of their pain problem and treatment	7. Discourage involvement in group discussions where pain complaints predominate, limiting healthy adult conversations

their family structure, work place, and community provides the focus of the nurse–patient psychotherapy encounter.

It should be noted that even though the psychological symptoms are reactive, they can in themselves produce significant distress in the patient. As described in earlier chapters, some chronic pain patients develop a severe major depressive illness. In working with the patient with major depression secondary to a chronic pain state, as with the patient with primary depression, relief of depressive symptoms may be necessary before grief work is initiated. It should be kept in mind that some patients turn to alcohol and drugs to treat their chronic pain and alleviate their psychological symptoms. As these patients work through the grieving process, they are more able to incorporate a healthier and more rational adaptation to their chronic pain and disability.

Accepting patients at their unique level of functioning and supporting them through the various stages of the grieving process will facilitate their ability to cope more effectively. Carey describes the six stages in this grieving process (10):

1. *Denial.* The patient refuses to believe that his pain can't be diagnosed or cured.
2. *Anger or depression.* The patient stops trying to cope and becomes dependent on others.
3. *Defiance.* The patient will do anything to get pain relief but refuses to change his lifestyle because of the pain.
4. *Withdrawal.* The patient refuses most pain relief measures and makes every effort to maintain his normal lifestyle.
5. *Seeking help.* The patient makes efforts to get relief from his pain and is willing to adjust his lifestyle to accommodate his pain.
6. *Coping.* The patient uses effective pain-relief strategies and resumes normal activities only when he can do them safely and without increasing pain. (p. 24)

As in structuring the milieu, the nurse takes a more active role in this supportive psychotherapy than on a traditional psychiatric unit. Again, the goals for this patient involve adaptation rather than personality reconstruction.

Patients with psychologically based pain are more limited in their ability to process the events of daily life. In the patient with chronic pain secondary to psychological causes (for example, somatoform disorder, hypochrondriasis, conversion disorder, psychogenic pain disorder, or generalized anxiety disorder), the above approach of adaptation and grief work will be met with resistance, exacerbation of physical complaints, psychological symptoms such as regression and acting-out behavior, or all of these. These patients use pain as a primary defense against underlying emotional conflict. In addition, many patients with psychologically based chronic pain have significant premorbid personality difficulties such as immature, dependent traits. If the pain defenses or coping behaviors are lessened in these patients due to effective treatment, one will quickly see regressed or acting-out behavior, since the personality structure is unable to adapt to life situations without the pain.

Thus, for those patients, the goals of hospitalization are not as intensely centered around ventilation of feelings and understanding of psychopathology. Rather, individual interaction with these patients should be structured around supporting their defenses. A very structured education and orientation approach is most helpful. Patients for whom dependency and anxiety are primary issues benefit by structured and time-limited hospitalizations. A short (several days to one week) hospitalization every six months or so will support such patients sufficiently to keep them functional and lessen the incidence of unnecessary medical or surgical hospitalizations and treatment. Patients with frank character disorders and histrionic personality structures are often more effectively treated on an outpatient basis.

As was stated in an earlier chapter, chronic pain complaints are frequently heard from patients with primary affective disorders. It should be kept in mind that in most depressed patients the chronic pain complaint will be alleviated as successful treatment of the depression occurs. The nurse should help the patient understand that the pain complaints are part of the depressive illness, and that these, like other biological and cognitive signs of depression, will abate with treatment.

Care Related to Specific Treatments

Effective nursing care of the chronic pain patient must also involve skilled care focused on the patients' pathophysiology. The importance of an in-depth nursing assessment has already been discussed. This assessment must be an on-going process, especially as it relates to physical findings. Our experience has shown that patients presenting with vague chronic pain complaints may be suffering from malignant disease. Initially, pain must be viewed as a symptom and its physical etiology pursued.

The pain nurse must have a good understanding of pain mechanisms and the neuroanatomy and physiology of nociception. A thorough discussion of these areas is contained in the section of this book, entitled "Basic Concepts," and in *Pain, A Nursing Approach to Assessment and Analysis* by Meinhart and McCaffery (11).

Medication

Nearly all chronic pain patients are treated pharmacologically. For this reason, it is important for the nurse to be knowledgeable about the variety of narcotic and nonnarcotic analgesics routinely used to treat pain. Nursing's responsibility for monitoring the safety and therapeutic responses to medication has grown with the development of more potent drugs and with the proliferation of new medications that have limited clinical track records. Indeed, in the area of chronic pain, one rationale for hospitalization frequently is to utilize expert nursing observation and documentation of responses to medications so that therapeutic levels can be determined.

The use of tricyclic antidepressants for the treatment of chronic pain is often based on trial and error. Few controlled studies that evaluate the efficacy of antidepressants have been reported (12). A review of those clinical studies that have used tricyclic antidepressants in chronic pain reveals that these medications are used in lower doses than is traditionally used for the treatment of major depression. It is important for the pain nurse to have an understanding of how these and other medications are applied. A review of the pharmacology, a good description of drug processing, analgesic actions, side effects, and drug interactions is contained in a recent nursing publication (10) and in Chapters 18, 20, and 21 of this book.

A difficult issue for many nurses, and, indeed, for all health-care professionals, is concern regarding narcotic abuse and addiction. Topics such as underutilization of narcotic medications due to misconceptions about drug dependence and addiction, respiratory depression, the half-life of narcotics, and the high variability of responses by individuals to narcotics have been repeatedly addressed. For example, Marks and Sachar (13) found that 73 percent of the 37 medical inpatients they interviewed suffered moderate or severe pain because insufficient narcotic analgesics had been administered. This study further explored physicians' attitudes and knowledge-base about narcotic analgesics. Also noted were indications of incorrect pharmacological information about the therapeutic dose range for meperidine. A general lack of understanding about addiction was also discovered to be common among physicians.

Moulin and Foley (14) reported that there has been, in general, a tendency to underutilize narcotic analgesics in patients with chronic pain because of a fear of the potential for abuse and/or addiction. They explain that much of this fear is unfounded and stems from the misconception that physical dependence and psychological dependence (addiction) are interchangeable terms. Physical dependence refers to the phenomenon of withdrawal that occurs following the abrupt discontinuation of a narcotic drug that has been administered chronically. This is a pharmacological response distinct from psychological dependence or addiction, in which the individual craves the drug for reasons other than pain relief and becomes overwhelmingly involved in its use and securing its supply. Since a person may be physically dependent on a drug without being psychologically addicted, in most cases our major concern should be that of providing adequate pain relief rather than worrying about drug abuse. As is well known, instances of abuse of narcotic analgesics by medically ill patients are extremely low.

Sriwatanakul and colleagues (15) studied postoperative patients and their caretakers and found that a significant number of patients suffered moderate or severe pain and were given only 70 percent of the maximal analgesic dose ordered, often at inflexible intervals. The questionnaires completed by physicians and nurses indicated that the staff's view of meperidine did not agree with the accepted pharmacological data regarding optimal dose and duration.

Though much is written to guide the nurse in the correct technical administration of medications and assessment for effectiveness, side effects and interactions, very little is available that emphasizes the importance of adequate analgesic dosages given at regularly timed intervals.

Nerve Blocks

Nursing care for the patient receiving a nerve block is dependent upon the type of block given (see Chapter 24 for a thorough discussion of nerve blocks). The most common type of therapeutic blocks utilized on an inpatient pain unit are local infiltration blocks, sympathetic blocks, and epidural blocks. A differential block is a common diagnostic tool.

Nerve blocks effect reversible interruption of nervous conduction. This is achieved by injecting a local anesthetic around a peripheral nerve or area of the spine (spinal cord). The effect of nerve blocks may be enhanced by the addition of other compounds; for example, narcotic corticosteroids. In addition to blocking nociceptive impulses, nerve blocks also interrupt motor and/or sympathetic reflexes.

In selected patients, permanent nerve blocks may be indicated. Such blocks achieve nonconduction by destroying nerve cells and/or fibers through chemical (alcohol, phenol) or physical (heat, cold) means. These blocks are usually reserved for patients with a limited life expectancy. They are also useful in the treatment of often painful spasticity.

Most nerve blocks can be performed on the floor in the treatment room. Necessary equipment consists of sterile needles and syringes and the drugs to be employed. Resuscitation equipment must be present: a suction apparatus; oxygen and the means to administer artificial ventilation (ventilation bag, airways, endotracheal intubation kit); intravenous fluids with administration sets including IV cannulae; and emergency drugs (such as diazepam, barbiturates, vasopressors, and muscle relaxants).

Complications or adverse side effects generally result from allergic reactions or high blood concentration of the drug. Allergic reactions may be mild or serious. A mild reaction consisting of vertigo, headache, tachycardia, or slight hypertension can be treated with reassurance. A more severe reaction that results in loss of consciousness, coma, severe hypotension, or respiratory depression must be treated medically with cardiopulmonary resuscitation.

The majority of side effects will be toxic reactions to high blood levels, usually caused by inadvertent intravascular injection or by the administration of excessive amounts of the drug. Initially, central nervous system excitation occurs, followed by depression. Clinical signs are excitement, incoherent speech, drowsiness, convulsions, and unconsciousness. Cardiovascular effects of high blood concentrations are hypotension, bradycardia, and cardiac arrest. The pain nurse must be familiar with these symptoms and be prepared to assist with resuscitation measures.

Local Infiltration Blocks. The local infiltration block is the simplest and safest kind of block. It is effective for patients with myofascial syndromes. The physician injects the trigger points with 3–10 ml of anesthetic solution. The injection is usually associated with short-lived (seconds) exacerbation of typical pain. Trigger injections should be followed by other treatment (for example, exercises) directed toward elimination of predisposing factors. Nursing care is minimal, primarily involving patient education and encouragement and the coordination of appropriate treatments after the block.

Sympathetic Blocks. A sympathetic block interrupts nervous conduction in the sympathetic system. Local anesthetic solutions injected into the stellate ganglion cause a block involving the upper body quadrant; those injected into the celiac plexus cause a block involving the abdomen; and those injected into the lumbar ganglia cause a block involving the lower body quadrant. Except for the stellate block, these injections are generally done with fluoroscopic assistance; thus, the patient is not on the unit for the procedure. Nursing care involves patient education, observation for untoward reactions and for effectiveness, and management of activity. These blocks are performed for patients with reflex sympathetic dystrophy or abdominal pain.

Epidural Blocks. Epidural analgesia involves continuous or intermittent administration of a local anesthetic, steroid, or narcotic analgesic into the epidural space surrounding the spinal cord. For nurses, this technique conjures up images of the delivery room and childbirth, as this has been the most common instance of use. More recently this procedure has been used in the treatment of chronic pain.

The most serious complication of an epidural narcotic block is respiratory depression. Depending on the narcotic employed, this can occur anytime up to 24 hours after injection. Frequent vital signs measurements and the use of an apnea monitor are important nursing assessment activities. The nurse should have naloxone readily available and should be prepared to initiate supportive measures such as oxygen administration, endotrachial intubation, and ventilatory assistance. Other complications are severe itching and urinary retention. Again, naloxone 0.4 mg administered IV, repeated every 10 minutes as needed, reverses these symptoms. However, it will also reverse the analgesia and may result in acute withdrawal symptoms of a habituated patient. Table 2 summarizes appropriate nursing care for a patient who has received a narcotic epidural block.

An epidural steroid block has less potential for complications. As with other blocks, nursing care consists of observation for effectiveness and complications as well as activity monitoring.

IV Chloroprocaine Blocks. As is noted further in Chapter 24, the intravenous administration of chloroprocaine has been shown to be effective in the treatment of specific pain disorders (16). Nursing care for patients receiving a chloroprocaine injection centers on prevention of complications and assessing effectiveness. Care should include keeping the patient on bed rest for 2 hours postprocedure, then up with assistance for the next 4 hours and assessing vital signs every 15 minutes for 1 hour after infusion, then every hour for the next 4 hours. Other assessments, such as level of consciousness, should be done while vital signs are assessed. A 0–10 pain rating should be done once each hour for five hours following the procedure to assess the effectiveness of the procedure.

Other Therapies

Other treatments such as transcutaneous electrical nerve stimulation (TENS), massage, application of heat and cold, exercise, biofeedback, relaxation, distraction, and guided imagery are reviewed in other chap-

Table 2. The Standard Nursing Care Following Narcotic Epidural Block as Practiced in our Pain Unit

1. Assess pain level
   (0 to 10 scale; 0 = no pain, 10 = as bad as it can be)
2. Apnea monitor for eight hours
3. Maintain patient IV for eight hours
4. Bedrest for eight hours, up with assistance for next two hours
5. Vital signs every five minutes for one-half hour, every fifteen minutes for next three hours, every one hour for five hours
6. One-to-one nursing observation for one hour after procedure
7. Monitor urinary output
8. Naloxone (Narcan) .4 mg IV or IM if respirations drop below six per minute. Call physician. Repeat naloxone every ten minutes as needed

ters of this book. The nurse's role in these therapies will vary somewhat depending upon the organization of the specific pain unit. Massage, heat and cold application, and exercises are generally performed by a physical therapist. It is important, however, for the nurse to know the basic principles related to these therapies and to be aware of the physical therapy treatment plan so that any components of the plan that are to be done on the unit can be carried out. The nurse can reinforce the need for the exercise program and reward compliance.

Many facilities employ an individual who functions as a TENS technician who provides the patient with the instrument and properly teaches him or her to use it. A TENS unit consists of a battery-powered generator that sends a mild electrical impulse through electrodes that have been placed on the skin near the pain site. The predominant theory on the mechanism of action asserts that electrical stimulation closes a gate in the spinal cord for pain-impulse transmission by overstimulating large afferent fibers (see Chapter 24). The nurse can help the patient to experiment with various electrode placements to find the optimal position for the individual patient. Frequently a slight shift of electrode placement will result in a significant improvement of pain. The frequency and intensity of stimulation can vary the level of pain relief as well; again, the nurse should help the patient to find the most effective instrument setting.

To be effective for chronic pain, the instrument may have to be worn for extended periods of time, often throughout the entire day, which may result in skin irritation at the electrode site. Varying electrode positions, using another brand of conductive jelly, changing the type of adhesive tape or electrode, or substituting hand cream for the conductive jelly are possible solutions for this annoying problem. Also, skin irritation can be effectively treated with a topical steroid cream. Transcutaneous stimulation has been successful in modulating the pain of myofascial syndrome and peripheral nerve injury; patients with central nervous system pain and with peripheral neuropathy have responded poorly, however (17).

In most facilities where biofeedback is utilized, trained technicians will instruct the patient in biofeedback techniques. When this is the case, the nurse's role is to reinforce the education that has been received and support the patient's use of the technique. In Chapter 19 biofeedback and its appropriate utilization as a pain management tool is described.

Cognitive strategies such as distraction, relaxation, and guided imagery are techniques that nurses have traditionally incorporated into their nursing care for patients experiencing pain. Tan (18) thoroughly reviewed the research literature that discusses the use and effectiveness of these coping skills. Distraction involves assisting patients to focus their attention on something other than pain. This refocused attention, concentrating on music, reading, or a conversation, for example, usually results in some reduction of pain intensity.

Relaxation effectively alters autonomic nervous system activity and thus diminishes a patient's pain. When utilized effectively, relaxation is accompanied by decreased blood pressure, heart rate, and muscle tension. Guided imagery encourages patients to create images that decease pain intensity by focusing their attention on images that are associated with feeling relaxed and peaceful. It is important to explain to patients that the ability to utilize these coping skills effectively does not indicate that their pain "is in their head." Patients, and even many health care professionals, erroneously believe that if one can effectively control or diminish pain by means of cognitive strategies, then the pain is psychogenic in origin. This is not so; cognitive strategies can be effectively employed to help pain even if caused by cancer. They are valuable components of a multimodal chronic pain treatment program.

Devices For Pain Relief

A simple device, such as a properly designed pillow, can significantly affect a patient's pain level. Most facilities have available, through either their physical therapy department or central supply department, items such as grabbers, coccygeal pillows, cervical pillows, body aligners, and egg-crate mattress pads. The nurse can assess a patient's need for these items and provide instruction on their proper use. A grabber is a device that allows patients to effectively extend their reaching capability without bending or stretching. A coccygeal pillow allows a patient with coccygodynia to sit more comfortably by eliminating pressure on the coccyx. A cervical pillow supports the cervical area in proper alignment while the patient is lying in bed. A body aligner supports the legs in the proper knee-bent position while lying on the back and reduces strain in the lumbar area. It can also be used as a brace to lean against while lying on either side. An egg-crate mattress pad provides a more comfortable surface upon which to lie while maintaining firmness in the mattress. This pad is especially effective in reducing the likelihood of a decubitus in a patient who spends a great deal of time in bed.

Patient Teaching

Patient teaching is becoming an increasingly important nursing function as a cost-saving measure (such as Medicare's system of payment by Diagnosis Related Groups) and are being utilized in the inpatient setting. As with any chronically ill patient, teaching is an integral aspect of the treatment provided to the chronic pain patient. By the time the typical patient is seen in a pain treatment facility, he or she has often had several unsuccessful surgical procedures and/or taken numerous pharmaceutical agents. Generally, we find that patients have been told, in a variety of direct and indirect ways, that their pain is not "real." A carefully planned teaching program is central to correcting the fears, misconceptions, and lack of trust in medical treatment that the chronic pain patient frequently experiences.

Doctors are often perceived, correctly or not, to be too busy to talk about the minutia of symptoms that chronic pain patients experience, even though such matters occupy a great deal of the patients' thoughts. Usually, patients ask their questions of the nurse before approaching the doctor or other health care professional with them.

It is important that the nurse working as a pain team member be well informed as to the causes and effects of the patient's illness. Furthermore, she must be knowledgeable about the full range of treatment modalities available to the patient. In many instances, it is the nurse who initiates a discussion with the chronic pain patient about his or her illness and treatment options. This is especially true for those patients who have become disillusioned with physicians and distrusting of whatever physicians may say. The nurse not only becomes a source of valuable information for the patient but also helps build realistic trust in the pain management team. With encouragement and support from the nurse, the patient then may have a frank discussion with the physician about diagnosis and prognosis. Sometimes the diagnosis and predicted outcome are below the patient's expectations. In these cases, the nurse working with the pain team can lend support to the patient.

In many instances, when a patient is undergoing a new treatment approach and suffering from some degree of psychological distress, information may have to be repeated on different occasions in order for the patient to fully grasp what is being said. The educational approach adopted by the nurse needs to be decided in collaboration with the treating physician and other members of the pain management team. Since chronic pain patients may have little, or conflicting, information about their illness or may have significant distortion of their illness due to a psychopathological disturbance, a clear empirical education approach by the team is essential. If not, destructive splitting of the treatment team will occur.

The knowledge that the nurse possesses, properly imparted to the patient, will increase the effectiveness of all treatments and will prepare the patient more effectively for discharge. For the chronic pain patient, perhaps the most important learning that occurs with effective patient–nurse "teaching sessions" does not occur in the formal, planned teaching-learning sessions, but rather happens in the less structured discussions that focus on coping. In these situations, the nurse not only offers information but also offers ways of being, ways of coping, and new possibilities. The experienced pain nurse has observed and understands the many ways of coping with chronic pain. She can offer the patient avenues of understanding, increased control, and acceptance.

REFERENCES

1. Hoffman RS: Operation of a medical-psychiatric unit in a general hospital setting. Gen Hosp Psychiatry 6:93–99, 1984
2. Fogel BS: A psychiatric unit becomes a psychiatric medical unit: administration and clinical implications. Gen Hosp Psychiatry 7:26–35, 1985
3. Pinsky JJ, Crue BL, Griffin S: Why a pain unit?, in Chronic Pain: Further Observations from City of Hope National Medical Center. Edited by Crue BL. New York, Spectrum Publications, 1979
4. American Nurses' Association Congress for Nursing Practice: Standards of Nursing Practice. Kansas City, American Nurses Association, 1973
5. Keefe FJ, Block AR: Development of an observation method for assessing pain behavior in chronic low back pain patients. Behavior Therapy 13:363–375, 1982
6. Krishnan KRR, France RD, Pelton S, et al: Chronic pain and depression, I: classification of depression in chronic low back pain patients. Pain 22:279–287, 1985
7. Houpt JL, Keefe FJ, Snipes MT: The Clinical Specialty Unit: the use of the psychiatry inpatient unit to treat chronic pain syndromes. Gen Hosp Psychiatry 6:65–70, 1984
8. Wilson RR, Aronoff GM: The therapeutic community in the treament of chronic pain. J Chronic Dis 32:477–481, 1979
9. Morse RH: Milieu psychotherapy, in Management of Patients with Chronic Pain. Edited by Brena SF, Chapman SL. New York, Spectrum Publications, 1983
10. Carey KW (Ed): Nursing Now Series: Pain. Springhouse, PA, Springhouse Corp, 1985
11. Meinhart NT, McCaffery M: Pain, A Nursing Approach to Assessment and Analysis. Norwalk, CT, Appleton-Century-Crofts, 1983
12. France RD, Houpt JL, Ellinwood EH: Therapeutic effects of anti-depressants in chronic pain. Gen Hosp Psychiatry 6:55–63, 1984
13. Marks RM, Sachar EJ: Undertreatment of medical inpatients with narcotic analgesics. Ann Intern Med 78:173–181, 1973
14. Moulin DE, Foley KM: Management of pain in patients with cancer. Psychiatric Annals 14:815–822, 1984
15. Sriwatanakul K, Weis OF, Alloza JL, et al: Analysis of narcotic analgesic usage in the treatment of postoperative pain. JAMA 250:926, 1983
16. Schnapp M, Mayo KS, North WC: Intravenous 2- chloroprocaine in treatment of chronic pain. Anesthesia and Analgesia Current Research 60:844–845, 1981
17. Long DM, Campbell JN, Guzer G: Transcutaneous electrical stimulation for relief of chronic pain. Advances in Pain Research Therapy. New York, Raven Press, 1976
18. Tan SY: Cognitive and cognitive-behavioral methods for pain control: a selected review. Pain 12:201–228, 1982

APPENDIX

NURSING PAIN ASSESSMENT

LOCATION
Mark on drawings the area of pain

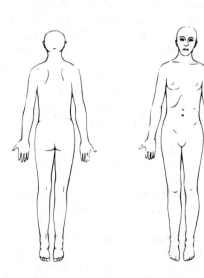

Indicate if pain is:
a) deep
b) superficial

If it is:
a) constant
b) intermittent

What type:
a) aching
b) burning
c) shooting
d) other

DURATION
Initial Onset _____

Duration of continuous pain _____

_____

INTENSITY (0-10 scale; 0 = no pain, 10 = pain as bad as it can be)
Present _____ Lowest _____ Highest _____ Average _____

CHARACTER
Have patient describe pain in his own words

_____

_____

Associated Symptoms _____

_____

_____

_____

FACTORS MODIFYING PAIN
What makes the pain better? _____

_____

_____

Which of these is most effective? _____

_____

_____

What has made the pain worse? _____

_____

_____

LIFESTYLE CHANGES
How has activity level changed? _____

_____

_____

What is pain preventing the patient from doing that he would really like to do? _____

_____

_____

What are present activities? _____

_____

_____

How have relationships been affected? _____

_____

_____

Chapter 24

Treatment of Chronic Pain by Local Modulation of Nociception

Bruno J. Urban, M.D.

Pain is conscious nociception associated with negative affective responses and distinct behaviors. In this context, nociception is defined as the sum of neural responses to noxious stimuli. The associated factors may feed into the original pain complaint sustaining it in spite of diminishing noxious stimulation (1).

Ideally, treatment of pain involves removing its underlying cause. Unfortunately, this is not always possible. There may be either little evidence for on-going noxious stimulation amenable to treatment (as, for example, in chronic low back pain), or tissue pathology may be such as to resist etiological therapy (for example, in cancer). Another possibility is that pain may originate without excitation of distal nociceptors within the central nervous system itself (for example, in phantom limb pain). Nevertheless, successful symptomatic treatment is possible in many of these cases. Treatment may be directed toward the elimination of aggravating factors originating from pain behaviors and affective responses, and toward modulation of nociception.

Modulation of nociception is based on the concept that nociception consists of the spatio-temporal integration of afferent impulses within the neuroanatomical substrate. Thus, pain should decrease—even in the presence of continuing noxious stimulation—if change can be effected in afferent impulses or in their pattern of summation. Change may consist of decreasing or increasing the number of impulses, or modulating their transmission pattern.

Successful pain moderation by modulating impulse transmission has been achieved for long periods of time by systemic administration of analgesics (for example, morphine). The use of analgesics and other medications modulating nociception is discussed in different chapters; this brief review attempts to summarize modulation of nociception locally by either decreasing or increasing the number of afferent impulses. Exceptions will be pituitary alcohol ablation and intravenous local anesthetic administration (chloroprocaine), which seem to exert their long-term effects via a general mechanism.

Classically, attempts at moderating pain by local manipulations of the nervous system consisted of impulse reduction. This can be accomplished reversibly by conduction block (nerve block) with local anesthetics (alone or enhanced with other drugs), or irreversibly by destruction of neural tissue involved in pain transmission with chemicals or in operation. Recently, impulse augmentation has been instituted to modulate nociception; this is achieved by adding impulses using electrical stimulation devices.

REVERSIBLE IMPULSE REDUCTION: NERVE BLOCK

Nerve blocks effect reversible interruption of nervous conduction. This is accomplished by inserting a needle through the skin to the selected nervous structure and injecting a measured amount of a local anesthetic. Local anesthetics are chemicals that inhibit neural excitation by preventing membrane depolarization. They are weak bases marketed in salt form. In solution they exist in charged and uncharged (base) form in a proportion dependent upon the pKa of the substance and the pH of the solution. The base diffuses more readily into the tissues; the charged salt is mainly responsible for receptor attachment. Tissue pH may affect local anesthetic effectiveness by altering the proportion of salt to base (2).

Clinically useful local anesthetics fall into two categories: ester compounds and amide compounds. The difference in chemical structure is biologically reflected in: 1) a different site of metabolism (ester compounds are hydrolyzed in plasma, amide compounds undergo enzymatic degradation in the liver); and 2) a different allergic potential (allergic reactions are almost completely absent with amide compounds). There is no cross-allergy between groups. Table 1 lists onset, duration, concentration, and total maximal dose of four frequently used local anesthetics. Procaine and chloroprocaine are esters, lidocaine and bupivacaine are amides. At present, lidocaine is probably the most commonly employed drug. To avoid systemic side effects it is mandatory not to exceed the recommended maximal doses. Duration of action may be extended by

Table 1. Commonly Used Local Anesthetics

Chemical Name (a common brand name)	Onset of Block	Duration of Block	Commonly Used Concentrations (%)			Total Maximal Dose in mg/kg Body Weight
			Infiltration	Field Block	Nerve Block	
procaine (Novocaine)	intermediate	short	0.5	0.75–1	1–2	15
chloroprocaine (Nesacaine)	fast	short	0.5	0.75–1	1–2	20
lidocaine (Xylocaine)	fast	intermediate	0.25	0.5–0.75	1–1.5	7
bupivacaine (Marcaine)	intermediate	very long	0.1	0.15–0.25	0.25–0.5	2.5

adding a vasoconstrictor to the anesthetic solution (usually adrenaline 1:200,000).

The application of nerve blocks to the treatment of pain is based on blocking nociceptive input producing temporary abolition of pain. This may allow for the investigation of the anatomical pathway of pain and help confirm a diagnosis. Alternatively, failure of the block to change pain perception may indicate a central origin of pain. To eliminate a placebo response as much as possible, consistent results should be obtained with a series of blocks, and there should be correlation between the pharmacologic action of the agent employed and the duration of pain relief. This is even more important when results are used in the decision process for specific treatment; for example, for neurodestructive operation. In the latter case, successful block also allows the patient to temporarily experience the neurologic deficit that will permanently follow the operation. Unfortunately, nerve blocks have little value as prognostic tools; for example, for dorsal rhizotomy no correlation was found between pain relief provided by paravertebral block and the long-term results of root section (3).

In addition to blocking nociceptive impulses, nerve blocks interrupt motor and/or sympathetic reflexes. Temporary analgesia, reflex interruption, and the clinical phenomenon that pain relief may outlast the duration of local anesthetic action constitute the rationale for treating chronic pain with repeated blocks (4). During the period of freedom from pain, other therapeutic modalities (for example, active and passive physical therapy) may be applied more successfully, shortening the process of rehabilitation. It is interesting to note that nerve blocks have also been found helpful with a contingency management program; symptomatic pain relief from blocks was used as reinforcement, contingent upon appropriate behavior (5). For certain diseases (reflex sympathetic dystrophy, myofascial syndrome) nerve blocks may be curative (6, 7).

The therapeutic effectiveness of specific nerve blocks may be enhanced by the addition and/or substitution of unrelated compounds.

Corticosteroids, alone or in combination with a local anesthetic, have been successfully applied to the management of musculoskeletal disorders and peripheral nerve entrapment syndromes (4). Injection into the peripheral nerve for the latter disease may cause degenerative changes in this nerve, thus effecting partial neurectomy (8). The epidural administration of crystalline suspensions of corticosteroids has been found useful in the treatment of low back pain with radiculopathy (9, 10). However, in spite of more than two decades of clinical use, there is still a paucity of information on this established treatment (11). The mechanism of action is not well understood but is supposed to rest in the reduction of edema in (or around) irritated nerve roots. Alternatively, corticosteroids may suppress ectopic neural discharges of the affected nerve root similar to their suppression of ectopic impulses originating in peripheral nerve neuroma (12).

Clinical reports have stressed the safety of the method and its lack of complications (11, 13). Animal investigation of one compound under conditions mimicking clinical usage concluded that significant histologic damage to neural tissue was not apparent with either light or electron microscope examination (14). In contrast, the subarachnoid injection of corticosteroids has a distinctly higher incidence of reported complications. They include meningitis, arachnoiditis, conus medullaris syndrome, and others. It seems prudent to avoid intrathecal steroid applications and even postpone their epidural use in cases where the subarachnoid space has inadvertently been entered (11, 13).

Narcotics have been applied directly to the spinal cord via the subarachnoid (spinal) or epidural route. When administered this way they effectively reduce pain without the motor and/or sympathetic blockade that follows local anesthetics (15). Clinically, dermatomal hypalgesia can be demonstrated (16). Side effects of spinal narcotics include respiratory depression, pruritus, nausea, vomiting, and urinary retention. Respiratory depression is the most serious complication. It has been more often reported after subarachnoid instillation; it may occasionally become life-threatening. Complications are completely reversible with naloxone; however, due to the short duration of action of this drug, repeated administration may be necessary.

Most experience with spinal narcotics has been obtained in acute (postoperative) pain states. Epidural morphine has most commonly been employed. The drug is prepared by diluting the selected amount of preservative-free morphine in preservative-free normal saline (usually 10 ml). Other narcotics are prepared similarly. The amount to be injected at one time varies; 8 to 10 mg morphine (or equipotent equivalent) may be needed to completely control severe postoperative abdominal pain. A dose-response curve obtained for pain following orthopedic operations suggests that there may be an optimal amount of epidural narcotic for a given painful lesion (17, 18).

Spinal narcotics have been successfully applied to the management of intractable pain of the terminally ill. This may be accomplished simply by injecting one or two doses of narcotic per day through an indwelling epidural catheter. Continuous long-term administration is possible with implanted catheter-perfusion systems (19). Both subarachnoid and epidural catheter placements have been utilized. Pain moderation was maintained over several months in patients with otherwise intractable pain caused by cancer (20). Reported side effects are notably absent; however, habituation does occur (21). There are no data as to the applicability of chronic spinal narcotic administration to pain states of nonmalignant etiology.

For treatment of pain, anesthetics are usually applied locally to the nerve. However, these dosages have also been administered systemically (intravenously) for the same purpose. Both ester and amide type agents have been employed with similar results (22, 23). Recently, chloroprocaine has been advocated because its rapid hydrolysis in plasma may decrease the occurrence and severity of toxic reactions (24). The mechanism of action is unknown. A general anesthetic mechanism does not seem to be the cause; denervation pain is reduced at blood levels of lidocaine which do not produce a general analgesic effect (23). Pain relief is maintained for several months in some cases. Patients suffering allodynia and spontaneous pain seem to respond more favorably (24).

Clinically, chloroprocaine is administered intravenously at a rate that produces mild signs of CNS toxicity (for example, tinnitus, slurred speech, lightheadedness, and others). We limit the total dose to 10 mg/kg body weight. Serious complications have not been reported; many patients remain sedated for several hours following administration, necessitating close observation. Responders show immediate pain reduction, which becomes further reduced with repeated treatments.

IRREVERSIBLE IMPULSE REDUCTION: NEUROLYSIS, OPERATION

Irreversible impulse reduction may be achieved by affecting destruction of selected neural tissue. This may be done either by substituting the local anesthetic used for nerve block with neurolytic agents, or by sectioning nerves during operation. Neurolysis may be effected by chemical or physical means. The two commonly employed chemicals are alcohol and phenol (25). Both are equally effective. Alcohol is used in a concentration of either 50 or 100 percent. Phenol is customarily employed in five to seven percent aqueous solution for peripheral block, and in a five percent solution in glycerine for subarachnoid (spinal) block (26). Alternatively, neurodestruction may be achieved by heating ($+80°C$) or cooling ($-60°C$) the tip of the needle resting in neural tissue with special instrumentation.

Chemical neurolysis presents an acceptable solution to neural destruction when injected into the subarachnoid space or into sympathetic ganglia (for example, the celiac block). When injected into peripheral nerves (with the possible exception of cranial nerves) its use may be followed by a painful neuritis, which may be more aggravating than the original pain complaint. For this reason and because of poor long-term results, permanent blocks are rarely applied to chronic pain of nonmalignant origin but are reserved for patients with limited life expectancy (27). Similarly, neurodestructive surgery is utilized less and less for pain states of nonmalignant etiology (28, 29). Exceptions may be percutaneous electrocoagulation of the trigeminal ganglion for tic douloureux, sympathectomy for causalgia and dorsal root entry zone lesions (DREZ) for specific pain syndromes; for example, brachial plexus avulsion (30–33).

In contrast, impulse reduction by neurodestruction should be considered early in the treatment of cancer pain. While the basic therapy consists of modulation of impulse transmission by time contingent administration of analgesics, evaluation for neuroablation should be performed either when medications become ineffective or when habituation becomes evident. Commonly used procedures include cordotomy, permanent nerve blocks or section, and chemical hypophysectomy.

Cordotomy is the operation of choice for unilateral cancer pain caudal to the nipple, but can be used for all somatic pain below the mandibles (34). The procedure effects destruction in the lateral spino-thalamic tract. It has been simplified to a percutaneous technique. An insulated needle is inserted under local anesthesia in the neck contralateral to the site of pain. It is advanced under radiographic control via the C_2 intervertebral foramen into the spinal cord and positioned so that the noninsulated tip rests in the anterior quadrant (spino-thalamic tract). Proper placement is accomplished by repeatedly checking with x-rays (fluoroscopy), impedance measurements, and electrical stimulation. Lesion of the tract is performed with radiofrequency current. Other percutaneous approaches have been described; section of the spino-thalamic tract following laminectomy is possible but carries a higher operative risk.

When performed on one side cordotomy results in analgesia (raised pain threshold) on the contra-lateral site of the body. Immediately following the operation 90 percent of patients consider themselves pain-free; this number decreases to 60 percent and 40 percent respectively at the one- and two-year follow-up evaluations. Return of pain after extended periods of time is a minor consideration in patients with limited life expectancy. The operation has a low complication rate, consisting mostly of ataxia paresis and bladder dysfunction. It may be performed in steps bilaterally but then carries the additional risk of sleep-induced apnea (about 3 percent of cases) (34).

Neurolytic blocks commonly applied to the management of cancer pain are: subarachnoid block, celiac plexus block, and block of cranial nerves.

Subarachnoid (spinal) blocks with a neurolytic chemical effects partial or complete rhizotomy/ganglionectomy. Appropriate positioning of the patient following spinal tap, combined with utilization of drugs lighter (alcohol) or heavier (phenol in glycerin) than cerebrospinal fluid (CSF), allows neurodestruction to be confined to the dorsal roots of preselected segments. Alcohol requires a separate needle to be placed for each root; hyperbaric phenol is injected through one needle and flows to the dependent roots. Duration of effect is highly variable; an average duration of nine months has been reported (26). Complications include headaches, weakness, numbness, painful paresthesia, and urinary and fecal incontinence. The incidence of permanent sequelae ranges from 1 to 13 percent (26). Because of the shorter duration of pain relief, chemical rhizotomy should be considered second to cordotomy. It may be used as adjunct to this operation when it is deemed inadvisable to perform it bilaterally. In this case cordotomy is performed to the body half with the most pain, chemical rhizotomy to the other half. Surgical rhizotomy has a higher complication rate; it is usually only applied to cancer patients with pain in a small area and longer life expectancy. Best results are obtained in pelvic neoplasms (35).

Permanent celiac plexus is probably the procedure of choice in controlling pain caused by pancreatic or other cancerous tumors of abdominal organs. The procedure consists of injection of up to 50 ml of 50 percent alcohol into the celiac plexus via two needles inserted from the back to this area. Following injection, the needles should be cleared of alcohol with air or fluid. This avoids contamination of somatic nerves during withdrawal of the needle. A diagnostic block with local anesthetic should always precede neurolytic injection and should have resulted in complete temporary abolition of pain.

Celiac alcohol injection produces the feeling of a "kick in the stomach"; it is followed by short-lived (seconds to minutes) intense burning. This has been used as a sign of proper needle placement. Nerve degeneration occurs gradually over several days; thus, the immediate effects of alcohol injection are usually not as pronounced as the effects of local anesthetic block. The patient should be apprised of this fact. Expected side effects are low intensity back pain lasting two to three days and—less frequent— transient orthostatic hypotension (up to one week); the side effects are treated symptomatically (22). An often welcome side effect consists in increased motility of the gut. Splanchnic nerve destruction will result in pain relief in more than 90 percent of patients; it may be expected to last for three to five months (occasionally one year) (25, 36). The block may be safely repeated on return of pain.

Neurolysis (or section) of cranial nerves has successfully been applied to control cancer pain of the head/neck region. Most often involved are the trigeminal and glossopharyngeal nerves. To encompass the entire area of tumor spread, the upper cervical nerves (C_2 and C_3) must often be treated in addition. Percutaneous radiofrequency electrocoagulation seems to be the method of choice at the present time. For the trigeminal nerve the procedure is identical to the one used for tic doloreux (30). The glossopharyngeal nerve may be approached with a needle in similar fashion, but directed toward the jugular foramen (37). The cervical nerves are easily accessible at their exit foramen.

Alcohol injection into the pituitary gland (neuroadenolysis) has been reported to result in prolonged pain relief in a large number of patients suffering from widespread metastatic cancer—excellent relief in 86 percent of patients (38); moderate relief in 42 percent; and partial relief in an additional 33 percent of patients (39). Most patients had cancer of the breast or prostate. The mechanism of action is unknown but seems to involve a general modulation of transmission of nervous impulses. It seems to be independent of endogenous opiates production, the amount of pituitary destruction, and subsequent hormonal dysfunction. It has been linked to a hypothalamic effect (40). Short-term electrical stimulation of the pituitary gland has produced similar though shorter lasting relief as subsequent pituitary alcoholisation in the same patients (41).

The procedure is carried out under light general anesthesia with the patient supine. Fluoroscopy is mandatory. After shrinking the mucosa with four percent topically applied cocaine or other drug, an 18-gauge thick-wall spinal needle (12 to 15 cm) is inserted through one nostril toward the pituitary fossa (through the sphneoid sinus). Repeat bi-plane fluoroscopy assures strict midline position aiming at a point about 2 mm inferior to the rim of the sella. A mallet is used to tap the needle in place just short of the posterior wall. Following negative aspiration 1 ml absolute alcohol is injected in increments of 0.1 ml, allowing for one minute intervals between doses. The size of the pupil is continuously monitored. If it decreases the injection is stopped; if it does not return to normal within three minutes the procedure should be abandoned.

Pain relief following the neuroadenolysis may occur rapidly or gradually over the next days. About 70 percent of patients may expect a good result (40). The procedure is equally effective in patients suffering metastatic pain from neoplasms originating from organs other than breast and prostate. Duration of pain relief varies widely; the majority of patients experience pain return within three months, though larger pain-free intervals have been observed. The operation has a definitive mortality and morbidity. Side effects and complications include transient headaches, hormonal deficiency, diabetes insipidus (often temporary), cerebrospinal fluid leak, and, infrequently, meningitis and defects of the third and second cranial nerves (blindness) (40).

IMPULSE AUGMENTATION: ELECTRICAL STIMULATION

Increasing afferent impulses with counterirritation has been used for a long time to modulate painful conditions; even the use of electrical current to this effect dates to antiquity (42). Intermittent intense stimulation is used in acupuncture and related therapy with often impressive results in cases of low back and myofascial pain (43). It has also been combined with electrical stimulation (hyperstimulation analgesia). Present technological progress has made continuous impulse augmentation by electrical stimulation devices practical (44). The simplest way to increase afferent impulses electrically consists of applying electrodes to the skin and connecting them to a suitable impulse generator (trans-cutaneous stimulation) (44, 45). Surface electrodes are made from flexible conductors. They are taped or glued close to the painful part of the body after skin resistance has been lowered by abrasive cleaning and application of electrolyte jelly. Flexible insulated wires connect the electrodes to a battery-powered generator, usually the size of a package of cigarettes (Figure 1). The user can independently vary frequency and intensity of stimulation; stimulation is perceived as light, repetitive shocks. The produced analgesia ceases shortly after discontinuation of stimulation. Thus, to be effective for chronic pain, the instrument has to be worn for an extended period of time, usually throughout the entire day. This may produce skin irritation at the electrode site, a minor but often annoying complication that may limit the effective use of the device. Transcutaneous stimulation has successfully moderated pain from a variety of conditions including causalgia, herpes zoster, low back pain, and others (45). It should be used early and not as a last resort.

Increase of impulses within one selected peripheral nerve may be achieved by implanting electrodes close to the nerve during operation. They are connected subcutaneously to a radio receiver, also buried, under the skin. Stimulation is supplied by a battery-powered transmitter coupled by means of a flexible antenna taped to the skin overlying the receiver. External controls allow the user to change the frequency and intensity of stimulation independently (Figure 1). Stimulation is per-

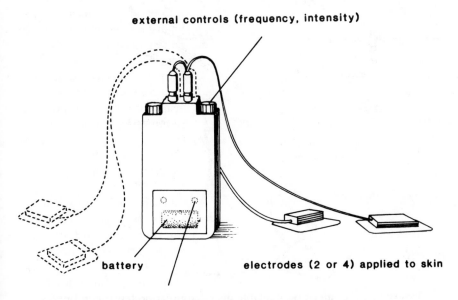

Figure 1. Diagram of transcutaneous nerve stimulator

ceived as paresthesia (tingling) in the dependent area of the particular nerve. Long-term pain modulation from peripheral nerve stimulation has been excellent in selected patients, where the electrodes could be placed central to the lesion producing the pain. Large series of studies are lacking (45). Stimulation of nerves of the arms seems to produce more satisfactory results than sciatic stimulation (46).

Impulse augmentation involving larger areas of the body is possible by electrical stimulation of the structures of the spinal cord (47). Originally, this was achieved by the surgical implantation of electrodes close to the dorsal columns during laminectomy. The electrodes are subcutaneously connected to an implanted radiofrequency receiver system activated by an external transmitter similar to peripheral nerve stimulators. External control of the frequency and intensity of stimulation is provided (Figure 2). Pain relief is linked to the production of paresthesia in the painful

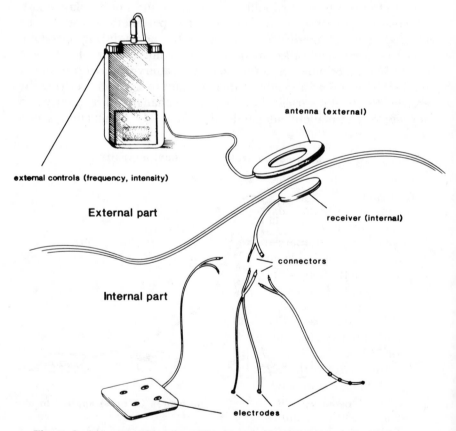

Figure 2. Diagram of implantable nerve stimulation (peripheral nerve stimulator and dorsal column stimulator)

part of the body (48). Long-term results demonstrated pain modulation in 30 percent of patients (49, 50). Retrospectively, three main problems were identified: 1) failure to achieve stimulation into the painful area of the body; 2) failure to derive pain relief from acceptable stimulation; and 3) failure to continue pain relief after initial success (49). This occurred in spite of careful patient selection and the use of various predictive tests, including transcutaneous stimulation. It seems that stimulation of the spinal cord over an extended period of time is necessary to predict the effect of this stimulation on pain moderation in the individual patient.

Electrical stimulation of the spinal cord can also be supplied by epidurally placed electrodes (Figure 2). When using flexible wire electrodes they can be inserted through needles into the epidural space without the need for laminectomy. The technique is similar to the placement of epidural catheters, which are routinely used for administration of continuous epidural anesthesia. The development of the percutaneous technique obviated the need for a major operation under general anesthesia, simplified the procedure, and produced acceptable cord stimulation (51–53). Thus, it constituted an ideal predictive test for a dorsal stimulator implant by laminectomy. Furthermore, since only local anesthesia is required, the electrodes could be manipulated to produce maximal paresthesia in the area of pain by observing the patient's response to trial stimulation during placement (54).

This solved the first main problem encountered with the open placement of dorsal column stimulators under general anesthesia. In an attempt to overcome the second main problem, epidural electrodes may be left partially exteriorized for trial stimulation extending over several days. This makes it possible to gain information on the effect of stimulation on pain before committing the patient to the implant. The third problem, that of failure to continue pain relief after initial success, has remained unsolved.

Internalizing percutaneously inserted epidural electrodes and connecting them to an implanted radio receiver allowed prorated (therapeutic) stimulation. Long-term results with percutaneous epidural stimulator implants demonstrated pain modulation in 30 to 50 percent of patients, similar to results from dorsal column stimulator implants by laminectomy (29, 54). The main complication consists of change of stimulation paresthesia, negating pain relief and necessitating operative revision (13, 54, 55). Side effects include often annoying paresthesia into nonpainful parts of the body. Combining a technique of percutaneous peripheral nerve stimulation with epidural stimulation shows promise of lowering side effects while producing equal pain moderation (56).

Finally, electrical stimulation may be applied directly to the brain, specifically, to the periventricular grey matter or to the internal capsule. At present this operation is carried out in few centers only; advantages, disadvantages, results, and complications have been reviewed recently (57). Short-term results are reported to show 90 percent good pain relief; long-term continued pain moderation is expected in 60 to 80 percent of patients (57).

CONCLUSION

A multidisciplinary approach to pain therapy is typically required. Specific procedures providing for reduction or augmentation of afferent nervous impulses may modulate pain, but rarely effect complete control in the chronic pain patient. Permanent neurodestruction and nerve stimulator implants have low overall success rates. They should be reserved for selected patients after exhaustion of all other therapeutic modalities, including alleviation of suffering and behavior modification. Augmentation procedures are preferred, as they do not produce a neurologic deficit.

APPENDIX: NERVE BLOCKS

Technical Aspects

Most blocks can be performed in a suitable office or clinic space; the facilities of an operating room are only rarely needed. Equipment consists of sterile needles and syringes, and the drugs to be employed; prepackaged sterilized block trays are commercially available. Resuscitation equipment must be present; that is, suction apparatus, oxygen and means to administer artificial ventilation (ventilation bag, airways, endotracheal intubation kit), intravenous fluids with administration sets (including IV cannulae), and emergency drugs (for example, diazepam, barbiturate, vasopressor, muscle relaxant). Contraindications to nerve blocks consist of allergies to the local anesthetic or its vehicle, infection in the area to be injected, bleeding tendencies, and lack of patient acceptance.

The procedure, including side effects and possible complications, is thoroughly explained to the patient. This is the best premedication; chemical sedation is not needed. If larger amounts of local anesthetic are to be injected or larger body areas are to be anesthetized, oral intake should be withheld for six to eight hours. Sterile precautions are observed. Other fundamentals of blocking technique include gentleness, knowledge of anatomy, frequent aspiration for blood, and awareness of maximal safe drug dosage. It is recommended that the operator talks with the patient throughout the procedure; this increases calmness and serves as a monitor. The use of local anesthetic skin wheal and field infiltration before insertion of larger gauge block needles renders the procedure almost completely painless.

Complications are rare; they consist of usually inconsequential sequelae of needle puncture (nerve, blood vessel) and side effects from the local anesthetic (25). The majority of the latter are comprised of toxic reactions to high blood levels usually caused by inadvertent intravascular injection or by administration of excessive amounts of drug. Initially, CNS excitation occurs; it is followed by depression. Clinical signs are excitement, incoherent speech, drowsiness, convulsions, and unconsciousness. Signs of nervous system depression may dominate. Cardiovascular effects of high blood concentrations are hypotension (general vasodilations, decreased myocardial contractility), sinus bradycardia, and, ultimately, cardiac arrest. Respiration is unaffected until overt CNS toxicity is present.

Other complications may be caused by allergic reactions. They are infrequent (probably less than one percent of all complications) and may be due to the preservative added to the local anesthetic solution. Treatment of all complications is symptomatic; the prognosis is good.

The performance of certain nerve blocks may be facilitated and success achieved by utilizing ancillary equipment when placing the needle. A nerve stimulator allows exact localization and identification of a peripheral nerve by producing contractions of its dependent muscles (58). The instrument delivers controllable repetitive electrical impulses (usually 1 or 2 Hz). Its groundlead is connected to an electrode pad placed on the patient's skin distant to the area of needle insertion. The active lead is clipped to the metal part of the needle. Stimulation is begun after the needle has been inserted according to anatomic landmarks and is presumed to rest in the vicinity of the selected nerve. It is gradually (gently) increased in intensity until distal motor response occurs (repetitive contractions of dependent muscles). The needle is repositioned so that minimal stimulation produces maximal response. Needles insulated but for the tip are helpful but not necessary. The use of a stimulator obviates the need to elecit painful paresthesia by repeated needle probing. Stimulation is painless in the clinical range.

Radiographic control (fluoroscopy with image intensification) increases accurate needle placement when a nerve is situated in close relation to distinct bony structures. In addition, fluoroscopy helps to avoid repeated unnecessary and painful needle contact with periosteum, decreases the time of the procedure, and, thus, patient discomfort. A 40 percent error in needle placement was documented radiographically when blocks were performed relying only on the classic methods of anatomic landmarks. (The highest incidence of faulty needle position occurred when attempting paravertebral somatic nerve block.) (59). An error of this magnitude is not acceptable, especially if the results of the block are to be used to confirm a diagnosis or therapeutic approach. In these cases verification of the blocked nerve with X-ray or stimulation techniques is mandatory.

Procedures

Applicable blocking procedures encompass the entire field of regional analgesia; they are detailed in standard textbooks (25, 60–62). Progressing from the CNS to the periphery, they consist of spinal (subarachnoid) block, epidural block, paravertebral somatic nerve block, sympathetic ganglion block, peripheral nerve block, and local infiltration. A complete description is beyond the scope of this chapter; the purpose of the following summary is to provide an outline of frequently used procedures.

Subarachnoid (Spinal) Block

The technique of spinal tap by midline approach is generally known. However, lateral approaches are often easier to perform and more comfortable for the patient (61). They may also have a reduced incidence of postspinal puncture headaches. The latter constitute the main complication and are caused by leakage of spinal fluid into the epidural space (low CSF pressure headache). Since the hole in the dura depends on the size of the needle, the use of small gauge needles is recommended. Below 22-gauge size is an introducer; that is, a larger needle placed in the interspinous ligament assures that the needle does not bend from its intended path. Postspinal puncture headache can almost always be managed conservatively (bedrest, increased fluid intake, mild analgesics). In resistant cases or when neurologic sequelae occur (for example, abducens paresis) closure of the persistent dural hole with an epidurally applied blood patch is indicated.

Utilizing the principle of differential blockade by the pharmacologic approach, graduated spinal anesthesia has been advocated for the evaluation of chronic lower back and extremity pain (63). In short, this test consists of sequential intrathecal instillations of normal saline (placebo) followed by equal volumes (usually 5 ml) of 0.2 percent, 0.5 percent, and 1 percent procaine at 10-minute intervals. If spinal anesthesia does not result, an additional dose of tetracaine is given. After each injection the patient is examined and subjective responses correlated with the produced neurologic deficit (for example, none, sympathetic, sensory, and motor block). Pain relief following the injection of normal saline is interpreted as placebo response or psychogenic pain, following 0.2 percent procaine as sympathetic pain, and so on. If pain persists unabated in the presence of a solid spinal block (as evidenced by paralysis) it is thought to be of central origin. Difficulties in interpretation arise from the inability to consistently block one fiber size only (for example, sympathetic block plus hypalgesia); the occurrence of spotty blocks (for example, in arachnoiditis); and the placebo response. Therapeutically, subarachnoid block with neurolytic agents or narcotics is utilized in the management of cancer pain and severe (painful) spasticity. In the latter case the patient is positioned so that the neurolytic solution preferentially flows to the central roots.

For chemical rhizotomy/ganglionectomy with hyperbaric phenol, midline spinal tap is performed with the patient lying on the painful side. An interspace in the middle of the spinal segments innervating the painful area is chosen. Alternatively, if the patient is tilted head-up, the needle is placed close to the cranial border of the selected segments. After free cerebrospinal fluid flow has been established, the patient is rotated backwards about 45°. Padding, braces, rotation of the table, and assistance help to maintain this position. The very viscous phenol is injected with a tuberculine syringe in increments of 0.1 to 0.2 ml. Occurrence and progress of segmental block is checked by the patient reporting warmth, tingling, and numbness in the affected dermatomes. Loss of sensation is confirmed by repeated pinscratch examination. During the first 10 minutes, spread may be further controlled by tilting the table head-up or head-down. The patient's position is maintained for 30 minutes following injection; bedrest is ordered for 24 hours.

The amount of phenol in glycerine needed for successful block varies with authors and site of injection. Larger volumes are needed in the cervical and upper thoracic space where the dural sleeves contain larger volumes. Maximal doses seem to be 2 ml in the cervico-thoracic space and 0.75 ml in the lumbar space. Since complications are dose-dependent, using smaller amounts and repeating the procedure, if necessary, is advised.

Epidural Block

For epidural block the local anesthetic solution is deposited in the extradural space resulting in nonconduction of the bathed spinal nerves/segments. Epidural puncture is possible and safe at any level from the cervical to the sacral area. Level of analgesia is predictable and depends mostly upon the mass of the anesthetic and the age of the patient, and, to a lesser extent, on volume and height of the patient (64). Segmental block refers to block of a limited number of adjacent segments. It is produced by tapping the epidural space in the approximate middle of these segments and injecting a calculated amount of drug.

Differential block is possible by a pharmacologic approach using dilute local anesthetic solutions; for example, sympathetic block of the lower extremities can be produced with little or no sensory or motor loss by lumbar epidural injection (4). Because of technical ease this is often preferred to sympathetic ganglion block for the treatment of reflex sympathetic dystrophies and vasospastic disorders of the lower extremities. Continuous block can be accomplished by inserting an indwelling epidural catheter (plastic tubing), through which repeated injections

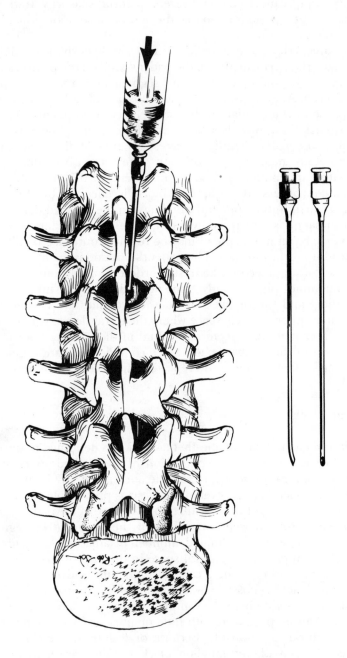

Figure 3. Diagram of epidural tap and Tuohy needles

are made. Other therapeutic applications consist of steroid block for radicular pain and narcotic block for severe postoperative or cancer pain.

Cervical, thoracic, or lumbar epidural puncture are usually performed in the lateral position with the body side to be affected preferentially placed down. Epidural tap in the prone position and sitting position is also possible. Tuohy type needles (usually 18-gauge, 7.5 to 10 cm) facilitate epidural puncture (Figure 3). A midline approach aims at the greatest distance between ligamentum flavum and dura (Figure 4). The needle is advanced steadily through subcutaneous tissues and ligaments; the yellow ligament is usually felt by its increased resistance to penetration. Entrance into the epidural space is accompanied by sudden decrease of resistance. Tap is facilitated and/or verified by the "negative pressure" method or by the "loss of resistance" method (25). In the former, a drop of fluid which has been placed in the hub of the needle is sucked inward when the epidural space is entered. In the latter, a glass syringe with an easily gliding (wetted) plunger is attached to the needle which is partially filled with air and/or fluid. Pressure is exerted against the plunger while the needle is advanced. Sudden discharge of the contents of the syringe occurs when the epidural space is entered (Figure 3).

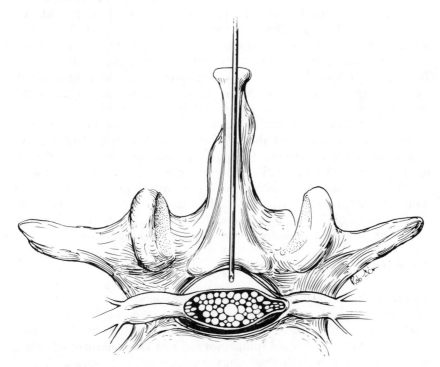

Figure 4. Diagram of epidural tap (transverse section)

Following negative aspiration and test injection, the calculated amount of local anesthetic or other agent is injected. When using steroids it is important to clear the needle with local anesthetic to avoid steroid deposition in its track.

Prolonged (continuous) epidural block is achieved by placing a catheter (plastic tube) in the epidural space (Figure 5). The curved directional point of the Tuohy needle imparts a bias allowing the catheter to travel according to the way the tip is oriented. However, coiling and other directional changes are common. For this reason the tubing should not be advanced more than 5 cm; if exact localization in the epidural space is required, fluoroscopy should be employed. Limiting the length of the catheter within the epidural space also decreases the incidence of laceration of vessels or dura. The needle is withdrawn over the catheter, which is fixed to the skin with a sterile dressing. It should be noted that the catheter should never be withdrawn through the needle, as this maneuver may cut it. If repositioning is necessary, both tubing and needle have to be removed together and the procedure repeated. Aspiration and test injection are repeated each time before administering the selected drug. Epidural catheters have been left in place for one week and longer without complications (25).

If the sacral nerves are to be blocked, the caudal approach to the epidural space is preferred. The patient is positioned prone with the sacrum elevated by a pillow and the legs rotated inward. The sacral hiatus is identified and anesthetized by local infiltration. The block needle (usually 22-gauge, 4 cm) is inserted at an approximate angle of 70° to 80° in midline between the sacral cornua until bone is contacted. Often loss of resistance is experienced when the sacrococcygeal membrane is pierced. Once within the caudal space, the needle is withdrawn from bony contact and further advanced, with its angle decreased to about 20° in the male and about 35° in the female. Following negative aspiration and test injection, the blocking solution is injected. Bilateral block from S_3 to S_5 can usually be accomplished with about 6 ml of local anesthetic solution; for example, one percent lidocaine. Steroid injections for sciatica have been found to be equally effective when given by the lumbar or caudal epidural route (10). This may be technically easier in patients who had undergone one or more back operations.

Paravertebral Somatic Nerve Block

This procedure effects nonconduction in the spinal nerve as it exits from the intervertebral foramen, resulting in analgesia of one dermatome. By blocking the nerves suspected to mediate pain, the pathway of pain may be narrowed to the involved spinal root and/or roots. Failure of adequate block to relieve pain is diagnostically conclusive. The procedure has no

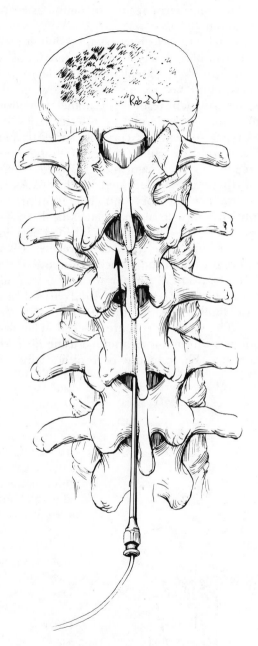

Figure 5. Diagram of epidural catheter insertion

prognostic value for long-term results of neurodestructive operations (for example, rhizotomy) (3).

Repeated paravertebral blocks have been used as adjuncts in the conservative management of a variety of painful conditions. We have given up this practice in favor of segmental (or continuous) epidural analgesia. Neurolytic injections into the mixed spinal nerve are generally contraindicated. For more permanent results, percutaneous neurodestruction by heating or cooling may be employed for selected cases.

Paravertebral block (except for cervical nerves) is performed by a posterior approach with the patient in the prone position. Twenty-two-gauge spinal needles or their equivalents (7.5 to 10 cm) are usually employed. Since they may be deflected by the tissues, verification of localization by x-ray is mandatory (59). The appropriate spinous processes are identified and a local anesthetic wheal is raised 3 to 4 cm lateral to the superior edge. The needle is inserted perpendicular to the skin until it impinges upon the transverse process. It is partially withdrawn and reinserted with a caudad inclination until it clears the transverse process. It is advanced further to a total length equaling the distance to the transverse process plus about 2 cm in the thoracic area or about 3 cm in the lumbar area (Figure 6). Final adjustments are made with fluoroscopy. The sacral nerves are blocked in similar fashion by a trans-sacral approach through the foramina using x-ray control for correct needle placement. Three ml one percent lidocaine are sufficient to block one nerve.

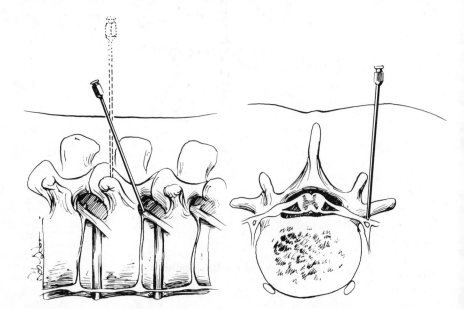

Figure 6. Diagram of paravertebral block

For cervical block the patient is placed in the supine position with the head turned to the side opposite to the one being blocked. The nerves lie beneath a line connecting the tip of the mastoid process with the anterior tubercle of C_6. The transverse processes of C_2 to C_5 can in most cases easily be palpated, identified, and marked about 0.5 cm below this line. A 22-gauge needle (4 to 5 cm) is inserted with a slight caudad tilt through a local anesthetic skin wheal to the transverse process to be blocked. Needle position on nerves innervating the upper extremity is most easily verified with the aid of a nerve stimulator. Careful aspiration is of particular importance during cervical nerve block because of the close proximity to vertebral artery and dural sleeves.

Sympathetic Ganglion Block

These procedures interrupt nervous conduction in the sympathetic system by an anatomic approach; the local anesthetic solution is placed at a site where the sympathetic nerves travel separated from the somatic nerves. This is in contrast to sympathetic block by the pharmacologic approach, which relies on preferential block of small fibers by a low concentration of the anesthetic, but is always associated with a certain degree of somatic block (for example, epidural block with less concentration of local anesthetic). The entire peripheral sympathetic network can be interrupted at three critical sites: stellate ganglion, celiac (splanchnic) plexus, and lumbar ganglia (4). Local anesthetic solutions injected into the vicinity of these structures will cause sympathetic block of one upper body quadrant, the abdomen, and of one lower body quadrant, respectively.

Stellate and lumbar sympathetic blocks are useful for diagnosis and treatment of reflex sympathetic dystrophy and vasospastic disease. They allow one to differentiate between mechanical and spastic obstruction of the circulation, and may be used prophylactically if vasospasm is expected to occur (for example, stellate block after upper extremity operation). A series of sympathetic blocks will confirm the diagnosis of causalgia and aid in evaluation for possible sympathectomy. In reflex sympathetic dystrophy, repeated blocks (or a continuous technique) may effect a cure. The decision to continue with block therapy is based upon duration and magnitude of pain relief. If pain relief outlasts local anesthetic action for increasing periods of time and pain returns to a lesser degree, blocks should be repeated. Other application of sympathetic blocks consists of differentiation between somatic and visceral pain. With neurolytic agents they effect palliative treatment for intractable pain secondary to cancer (for example, celiac plexus block for pancreatic cancer).

Stellate ganglion block is easily and safely performed by an anterior paratracheal approach at the level of C_6. This avoids the possibility of pneumothorax, which may occur after injection of the ganglion at C_7. The patient rests supine with the head tilted backward. The anterior tubercle of C_6 is identified on the medial border of the sternocleidomastoid muscle. It is usually at the level of the cricoid cartilage (except in thin, long-necked persons). A finger is placed on the tubercle and gently contracts the sternocleidomastoid muscle and carotid sheath laterally (Figure 7). (The neck muscles can be relaxed by asking the patient to slightly open his or her mouth.) A regular 22-gauge needle (4 to 5 cm) attached to a 10 ml syringe filled with the local anesthetic solution (for example, one percent lidocaine) is inserted to the tubercle (Figure 7). Following negative aspiration and test dose, the local anesthetic is injected. As with cervical nerve blocks, careful aspiration is particularly important because of the proximity of major vessels and the dural sleeves. Ten ml solution will spread to affect the sympathetic chain from the middle cervical ganglion to the fourth or fifth thoracic ganglion (4). Spread may be facilitated by elevating the head after needle removal.

Successful block is clinically evident by the occurrence of Horner's syndrome, absence of sweating, increased temperature of the hand, and other signs of sympathetic paralysis. If necessary it can be documented by measuring finger temperature, finger pulse pressure (plethysmograph), psychogalvanic skin reflex, or observing the absence of skin wrinkling in the blocked hand after immersion of both hands into warm water for 20 minutes. A common side effect consists of transient hoarseness caused by anesthetic spill-over to the recurrent laryngeal nerve. (For this reason, bilateral stellate block should not be performed.) Other rare complications include partial or complete brachial plexus block, phrenic nerve block, and asthma attacks.

Lumbar sympathetic ganglion block can be performed in the lateral or prone position. We prefer the patient prone and insert 20-gauge spinal needles (10 to 12.5 cm) with fluoroscopic assistance. The second or third lumbar spine is identified. A local anesthetic wheal is raised 4.5 to 5 cm lateral to the middle of the selected spine. The needle is inserted through this wheal with cephalad inclination to the transverse process. The sympathetic ganglion is situated about 3.5 to 4 cm deeper. The needle is withdrawn to the subcutaneous tissue and reinserted with downward and slightly inward direction to this predetermined depth (Figure 8). Should the vertebral body be encountered first, the needle is partially withdrawn and advanced in more perpendicular fashion so that it slips off the bone. Final adjustments of position are made with fluoroscopic control; the tip of the needle should rest just antero-lateral to the vertebral body.

Injection of 10 ml of anesthetic solution (for example, one percent lidocaine) will result in complete sympathetic block of the lower extremity if the needle has been properly placed at the L_2 (or L_3) area.

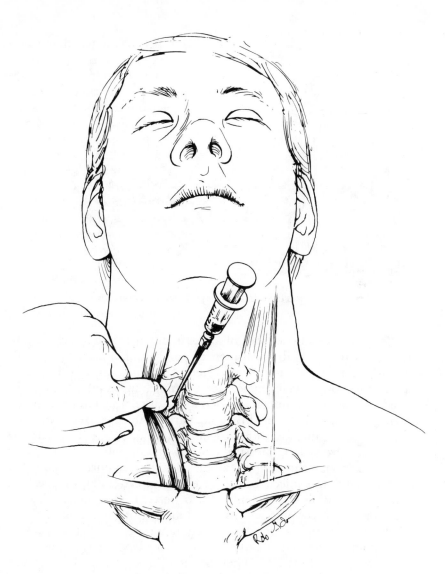

Figure 7. Stellate ganglion block

Prolonged block can be accomplished by inserting a catheter but may be managed more easily by a lumbar epidural approach. Neurolytic injection is infrequently used, though excellent results have been reported (65). If it is considered, a more lateral approach is recommended (Figure 8) (66, 67). We have come to prefer this lateral approach, as it additionally helps avoid needle contact with the lumbar nerve (peripheral paresthesia).

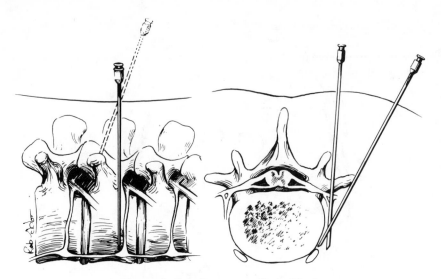

Figure 8. Lumbar sympathetic block

Prolonged sympathetic block of an extremity may also be achieved by intravenous regional administration of guanethidine (Bier block) (68). Only adrenergic mediated sympathetic functions are affected; cholinergic functions remain intact (for example, sweating) (69). For the procedure a plastic cannula is inserted into a distal vein and a pneumatic Tourniquet applied to the proximal part of the diseased extremity. Following exsanguination with an Esmarch bandage, the Tourniquet is inflated to above systolic pressure (usually 250 or 350 Torr for arm or leg, respectively). Guanethidine (20 mg) dissolved in normal saline or a lidocaine solution is injected into the bloodless extremity. We prefer to dilute guanethidine with 40 ml of 0.25 percent lidocaine, as this decreases patient discomfort. Tourniquet time is 15 to 20 minutes.

No serious complications have been reported for Bier block with guanethidine. Increased bloodflow of the treated extremity can be documented for three days (69). Therapeutic effects on pain, edema, and other signs of reflex sympathetic dystrophy are equal to those obtained with classical sympathetic nerve block (70). However, since the effects of the intravenous regional method are longer lasting, fewer blocks are required for equal results.

Celiac (splanchnic) plexus block is performed with the patient in prone position. We always use fluoroscopic control. The 12th ribs and the first lumbar spine are identified. A flat triangle is constructed on the skin. The base is on a horizontal line drawn through the caudal edge of the first lumbar spine extending 6.5 to 7.5 cm to each side of midline. The sides connect the base to the cranial edge of this spine; they project the pathway of the needles. The lateral tips of the triangle should lie in the region of the angle of the ribs just lateral to the sacrospinalis muscles (Figure 9). Following local infiltration a 20-gauge spinal needle (10 to 15 cm) is introduced with a 45° angle to the skin at the lateral tip of the triangle. It is advanced along a line projected by the side of the triangle

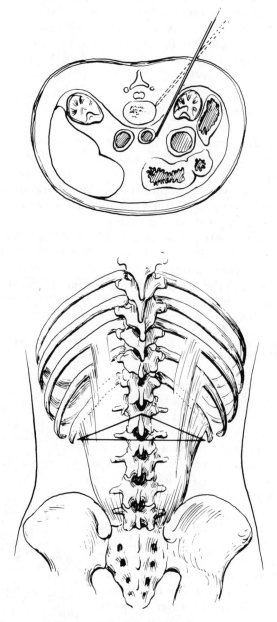

Figure 9. Celiac ganglion block

until it impinges upon the first lumbar vertebral body. The needle is withdrawn to the subcutaneous tissue and reinserted with an increased angle (about 60°) until it passes the body and rests anterior in the areolar tissue containing the plexus (Figure 9). Fluoroscopy allows one to direct the needle so that more than two passes rarely are necessary. The procedure is repeated on the other side; placement of two needles seems to assure more complete block. After negative aspiration 20 ml anesthetic solution (for example, 0.25 to 0.5 percent lidocaine) are injected through each needle; for neurolysis an equal amount of 50 percent alcohol is used.

Peripheral Nerve Block

These procedures temporarily interrupt conduction in one or more peripheral nerves. They may be helpful in establishing the pathway of pain and determining a peripheral etiology. This is of particular importance if a peripheral nerve stimulator implant is considered for treatment. Peripheral nerve blocks allow one to distinguish between different neuralgias presenting with similar symptoms, between somatic and visceral pain projected to the same area, and help in the diagnosis of nerve entrapment syndromes. Repeated blocks are used to manage self-limited painful disorders (for example, intercostal blocks for rib fractures). Neurolytic injections into the peripheral nerve should be avoided because of a high incidence of postinjection neuritis. The description of individual nerve blocks is beyond the scope of this chapter.

Local Infiltration

Local infiltration constitutes the simplest and safest block. Local anesthetic injection of trigger points is used to treat patients with myofascial syndromes, painful scars, and other musculoskeletal disorders (4, 7, 22). Myofascial syndrome refers to a condition characterized by: 1) a painful trigger point in muscle or connective tissue; 2) a predictable pain pattern (often associated with stiffness, muscle spasms, and so on); and 3) the absence of local neurologic findings. Trigger points are confirmed by palpation; their localization is constant for particular pain patterns. Anesthetic infiltration is usually performed with 25-gauge needles (1.5 to 2.5 cm) using 3 to 10 ml solution (for example, one percent lidocaine); the injection is usually associated with short-lived exacerbation (seconds) of typical pain. Trigger injections should be integrated with other treatments (such as exercise) directed toward elimination of predisposing factors. However, they are also helpful in alleviating pain in the patients with incurable disease (for example, permanent neurologic deficit, cancer). Particularly, cancer patients are often subject to myofascial syndromes because of generalized muscle wasting, prolonged convalescence, and mutilating operations.

REFERENCES

1. Fordyce WE: Environmental factors in the genesis of low back pain, in Advances in Pain Research Therapy, vol. 3. Edited by Bonica JJ, Liebeskind JC, Albe-Fessard D. New York, Raven Press, 1979
2. de Jong RH: Physiology and Pharmacology of Local Anesthesia. Springfield, IL, Charles C Thomas, 1970
3. Loeser JD: Dorsal rhizotomy: indications and results, in Advances in Neurology, vol. 4. Edited by Bonica JJ. New York, Raven Press, 1974
4. Bonica JJ: Clinical Applications of Diagnostic and Therapeutic Nerve Blocks. Springfield IL, Charles C Thomas, 1959
5. Brena SF, Unikel IP: Serve blocks and contingency management in chronic pain states, in Advances in Pain Research Therapy, vol. 1 Edited by Bonica JJ, Albe-Fessard D. New York, Raven Press, 1976
6. Bonica JJ: Causalgia and other reflex sympathetic dystrophies, in Advances in Pain Research Therapy, vol. 3. Edited by Bonica JJ, Liebeskind JC, Albe-Fessard D. New York, Raven Press, 1979
7. Travell J: Myofascial trigger points: clinical view, in Advances in Pain Research Therapy, vol. 1. Edited by Bonica JJ, Albe-Fessard D. New York, Raven Press, 1976
8. Wood KM, Arguelles J, Norenberg MD: Degenerative lesions in rat sciatic nerves after local injections of methylprednisolone in sterile aqueous suspension. Reg Anaesth 5:13–15, 1980
9. Dilke TF, Burry HC, Grahame R: Extradural corticosteroid injection: management of lumbar nerve root compression. Br Med J 2:635–637, 1973
10. Breivik H, Hesla PE, Molnar I, et al: Treatment of chronic low back pain and sciatica: comparison of caudal epidural injection of bupivacaine and methylprednisolone with bupivacaine followed by saline, in Advances in Pain Research Therapy, vol. 1. Edited by Bonica JJ, Albe-Fessard D. New York, Raven Press, 1976
11. Kepes ER, Duncalf D: Treatment of backache with spinal injections of local anesthetics, spinal and systemic steroids: a review. Pain 22:33–47, 1985
12. Devor M. Govrin-Lippmann R, Raber P: Corticosteroids suppress ectopic neural discharges originating in experimental neuroma. Pain 22:127–137, 1985
13. Urban BJ: Complications of spinal steroids and spinal stimulators, in Anaesthesiology. Edited by Rugheimer E, Zindler M. Excerpta Medica International Congress Series 538:953–955, 1981
14. Delaney TJ, Rowlinson JC, Carron H: Epidural steroid effects on nerves and meninges. Anesthesia and Analgesia Current Research 59:610–614, 1980
15. Yaksh TL: Spinal opiate analgesia: characteristics and principles of action. Pain 11:293–346, 1981
16. Bromage PR, Camporesi EM, Durant PAC, et al: Rostral spread of epidural morphine. Anesthesiology 56:431–436, 1982

17. Martin R, Salbaing J, Blaise G, et al: Epidural morphine for postoperative pain relief: a dose response curve. Anesthesiology 56:423–426, 1982

18. Lanz E, Kehrberger E, Theiss D: Epidural morphine: a clinical double-blind study of dosage. Anesthesia and Analgesia Current Research 64:786–791, 1985

19. Coombs DW, Saunders RL, Gaylor M, et al: Epidural narcotic infusion reservoir: implantation technique and efficacy. Anesthesiology 56:469–473, 1982

20. Poletti CE, Cohen AM, Todd DP, et al: Cancer pain relieved by long-term epidural morphine with permanent indwelling systems for self-administration. J Neurosurg 55:581–584, 1981

21. Greenberg HS, Taren J, Ensminger WD, et al: Benefit from and tolerance to continuous intrathecal infusion of morphine for intractable cancer pain. J Neurosurg 57:360–364, 1982

22. Bonica JJ: The management of pain. Philadelphia, Lea and Febinger, 1953

23. Boas RA, Covino BG, Shahnarian A: Analgesic responses to i.v. lignocaine. Br J Anaesth 54:501–505, 1982

24. Schnapp M, Mayo KS, North WC: Intravenous 2-chloroprocaine in treatment of chronic pain. Anesthesia and Analgesia Current Research 60:844–845, 1981

25. Moore DC: Regional Block: A Handbook for Use in the Clinical Practice of Medicine and Surgery, 4th edition. Springfield, IL, Charles C Thomas, 1965

26. Wood KM: The use of phenol as a neurolytic agent: a review. Pain 5:205–229, 1978

27. Katz J: Current role of neurolytic agents, in Advances in Neurology, vol. 4. Edited by Bonica JJ. New York, Raven Press, 1979

28. Loeser JD: Neurosurgical control of chronic pain. Arch Surg 112:880–883, 1977

29. Long DM: Surgical therapy of chronic pain. Neurosurgery 6:317–328, 1980

30. Nugent GR: Trigeminal neuralgia: treatment by percutaneous electrocoagulation, in Neurosurgery. Edited by Wilkins RH, Rengachary SS. New York, McGraw-Hill, 1985

31. Bay JW, Dohn DF: Surgical sympathectomy, in Neurosurgery. Edited by Wilkins RH, Rengachary SS. New York, McGraw-Hill, 1985

32. Nashold BS, Urban BJ, Zorub DS: Phantom pain relief by focal destruction of the substantia gelatinosa of Rolando, in Advances in Pain Research Therapy, vol. 1. Edited by Bonica JJ, Albe-Fessard D. New York, Raven Press, 1976

33. Nashold BS, Higgins AC, Blumenkopf B: Dorsal root entry zone lesions for pain relief, in Neurosurgery. Edited by Wilkins RH, Rengachary SS. New York, McGraw-Hill, 1985

34. Rosomoff HL: Percutaneous spinothalamic cordotomy, in Neurosurgery. Edited by Wilkins RH, Rengachary SS. New York, McGraw-Hill, 1985

35. Harris BA: Dorsal rhizotomy, in Neurosurgery. Edited by Wilkins RH, Rengachary SS. New York, McGraw-Hill, 1985

36. Thompson GE, Moore DC, Bridenbaugh LD, et al: Abdominal pain and alcohol celiac plexus nerve block. Anesthesia and Analgesia Current Research 56:1–5, 1977

37. Pagura JR, Schnapp M, Passarelli P: Percutaneous radiofrequency glossopharyngeal rhizotomy for cancer pain. Appl Neurophysiol 46:154–159, 1983

38. Moricca G: Neuroadenolysis for diffuse unbearable cancer pain, in Advances in Pain Research Therapy, vol. 1. Edited by Bonica JJ, Albe-Fessard D. New York, Raven Press, 1976

39. Lipton S, Miles JB, Williams NE: Pituitary injection of alcohol for inoperable and intractable cancer pain, in Advances in Pain Research Therapy, vol. 3. Edited by Bonica JJ, Liebeskind JC, Albe-Fessard D. New York, Raven Press, 1979

40. Miles J: Pituitary destruction, in Textbook of Pain. Edited by Wall PD, Melzack R. Edinburgh, Churchill Livingstone, 1984

41. Yanagida H, Corssen G, Trowborst A, et al: Relief of cancer pain in man: alcohol induced neuroadenolysis vs. electrical stimulation of the pituitary gland. Pain 19:133–141, 1984

42. Kane K, Taub A: A history of local electrical analgesia. Pain 1:125–138, 1975

43. Melzack R: Acupuncture and related forms of folk medicine, in Textbook of Pain. Edited by Wall, PD, Melzack R. Edinburgh, Churchill Livingstone, 1984

44. Long DM: Electrical stimulation for control of pain. Arch Surg 112:884–888, 1977

45. Woolf CJ: Transcutaneous and implanted nerve stimulation, in Textbook of Pain. Edited by Wall PD, Melzack R. Edinburgh, Churchill Livingstone, 1984

46. Nashold BS: Peripheral nerve stimulation for pain. J Neurosurg 53:132–133, 1980

47. Shealy CN, Mortimer JT, Reswick JB: Electrical inhibition of pain by stimulation of the dorsal columns: preliminary clinical report. Anesthesia and Analgesia Current Research 46:489–491, 1967

48. Nashold BS, Friedman H: Dorsal column stimulation for control of pain: preliminary report on 30 patients. J Neurosurg 36:590–597, 1972

49. Sweet WH, Wepsic JG: Electrical stimulation for suppression of pain in man, in Neural Organization and its Relevance to Prosthetics. Edited by Fields WS. New York, Intercontinental Medical Books, 1973

50. Nashold BS: Electrical stimulation of the skin, peripheral nerves, or dorsal column for pain relief, in Current Controversies in Neurosurgery. Edited by Morley TB. Philadelphia, WB Saunders, 1976

51. Shimoji K, Kitamure H, Ikezono E, et al: Spinal hypalgesia and analgesia by low-frequency electrical stimulation in the epidural space. Anesthesiology 41:91–94, 1974

52. Cook AW: Electrical stimulation in multiple sclerosis. Hosp Pract 11:51–58, 1976

53. Zumpano BJ, Saunders RL: Percutaneous epidural dorsal column stimulation: technical note. J Neurosurg 45:459–460, 1976

54. Urban BJ, Nashold BS: Percutaneous epidural stimulation of the spinal cord for relief of pain: long-term results. J Neurosurg 48:323–328, 1978

55. Young RF: Evaluation of dorsal column stimulation in the treatment of chronic pain. Neurosurgery 3:373–379, 1978

56. Urban BJ, Nashold BS: Combined epidural and peripheral nerve stimulation for relief of pain: description of technique and preliminary results. J Neurosurg 57:365–369, 1982

57. Richardson DE: Deep brain stimulation for pain relief, in Neurosurgery. Edited by Wilkins RH, Rengachary SS. New York, McGraw-Hill, 1985

58. Raj PP, Rosenblatt R, Montgomery SJ: Use of the nerve stimulator for peripheral blocks. Reg Anesth 5:14–21, 1980

59. Ferrer-Brechner T, Brechner VL: Accuracy of needle placement during diagnostic and therapeutic nerve blocks, in Advances in Pain Research Therapy, vol. 1. Edited by Bonica JJ, Albe-Fessard D. New York, Raven Press, 1976

60. Erikson E: Illustrated Handbook in Local Anesthesia. Chicago, Year Book Medical Publishers, 1969

61. Adriani J: Labat's Regional Anesthesia: Techniques and Clinical Applications, 3rd edition. Philadelphia, WB Saunders, 1967

62. Neural blockade, in Clinical Anesthesia and Management of Pain. Edited by Cousins MJ, Bridenbaugh PO. Philadelphia, JB Lippincott, 1980

63. McCollum DE, Stephens CR: The use of graduated spinal anesthesia in the differential diagnosis of pain of the back and lower extremities. South Med J 57:410–416, 1964

64. Bromage PR: Physiology and pharmacology of epidural analgesia. Anesthesiology 28:592–622, 1967

65. Boas RA, Hatangdi VS, Richards EG: Lumbar sympathectomy—a percutaneous chemical technique, in Advances in Pain Research Therapy, vol. 1. Edited by Bonica JJ, Albe-Fessard D. New York, Raven Press, 1976

66. Reid W, Watt JK, Grag TG: Phenol injection of the sympathetic chain. Br J Surg 57:45–50, 1970

67. Hatangdi VS, Boas RA: Lumbar sympathectomy: a simple needle technique. Br J Anaesth 57:285–288, 1985

68. Hannington-Kiff, JG: Intravenous regional sympathetic block with guanethidine. Lancet 1:1019–1020, 1974

69. McKain CW, Urban BJ, Goldner JL: The effects of intravenous regional guanethidine and reserpine: a controlled study. J Bone Joint Surg 65-A:808–811, 1983

70. Bonelli S, Lonoscente F, Movilia PG, et al: Regional intravenous guanethidine vs. stellate ganglion block in reflex sympathetic dystrophies: a randomized trial. Pain 16:297–307, 1983

Chapter **25**

Management of
Cancer Pain

Randal D. France, M.D.
K. Ranga Rama Krishnan, M.D.

The treatment of cancer pain depends on the cause of the pain syndrome produced by the cancer or treatment of the cancer, stage of the illness, psychological state of the patient, and nature of the specific therapeutic approaches. The most effective treatment for cancer pain is the treatment of the underlying causes. Failing this, cancer pain treatment is aimed at the symptomatic relief of the pain by analgesic medications, nerve blocks, neurosurgical procedures, neuroaugmentative techniques, behavioral methods, and supportive care. Foley (1) has stated that management of cancer pain requires specific understanding in the following areas: knowledge of pain syndromes that are common in cancer and their pathophysiological mechanism, psychological health of the patient, and the indications and limitations of the available treatments. A number of authors (1–7) have advocated a multidisciplinary approach to provide the most effective treatment for the patient with cancer pain using a variety of treatments. The overall goal for treatment of the terminally ill cancer patient with pain is to control the pain so the patient can achieve the highest level of function (8).

As noted in the earlier section on cancer pain, the pain can result from many causes. Patients may have pain as part of the initial presentation of the cancer or reoccurrence of the cancer after a period of remission. The treatment in these patients is aimed at the causes of the cancer (that is, removal of a tumor compressing a peripheral nerve). Patients undergoing chemotherapy or radiation may experience pain as a result of the treatment itself. The pain is usually self-limited and can be controlled with symptomatic treatment (analgesic medications). The treatment for the above types of cancer pain is directed toward the causes of the pain, or toward symptomatic relief for acute cancer pain occurring with cancer treatment. In other cancer patients, the pain persists. The causes of this pain are related to a progression of the cancer or to the cancer treatment by chemotherapy or radiation. In this group of patients, various treatments are used to control the pain.

Psychological factors tend to modify the pain and treatment course. Therefore, an assessment of the patient's present psychological state, premorbid personality, social support system, and presence of a psychopathological disorder are important. The most common psychological disturbances in cancer patients are depression and anxiety (9–13). Patients with a prior history of personality disorder or psychiatric disorder such as somatoform disorder, psychogenic pain disorder, substance abuse, hypochondriasis, or conversion disorder have an increased likelihood of having an exaggerated response to cancer pain. This may be demonstrated by medication abuse, limited function which is out of proportion to their physical state, or somatization. Care of these patients is extremely difficult. The physician should not withhold analgesic medications solely on the basis of the premorbid personality of the patient.

Effective treatment of these patients means a collaborative effort attending to both the psychological and medical needs of these patients.

MEDICATION MANAGEMENT

Analgesic medication is the mainstay of treatment for the cancer pain patient (1, 5, 8, 14–16). Drug management is initiated with nonopioid analgesics for mild to moderate cancer pain. These drugs have a limit to their analgesic effect. In addition, their use is restricted by gastrointestinal and hematological side effects. In these drugs tolerance and physical dependency do not occur as it does with opioid analgesics. For further discussion on nonopioid analgesics, see Chapter 20. For moderate to severe cancer pain, opioid analgesics are the drugs of choice.

It is generally advisable to start with a less potent opioid analgesic (propoxyphene, codeine) and progress to more potent drugs (methadone, oxycodone, morphine) as the need arises. The route of administration should conform with the patient's need. After an effective dose range has been established, the drug should be given on a regular basis (time contingent) as opposed to an as needed schedule (prn). For a more detailed discussion on the pharmacology in clinical use of opioid analgesics, refer to Chapter 20. As the pain becomes more intense, adjuvant medications are added to provide additional analgesia. Side effects of the medications (sedation, constipation, nausea and vomiting, respiratory depression) are monitored and treated.

Adjuvant medications include hydroxyzine, amphetamines, antidepressants, neuroleptics, and anticonvulsants. As noted in the chapter on opioid analgesics, hydroxyzine and opioid analgesics provide more pain relief than does the opioid analgesic alone. Likewise, dextroamphetamine (5–10 mg daily) increases the analgesic effect of opioid analgesics (17). Neuroleptics, both phenothiazines (18–22) and butyrophenones (23–26), have been reported to have analgesic activity or enhance opioid analgesia. No controlled studies have confirmed these initial observations. These drugs, however, are very effective at controlling nausea and vomiting that are common symptoms due to the patient's illness or treatment in cancer pain patients. In patients with bone pain from metastatic breast cancer, L-dopa (1500–3000 mg daily) was effective in decreasing the pain (27–29). The apparent mechanism is the suppression of prolactin by L-dopa. Anticonvulsants are also reported to be effective for cancer pain (30).

Antidepressants have been used alone (31, 32), in combination with a neuroleptic (33), or in combination with an opioid analgesic (34) to treat cancer pain. There are no controlled studies on the efficacy of antidepressants in the control of cancer pain. Imipramine (32, 35–42) and clomipramine (43–47) have been reported in case studies to be effective in the control of cancer pain. The dose range for imipramine is 25–150 mg daily and for clomipramine is 30–150 mg daily. The route of administration is either oral or parenteral. It is difficult to assess the analgesic effects of antidepressant medications in cancer pain, since no control studies have been done. As with the studies evaluating the efficacy of antidepressants in chronic pain due to nonmalignant causes, it is important to control for the type of cancer pain, presence or absence of psychopathological disorders, dose of medications, and presence or absence of other treatments. Enhancement of opioid analgesics by antidepressants needs further clarification by controlled studies. For a more detailed discussion of the clinical use of antidepressants in chronic pain, refer to Chapter 18. Minor tranquilizers do not enhance the analgesia produced by opioid drugs. These drugs, in combination with opioid analgesics, increase sedation, which in most cases, is not a desirable effect.

PSYCHOLOGICAL AND BEHAVIORAL TREATMENTS

Sortive psychotherapy can be useful for patients with cancer pain, since these patients have significant amounts of hopelessness and despair that may be based on unrealistic fears. Cancer pain magnifies the severity of the illness to the patient. In some cases, the cancer pain may indeed be an accurate barometer of the progression of the disease; but in other cases, it may represent altered pathophysiology caused by the cancer but not related to the progression of the disease (nerve damage secondary to radiation). In addition, the pain complaint in a cancer patient may represent an underlying psychopathological state (depression) or defense against the multiple conflicts and stresses facing the patient with cancer. It is therefore valuable for the treating physician to recognize the cause of the pain and formulate physical and psychological care appropriate to the underlying problem. It should be kept in mind that the patient with cancer pain will benefit little from intensive psychotherapy designed to explore and modify characterological coping mechanisms. The psychological approach to the patient who is using pain as a defense is to support other healthier defenses and provide realistic reassurance that the various problems facing the patient will be addressed and cared for. Issues that commonly arise in these patients that need to be addressed through supportive psychotherapy include the patient's concern about bodily changes, anger, and increased dependency caused by the progression of the illness.

The advantage of individual psychotherapy for the cancer patient is the patient's avoiding the suppression of important emotional issues out of a desire to protect family and friends. The disadvantages of individual psychotherapy for the cancer patient includes: 1) cost and time concerns;

2) limited exposure to patients who have successfully coped with their cancer; and 3) stigma that the cancer patient is weak if he or she needs psychotherapy to cope.

In addition to individual supportive psychotherapy, professionally led support groups and self-help groups are playing an increasingly significant role in the psychological care of oncology patients and their families. Several controlled studies have documented that cancer patients receiving group therapy have less mood disturbance, fewer maladaptive coping responses, and improved self-concept as compared to patients without this intervention (48–50). Issues frequently discussed in groups with the terminally ill include: 1) concern over physical changes from the cancer and its treatment; 2) fear of dying; 3) fear of pain; and 4) fear of loss of control of oneself (51–53). Given the benefits of group therapy for the patients, the cancer patient with pain may achieve better control of the pain through improved psychological adaptation and lessening of psychological distress. In addition to the supportive psychotherapy, the group setting can also be used for educational presentations and teaching of stress management and relaxation techniques (54).

Self-help groups are defined as groups of individuals with similar problems and needs, who organize to promote support and education for the common problem without professional intervention. The functions of a self-help group include: 1) to provide special information and coping techniques proven to be beneficial by other group members; 2) to encourage compliance with medical regimens; 3) to assist the patient in resuming a more active role; and 4) to educate health caregivers and the public about the special needs of the group. Given these functions and the needs of cancer patients and their families, self-help groups are often reported to be helpful (55–60). Helplessness, grief, dying, and problems of everyday living are noted themes continuously reviewed in these groups despite a change in membership (55, 58, 61). Potential negative effects from a self-help group include: 1) they can intensify resentment of health caregivers; 2) they can foster a delay in the rehabilitation of a patient who uses the support of the group to avoid participation with their families and their own social settings; and 3) they can lead to overidentification of the helpers in the group with the patients being helped. There are abundant anecdotal reports claiming efficacy in promoting improved adaptation in the cancer patient, but controlled studies are lacking.

Hypnosis is used to manage cancer pain as part of an interval treatment approach (62–65). Since anxiety symptoms are common in patients with both cancer and chronic pain, progressive relaxation, with or without biofeedback techniques, can be useful (66). With these techniques, anxiety control occurs without the use of medications that cause sedation and mental dullness. Surface electromyography biofeedback can be

useful in treating the physical symptoms of anxiety or associated physiological response to pain such as increased muscle tension. As patients
learn and apply these techniques, their fears of helplessness will decrease
as they themselves can control their pain level by using a self-reliant
treatment as opposed to passively taking medications. Analgesic medications should be given on a time contingent basis to avoid reinforcing pain
behaviors by the administration on an as-needed basis. A regular schedule of the analgesic will mean that the patient is receiving the drug
independent of the pain complaint. Using this approach, the administration of the pain medication will not serve to reinforce the pain behavior.

NERVE BLOCKS

After a diagnostic evaluation of the cancer pain (and when there is no
indication for causative therapy), nerve blocks can be useful when the
pain is localized to well defined body areas (67, 68). Local anesthetic
agents can be used for temporary relief or as diagnostic nerve blocks
(69). Destruction of peripheral nerves by neurolytic agents (phenol or
alcohol) is used for permanent nerve blocks (3, 70). Permanent nerve
blocks are performed after pain relief occurs with a diagnostic nerve
block. It should be kept in mind that permanent nerve blocks of peripheral nerves not only diminish sensory input but motor control as
well. Sympathetic nerve blocks are used to control burning pain of the
head (3, 68) and extremities. Blocks of the stellate ganglion control
sympathetic dystrophy in the upper extremities, and lumbar sympathetic
blocks control burning pain in the lower extremities and vascular insufficiency to the lower extremities. Sympathetic blocks of the celiac plexus
are used to control midabdominal pain caused by cancer of the abdominal viscera (71). This block is not effective for pain from cancer of the
lower abdominal viscera. Permanent nerve blocks to control pain in the
lower abdomen or pelvis involve injection of neurolytic agents epidurally
or in the subarachnoid space. The incidence of complications, including
incontinence of urine and feces and some motor paralysis in the lower
extremities, precludes its use in many cases (72). Epidural infusion of
opioid analgesics has the advantage of providing selective analgesia
without the loss of motor function (73–75). Tolerance to the analgesic
effects of opioids is not avoided by this technique.

NEUROSURGICAL APPROACHES

Neuroablative surgical procedures can be beneficial in selected patients
with cancer pain who are physically able to undergo a neurosurgical
procedure, and for whom the neurological deficit from the procedure
does not result in significant impairment. Rhizotomy of sensory spinal

nerve roots is used for localized pain in the trunk when a few segments are involved and spread of the tumor is unlikely. This technique is avoided in the extremities since this will result in a loss of proprioception. The disadvantage to rhizotomy is that the pain will recur. Cordotomy involves the interruption of the spinalthalamic tract in either the cervical or thoracic regions. It may be performed open (76) and closed (77). It is useful in managing unilateral cancer pain. This technique is not useful for diffused or bilateral cancer pain. In most patients who undergo a cordotomy for pain control, the pain generally recurs within a year in most patients. Transsphenoidal hypophysectomy (78, 79) or chemical hypophysectomy (alcohol injection into the sella turcica by the transsphenoidal route) (80–83) can produce significant pain relief in cancer pain from metastatic bone lesions, especially hormone dependent malignancies of breasts and prostate. Recently, this procedure has been shown to be effective in the disseminated neoplasms of any kind (78, 80).

Transcutaneous electrical stimulation by electrodes applied to the skin in the areas of cancer pain may produce some control of the pain (84). Electrical stimulation of the dorsal columns or peripheral nerves has recently been tried in cancer pain, but clinical experience is lacking (85).

In summary, the management of cancer pain is a multidisciplinary approach using a combination of the above described treatments. However, before any one of the treatments is used, a careful diagnostic assessment of the cancer pain is done to determine which treatment are appropriate. As with many of the treatments, side effects or resulting complications from the procedure must be weighed against the beneficial effects of the treatment and impairment to the patient who has limited function from the cancer itself. The psychological health of the cancer pain patient must be considered before these complex treatments are initiated. Psychological support of the cancer patient with pain will undoubtedly improve the outcome of physical treatments as seen in the treatment approach of chronic pain due to nonmalignant causes.

REFERENCES

1. Foley KM: The treatment of cancer pain. N Engl J Med 313:84–95, 1985
2. Bonica JJ: Introduction to management of pain of advanced cancer, in Advances in Pain Research and Therapy, vol. 2. Edited by Bonica JJ, Ventafridda V. New York, Raven Press, 1979
3. Black P: Management of cancer pain: an overview. Neurosurgery 5:507–518, 1979
4. Moulin DE, Foley KM: Management of pain in patients with cancer. Psychiatric Annals 14:815–822, 1984
5. Shimm DS, Logue GL, Maltbie AA, et al: Medical management of chronic cancer pain. JAMA 241:2408–2412, 1979

6. Twycross RG, Lack SA: Symptom Control in Far Advanced Cancer: Pain Relief. London, Pitman, 1983
7. Bonica JJ: Cancer pain: importance of the problem, in Advances in Pain Research and Therapy, vol. 2. Proceedings of the International Symposium on Pain in Advanced Cancer. Edited by Bonica JJ, Ventafridda V. New York, Raven Press, 1979
8. McGivney WT, Crooks GM: The care of patients with severe chronic pain in terminal illness. JAMA 251:1182–1188, 1984
9. Peteet JR: Depression in cancer patients. JAMA 241:1487–1489, 1979
10. Silberfarb PM, Philibert D, Levine PM: Psychosocial aspects of neoplastic disease, II: affective and cognitive effects of chemotherapy in cancer patients. Am J Psychiatry 137:597–601, 1980
11. Derogatis LR, Morrow GR, Etting J, et al: The prevalence of psychiatric disorders among cancer patients. JAMA 249:751–757, 1983
12. Levine PM, Silberfarb PM, Lipowski ZJ: Mental disorders in cancer patients. Cancer 42:1385–1391, 1978
13. Massie MJ, Holland JC: Diagnosis and treatment of depression in the cancer patient. J Clin Psychiatry 45:25–28, 1984
14. Moertel CG: Treatment of cancer pain with orally administered medications. JAMA 244:2448–2450, 1980
15. Beaver WT: Management of cancer pain with parenteral medication. JAMA 244:2653–2657, 1980
16. Gybels J, Adreaensen H, Cosyns P: Treatment of pain in patients with advanced cancer. European Journal of Cancer 12:341–351, 1971
17. Forrest WH, Brown BW, Brown CR, et al: Dextroamphetamine with morphine for the treatment of postoperative pain. N Engl J Med 296:712–715, 1977
18. Adler, RH: Psychotropic agents in the management of chronic pain. J Human Stress 4:13–17, 1978
19. Sadove MS, Levin MJ, Rose RF, et al: Chlorpramazine and narcotics in the management of pain of malignant lesions. JAMA 155:626–628, 1954
20. Beaver WT, Wallenstein SL, Houde RW, et al: A comparison of the analgesic effect of methotrimeprazine and morphine in patients with cancer. Clin Pharmacol Ther 7:436–446, 1966
21. Sigwald J, Boutlier D, et al: Analgesic action of phenothiazines, I: treatment of severe or intractable pains by levomepromazine. Therapie 14:978–984, 1959
22. Bloomfield S, Simard-Savoie S, Bernier J, et al: Comparative analgesic activity of levomepromazine and morphine in patients with chronic pain. Can Med Assoc J 90:1156–1159, 1964
23. Maltbie AA, Cavenar JO: Haloperidol and analgesia: care reports: Milit Med 142:946–948, 1977
24. Cavenar JO, Maltbie AA: Another indication of haloperidol. Psychosomatics 17:128–130, 1976
25. Maltbie AA, Cavenar JO, Sullivan JL, et al: Analgesia and haloperidol: a hypothesis. J Clin Psychiatry 40:323–325, 1979
26. Hanks GW, Thomas PT, Trueman T, et al: The myth of haloperidol potentiation. Lancet 2:523–524, 1983

27. Minton JP: The response of breast cancer patients with bone pain to L-dopa. Cancer 33:358–362, 1974
28. Nixon DW: Use of L-dopa to relieve pain from bone metastases. N Engl J Med 292:647, 1975
29. Dickey RP, Minton JP: L-dopa relief of bone pain from breast cancer. N Engl J Med 286:843, 1972
30. Swerdlow M: Anticonvulsant drugs and chronic apin. Clin Neuropharmacol 7:51–82, 1984
31. Saunders C: The treatment of intractable pain in terminal cancer. Proceedings of the Royal Society of Medicine 56:295–297, 1963
32. Buttaro CA, Selvestri D, Turchetti A: Gull'azione antalgica dell'imipramina in oncologia. Minerva Medica 61:485–488, 1970
33. Kocher R: The use of psychotropic drugs in the treatment of chronic, severe pains. Eur Neurol 14:458–464, 1976
34. Walsh TD: Antidepressants in chronic pain. Clin Neuropharmacol 6:271–295, 1983
35. Hughes A, Chauvergne J, Lessilour J, et al: L'imipramine utilisee comme antalgigue majeur en carcinologie. La Presse Medicale 27:1073–1074, 1973
36. Stendardo B: The analgesic properties of imipramine in oncology. Riforma Medicale 44:3–12, 1964
37. Bortz W: The treatment of severe pain of carcinoma patients. Medizinische Welt (Stuttgart) 18:2126–2127, 1967
38. Deutschmann W: Tofranil in the treatment of pain in cancer cases. Medizinische Welt (Stuttgart) 22:1346–1350, 1971
39. Monkemeier, K, Steffen U: Imipramine in the treatment of pain in malignant diseases. Medizinische Klinik (Munchen) 65:213–215, 1970
40. Paschetta V: Comparative results with drugs for pain in cancer. Nice Medicale 1:26–29, 1963
41. Parolin AR: The treatment of pain and anxiety in advanced carcinoma. Medical Practice (Buenos Aires) 21:3–5, 1966
42. Tateno I: The therapeutic effects of Tofranil in the treatment of pain in malignant disease. New Drugs Clinic 18:1723–1727, 1969
43. Beaumont G, Seldrup J: Comparative trial of clomipramine and placebo in the treatment of terminal pain. J Int Med Res 8:67–69, 1980
44. Serin D: Contribution to the study of the analgesic effects of an antidepressant in the treatment of cancer. Lyon Medicale 232:483–487, 1974
45. Adjan M: The treatment of pain in terminal cancer. Therapie der Gegenwart 109:1620–1627, 1970
46. Bresson P: Contribution to the study of the analgesic action of a major antidepressant. Clermont Medical 19:89–91, 1971
47. Mascles JC: Clinical trial of anafronil in the treatment of 35 patients with cancer. Progress in Medicine 104:163–164, 1976
48. Ferlic M, Goldman A, Kennedy BJ: Group counselling in adult patients with advanced cancer. Cancer 43:760–766, 1979
49. Spiegel D, Bloom JR, Yalom I: Group support for patients with metastatic cancer. Arch Gen Psychiatry 38:527–533, 1981
50. Heinrick RL, Schag CC: Stress and activity management: group treatment for cancer patients and spouses. J Consult Clin Psychol 53:439–446, 1985

51. Yalom I, Greaves C: Group therapy with the terminally ill. Am J Psychiatry 134:396–400, 1977
52. Herzoff NE: A therapeutic group for cancer patients and their families. Cancer Nursing 2:469–474, 1979
53. Kelly PP, Ashby GC: Group approaches for cancer patients; establishing a group. Am J Nursing 79:914–915, 1979
54. Joseph CD: Psychological supportive therapy for cancer patients. Indian J Cancer 20:268–270, 1983
55. Adams J: Mutual-help groups: enhancing the coping ability of oncology clients. Cancer Nursing 2:95–98, 1979
56 Comartin MA: Self-help for the cancer patient. Canadian Nurse 79:42–44, 1983
57. Maisiak R, Cain M, Yarbro CH, et al: Evaluation of TOUCH: an oncology self-help group. Oncology Nursing Forum 8:20–25, 1981
58. Parsell S, Tageareni EM: Cancer patients help each other. Am J Nursing 74:650–651, 1974
59. Mantell JE, Alexander ES, Kleiman MA: Social work and self-help groups. Health and Social Work 1:87–100, 1976
60. Colman KC, Welsh J: Tak tent: an experiment in self-help for cancer patients. The Practitioner 228:585–587, 1984
61. Whitman HH, Gustafson JP, Coleman FW: Group approaches for cancer pain: leaders and members. Am J Nursing 79:910–913, 1979
62. Koerner ME: Using hypnosis to relieve pain of terminal cancer. Hypnosis Quarterly 20:39–46, 1977
63. Barber J, Gitelson J: Cancer pain: psychological management using hypnosis. Cancer 30:130–135, 1980
64. Sacerdote P: Theory and practice of pain control in malignancy and other protracted or recurring painful illnesses. Int J Clin Exp Hypn 18:160–180, 1970
65. Orne MT: Pain suppression by hypnosis and related phenomena. Adv Neurol 4:563–572, 1974
66. Turk DC, Meichenbaum DH, Berman WH: Application of biofeedback for the regulation of pain: a critical review. Psychol Bull 86:1322–1328, 1979
67. Bonica JJ: The Management of Pain. Philadelphia, Lea and Febiger, 1953
68. Gerbershagen HU: Blocks with local anesthetics in the treatment of cancer pain, in Advances in Pain Research and Therapy, vol. 2. Edited by Bonica JJ, Ventafridda V. New York, Raven Press, 1979
69. Urban BJ: Diagnostic and therapuetic nerve blocks, in Neurosurgery. Edited by Wilkins RH, Rengachary SS. New York, McGraw-Hill, 1985
70. Arner S: The role of nerve blocks in the treatment of cancer pain. Acta Anaesthesiol Scand 74:104–108, 1982
71. Moore DC: Celiac (splanchnic) plexus block with alcohol for cancer pain of the upper intra-abdominal viscera, in Advances in Pain Research and Therapy, vol. 2. Edited by Bonica JJ, Ventafridda V. New York, Raven Press, 1979
72. Moore DC: Role of nerve block with neurolytic solutions for pelvic visceral cancer pain, in Advances in Pain Research and Therapy, vol. 2. Edited by Bonica JJ, Ventafridda V. New York, Raven Press, 1979
73. Yaksh TL: Spinal opiate analgesics: characteristics and principles of action.

Pain 11:293–346, 1981

74. Coombs DW, Saunders RL, Gaylor MS, et al: Relief of continuous chronic pain by intraspinal narcotics infusion via an implanted reservoir. JAMA 250:2336–2339, 1983

75. Coombs DW, Saunders RL, Gaylor MS, et al: Epidural narcotic infusion reservoir implant technique and efficacy. Anesthesiology 56:469–473, 1982

76. Papo I: Open cordotomy in the treatment of cancer pain, in Advances in Pain Research and Therapy, vol 2. Edited by Bonica JJ, Ventafridda V. New York, Raven Press, 1979

77. Lipton S: Percutaneous cervical cordotomy, in Advances in Pain Research and Therapy, vol 2. Edited by Bonica JJ, Ventafridda V. New York, Raven Press, 1979

78. Tindall GT, Nixon DW, Christy JH, et al: Pain relief in metastatic cancer other than breast and prostate gland following transsphenoidal hypophysectomy: a preliminary report. J Neurosurg 47:659:662, 1977

79. Van Gilder JC, Goldenberg IS: Hypophysectomy in metastatic breast cancer. Arch Surg 110:293–295, 1975

80. Moricca G: Chemical hypophysectomy for cancer pain. Adv Neurol 4:707–714, 1974

81. Madrid JL: Chemical hypophysectomy, in Advances in Pain Research and Therapy, vol 2. Edited by Bonica JJ, Ventafridda V. New York, Raven Press, 1979

82. Miles J: Chemical hypophysectomy, in Advances in Pain Research and Therapy, vol 2. Edited by Bonica JJ, Ventafridda V. New York, Raven Press, 1979

83. Trouwborst A, Yanagida H, Erdmann W, et al: Mechanism of neuroadenolysis of the pituitary for cancer pain control. Appl Neurophysiol 47:97–110, 1984

84. Loeser JD, Black RG, Christman A: Relief of pain by transcutaneous stimulation. J Neurosurg 42:308–314, 1975

85. Loeser JD: Dorsal column and peripheral nerve stimulation for relief of cancer pain, in Advances in Pain Research and Therapy, vol. 2. Edited by Bonica JJ, Ventafridda V. New York, Raven Press, 1979

Index

549